Diabetes an Health Disparities

Community-Based
Approaches for Racial
and Ethnic Populations

Leandris C. Liburd, PhD, MPH, serves as Chief of the Community Health and Program Services Branch within the Division of Adult and Community Health at the U.S. Centers for Disease Control and Prevention (CDC) in Atlanta. In this role, Dr. Liburd directs public health programs addressing community health promotion and the elimination of health disparities, including CDC's flagship health disparities program REACH U.S., the acronym for Racial and Ethnic Approaches to Community Health across the U.S. Prior to joining the Division of Adult and Community Health in 2004, Dr. Liburd spent 12 years in the Division of Diabetes Translation at CDC as a Community Interventionist and later as Chief of the Community Interventions Section. During her tenure in the Division of Diabetes Translation, her work focused on developing community models for diabetes prevention and control programs in racial and ethnic communities in the continental U.S., in the Pacific Rim, along the U.S.-Mexico border, and for American Indian tribes in the Southwest. She has written extensively on community-based public health approaches to chronic disease prevention and control, the influence of culture and gender on health beliefs and behaviors, and the elimination of health disparities. Her principal research interests are focused on understanding the intersection of race, class, and gender in chronic disease risks, management, and prevention. A native of Richmond, VA, Dr. Liburd holds a BA degree from the University of Michigan at Ann Arbor, a MPH in health education from the University of North Carolina at Chapel Hill, and a MA in cultural anthropology and PhD in medical anthropology from Emory University.

Diabetes and Health Disparities

*Community-Based Approaches
for Racial and Ethnic Populations*

LEANDRIS C. LIBURD, PhD

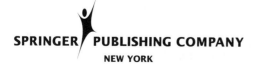

SPRINGER PUBLISHING COMPANY

NEW YORK

Springer Publishing Company, LLC
11 West 42nd Street
New York, NY 10036
www.springerpub.com

Acquisitions Editor: Jennifer Perillo
Project Manager: Judy Worrell
Cover Design: TG Design
Composition: Six Red Marbles

Disclaimer: The findings and conclusions in this book are those of the authors and do not necessarily represent the official position of the Centers for Disease Control and Prevention.

Ebook ISBN: 978-0826-10129-7
09 10 11 12 13 / 5 4 3 2 1

The author and the publisher of this Work have made every effort to use sources believed to be reliable to provide information that is accurate and compatible with the standards generally accepted at the time of publication. The author and publisher shall not be liable for any special, consequential, or exemplary damages resulting, in whole or in part, from the readers' use of, or reliance on, the information contained in this book. The publisher has no responsibility for the persistence or accuracy of URLs for external or third-party Internet Web sites referred to in this publication and does not guarantee that any content on such Web sites is, or will remain, accurate or appropriate.

Library of Congress Cataloging-in-Publication Data
Diabetes and health disparities : community-based approaches for racial and ethnic populations / [edited by] Leandris C. Liburd.
    p. ; cm.
Includes bibliographical references and index.
ISBN 978-0-8261-0128-0
1. Diabetes—United States—Epidemiology.   2. Minorities—United States—Diseases.   I. Liburd, Leandris C.
    [DNLM: 1. Diabetes Mellitus—ethnology—United States.   2. Community Networks—United States.   3. Diabetes Mellitus—prevention & control—United States.   4. Government Programs—United States.   5. Health Status Disparities—United States.   6. Healthcare Disparities—United States. WK 810 D53719 2009]
    RA645.D5D4925   2009
    616.4'62—dc22

                                                                            2009029807

Printed in the United States of America by Hamilton Printing.

For my teachers:
Miss Ruth Taylor
Professor Walter Allen
Dr. John W. Hatch
Dr. Peter J. Brown
Thanks for believing in me.

—Leandris C. Liburd

Contents

Contributors

Nia Aitaoto, MPH, MS
Program Coordinator
Pacific Diabetes Education Program
Papa Ola Lōkahi
Honolulu, HI

Emily E. Anderson, PhD, MPH
Project Director
Illinois Prevention Research Center
School of Public Health
University of Illinois at Chicago
Chicago, IL

Jose O. Arrom, MA
Project Coordinator
Midwest Latino Health Research,
Training and Policy Center
University of Illinois at Chicago
Chicago, IL

Jeff Bachar, MPH
Principal Investigator
Cherokee Choices/REACH U.S.
Eastern Band of Cherokee Indians
Cherokee, NC

Gloria L. Beckles, MD
Visiting Scientist
Division of Diabetes Translation
National Center for Chronic Disease
Prevention and Health Promotion
Centers for Disease Control and
Prevention
Atlanta, GA

Elaine S. Belansky, PhD
Assistant Director
Community and Behavioral Health
Rocky Mountain Prevention Research
Center
Colorado School of Public Health
University of Colorado
Denver, CO

Neal Bosanko
Director
South Chicago Chamber of Commerce
Chicago, IL

Janice V. Bowie, PhD, MPH
Associate Professor
Department of Health, Behavior and
Society
Hopkins Center for Health Disparities
Solutions
Johns Hopkins Bloomberg School of
Public Health
Baltimore, MD

Kathryn L. Braun, DrPH
Professor & Director
Center on Aging
Cancer Research Center of Hawaii
University of Hawaii
Honolulu, HI

Barbara Carlson, MLIS, AHIP
Librarian
REACH Charleston and Georgetown
Diabetes Coalition
Medical University of South Carolina
College of Nursing
Charleston, SC

Lemyra DeBruyn, PhD
Regulatory Director
U.S. Public Health Service
Native Diabetes Wellness Program
Division of Diabetes Translation
National Center for Chronic Disease
Prevention and Health Promotion
Centers for Disease Control and
Prevention
Albuquerque, NM

Carolee Dodge-Francis, EdD
Professor
American Indian Research and
Education Center
School of Public HealthCommunity
Health Sciences
University of Nevada, Las Vegas
Las Vegas, NV

Linda S. Geiss, MA
Surveillance Section Chief
Division of Diabetes Translation
National Center for Chronic Disease
Prevention and Health Promotion
Centers for Disease Control and
Prevention
Atlanta, GA

Aida L. Giachello, PhD
Associate Professor
Jane Addams College of Social Work
Midwest Latino Health Research,
Training and Policy Center
University of Illinois at Chicago
Chicago, IL

John W. Hatch, DrPH, MSW
Professor Emeritus
Project DIRECT
Department of Public Health
Education
North Carolina Central University
School of Public Health
University of North Carolina
Health and Human Services Program
General Baptist State Convention of
North Carolina
Durham, NC

Carolyn Jenkins, DrPH, APRN-BC-ADM, RN, RD, LD, FAAN
Ann Darlington Edwards Endowed
Chair and Professor
REACH Charleston and Georgetown
Diabetes Coalition
College of Nursing
Medical University of South Carolina
Charleston, SC

Florene Linnen
Founder
Georgetown Diabetes CORE Group
REACH Charleston and Georgetown
Diabetes Coalition
College of Nursing
Medical University of South Carolina
Charleston, SC

Gayenell Magwood, PhD
Assistant Professor and
Co-Investigator
REACH Charleston and Georgetown
Diabetes Coalition
College of Nursing
Medical University of South Carolina
Charleston, SC

Kelly Moore, MD
Associate Professor
Health Sciences Center
University of Colorado Denver
American Indian and Alaska Native
Programs
REACH U.S. Center of Excellence for
Eliminating Disparities
Centers for Disease Control and
Prevention
Denver, CO

Amanda M. Navarro, DrPH, MPH
Health Policy Analyst
Division of Adult and Community
Health
National Center for Chronic Disease
Prevention and Health Promotion
Centers for Disease Control and
Prevention
Atlanta, GA

Joyce C. Page, MPH, MSPH
Director
Project DIRECT
Diabetes Prevention and Control
Program
North Carolina Department of Health
and Human Services
Raleigh, NC

Meda E. Pavkov, MD, PhD
Senior Service Fellow
Division of Diabetes Translation
National Center for Chronic Disease
Prevention and Health Promotion
Centers for Disease Control and
Prevention
Atlanta, GA

Dinah Ramirez
Executive Director
Healthy Southeast Chicago
Chicago, IL

Laverne Reid, PhD, MPH
Project DIRECT Associate Dean
College of Behavioral and Social
Science
North Carolina Central University
Durham, NC

Mark D. Rivera, PhD
Health Scientist
Division of Adult and Community
Health
National Center for Chronic Disease
Prevention and Health Promotion
Centers for Disease Control and
Prevention
Atlanta, GA

Laurie Ruggiero, PhD
Professor & Co-Investigator
Illinois Prevention Research Center
School of Public Health
University of Illinois at Chicago
Chicago, IL

Virginia Thomas, BS
Community Health Advisor
REACH Charleston and Georgetown
Diabetes Coalition
College of Nursing
Medical University of South Carolina
Charleston, SC

JoAnn U. Tsark, MPH
Program Director
'Imi Hale – Native Hawaiian Cancer
Network
Papa Ola Lōkahi
Honolulu, HI

Pattie J. Tucker, DrPH, RN
Lead Health Scientist
Division of Adult and Community
Health
National Center for Chronic Disease
Prevention and Health Promotion
Centers for Disease Control and
Prevention
Atlanta, GA

Lucille H. Webb, MEd
President
Strengthening the Black Family
Project DIRECT
Raleigh, NC

Desmond E. Williams, MD, PhD
Senior Service Fellow
Division of Diabetes Translation
National Center for Chronic Disease
Prevention and Health Promotion
Centers for Disease Control and
Prevention
Atlanta, GA

Foreword[1]

Diabetes is exacting a serious toll in the United States and around the world as a leading cause of blindness, amputations, and kidney failure and as a major risk factor for heart disease and stroke. Those hardest hit by diabetes are often those who also face health disparities. In this edition of *Diabetes and Health Disparities: Community-Based Approaches for Racial and Ethnic Populations*, Liburd and colleagues provide the reader with a comprehensive review of the literature related to the epidemiology; anthropologic research; literature from public health, social science, and community-based interventions and evaluation; and case studies from the field to provide a broad-based public health framework to address racial and ethnic disparities in diabetes.

A key component to a comprehensive approach to eliminating disparities and achieving health equity is addressing the socioecological model, which embraces individual, interpersonal, organizational, and public policy influences on health. A unique aspect of this work is the importance of addressing the root causes or upstream determinants of health, including the social determinants of health and the role of racially or ethnically based discrimination, in its personally mediated, internalized, and institutional forms. The authors provide key examples and frameworks that are integral to future community efforts aimed at addressing and eliminating disparities in health.

Racial and ethnic disparities in health are certainly not new; in 1898 W. E. B. Dubois wrote *The Philadelphia Negro*, the first comprehensive documentation of the health status of a racial minority group in the United States. Dubois documented the high rates of infectious and chronic diseases among African Americans residing in Philadelphia. He noted that the health status of African Americans was not solely individually

---

[1] Disclaimer: The findings and conclusions in this foreword are those of the authors and do not necessarily represent the official position of the Centers for Disease Control and Prevention.

mediated but that there were also community, environmental, and institutional factors that impacted the health of communities of color. He concluded with a call to action, writing, "We must endeavor to eliminate, as much as possible, the problem elements that make a difference in health among people" (Dubois, 1898). It is this very broad-based embrace that Liburd and colleagues emphasize in *Diabetes and Health Disparities*. The authors note the need to address the structural influences on health through policies and other practices that impact where people live, work, worship, and play and that help to eliminate, as much as possible, disparities in diabetes. Public health workers involved in diabetes prevention and control in racial and ethnic communities must support and partner with community institutions whose mission supports achieving health equity.

The work of eliminating health disparities must be part of the nation's core efforts in the prevention and control of diabetes. What Liburd and colleagues provide in this edition is a framework for all practitioners—not only public health practitioners but also researchers, policy makers, community organizers, clinicians, and community institutions involved in diabetes prevention and control. The recommendations and tools provided here are keys to the success of future research and programmatic efforts.

Wayne H. Giles, MD, MS
Ann Albright, PhD, RD
Division of Adult and Community Health
and Division of Diabetes Translation
National Center for Chronic Disease
Prevention and Health Promotion
Centers for Disease Control and Prevention

REFERENCES

Dubois, W. E. B. (1898). *The Philadelphia Negro*. Philadelphia: University of Pennsylvania.

Preface

The publication of *Diabetes and Health Disparities: Community-Based Approaches for Racial and Ethnic Populations* marks a significant milestone in my professional public health journey. The conceptual and applied premises of this text are grounded in the rich traditions of community public health, the keen influence of clinical medicine, and the promise of better health outcomes through a population approach to the determinants of health. The content moreover reflects an orientation to public health and the elimination of health disparities, which has guided different stages of my work at the Centers for Disease Control and Prevention (CDC) over the past 2 decades.

In 1987 I began my career at the CDC in the Division of Health Education within the Center for Health Promotion and Education. I was recruited to the agency during the political period of a national interest in minority health that stemmed from the 1985 Task Force Report on Black and Minority Health commissioned by then Secretary of Health and Human Services Margaret Heckler. This report of excess deaths experienced by African Americans and other disadvantaged ethnic groups in the U.S. would institutionalize a federal commitment to address health disparities from the late 1980s to the present. I have counted it a privilege to devote my career in public health to trying to make a difference in communities of color. I have observed and participated in the development and implementation of a multitude of community-based and policy interventions, but none have been adequate to close the gap in the growing burden of type 2 diabetes.

After 17 years of public health practice, I returned to school in 2000 to pursue a doctorate in medical anthropology. I had reached a point in my career where I had exhausted my understandings of how to achieve behavior change for better health—the presiding ideology for chronic disease prevention and control in public health at that time. Having grown up in de facto segregation in the southeastern region of the United States, I experienced firsthand the social and economic conditions that tend toward disease and premature mortality. As I entered college in pursuit of a health career, I believed that if people *knew* better, they would do better, as based on many anecdotal experiences I could recount from my indigenous inner-city community. The first lesson I learned in my graduate public health training was that "knowledge is necessary, but not sufficient for behavior change"—thereby debunking my original hypothesis. What then is sufficient for behavior change? Is behavior change what we should be pursuing as public health professionals? As I entered the doctoral program in medical anthropology, my answer to these questions was summed up in three words: *I'm not sure.* I have spent my entire professional career trying to better understand the complexity of human behavior and most recently, the power of culture, history, the social and material context, and local and global political economies in both the creation of risks for and the ability to respond to chronic diseases, particularly diabetes.

Diabetes can be fairly described as a "whole life" disease in that few areas of one's life is not either influenced by or implicated in the manifestation and control of the disease. *Diabetes and Health Disparities* is written to invert the traditional biomedical view of type 2 diabetes, which privileges the body and individual agency in diabetes prevention and control to a focus on the macro-social context that constructs risks for the development of chronic diseases, as well as opportunities for health and wellness. Ideally, the reader will walk away with a more balanced view of the multiple dimensions of what is needed to eliminate diabetes disparities in racial and ethnic populations in the U.S. and internationally. *Diabetes and Health Disparities* comes at a time when the global public health community is mobilizing with a renewed determination to address the social determinants of health equity. Whereas the associations between social and economic conditions and health are well established, the evidence base for what works to reverse these negative social determinants is weak. It is my aim that the conceptual frameworks and case studies provided in this text will build confidence and inspire creativity and political will to invest in even more robust community-based approaches that will eliminate disparities in diabetes and other chronic diseases disproportionately affecting racial and ethnic communities.

Diabetes and Health Disparities is written for teachers, students, professionals, community leaders, policymakers, and others interested in joining the growing movement to eliminate health disparities and achieve health equity for all. I am hopeful this text will be used by academic institutions, schools of public health, sister federal agencies, state and local health departments, community-based organizations, and national organizations committed to a society where health equity is valued and considered in all policies that affect life and well-being.

Acknowledgments

This text would not have been possible without the support and contributions of numerous people. For each of them, I am eternally grateful. I am especially thankful for the hard work and commitment of Amanda Navarro, who started this project with me and was invaluable in fulfilling the many coordinating and writing roles she played in the development of this book. For Mark Rivera and Pattie Tucker, I extend my heartfelt thanks for their willingness to add writing the evaluation chapter to an already overextended workload. This is the kind of dedication that characterizes the leadership and fortitude in our branch. To Tracy Perkins, I will be forever impressed by her initiative in asking to write some of the Editor's Notes that precede the case studies. I also owe a huge debt of gratitude to the authors and co-authors of the case studies included in this book that demonstrate the vision, courage, and tenacity needed to implement effective community-based diabetes programs in communities of color. Thanks for taking the time and effort to tell your stories for others to benefit.

I must acknowledge my personal cheering squad: my family and closest friends, who have supported me in word and deed over the 14 months that I was engaged in this project. Space will not allow me to name everyone, but my life is richer because of all of you. I must say that words cannot express my gratitude to Janice Bowie, who not only had to hear about the book over and over again, but agreed to co-author a chapter with me during a time when I could not muster the strength to meet all of the demands that were before me. To my friends Yvonne Saunders-Brown and Brenda Hurley, thanks for checking on me and the many expressions of friendship while I was spending weekends at work. To my sisters, Ruth and Rosalyn, and my children, Ronald, Kimberly, and Joy, thanks for always supporting me in my professional pursuits.

Special thanks to Jennifer Perillo and Springer Publishing Company for seeing the merits of this volume; Harry Chambers and Peter Brown for challenging my hesitations and encouraging me to pursue this opportunity; George Armelagos, Chair of the Department of Anthropology at Emory University, for extending an adjunct faculty appointment to me in support of this project; Wayne Giles, Kurt Greenlund, and Laurie Elam-Evans in the Division of Adult and Community Health for your support, endurance, and scientific oversight; Eduardo Simoes, Joann Grumbaum, and the Prevention Research Centers Program for gladly agreeing to collaborate with me in identifying case studies for the book; the Division of Diabetes Translation and my colleagues who immediately saw the value of this book, Ann Albright, Angela Green-Phillips, Desmond Williams, and Barbara Park; the Branch Management Team of the Community Health and Program Services Branch for your patience and perseverance during this and other distractions that competed with my ability to attend more fully to the day-to-day issues of the branch— you continue to be my "dream team" through it all; to the members of the Community Health and Program Services Branch, the hardest working people in public health, I hope you see some of your work and technical assistance in these pages.

Background and Conceptual Frameworks

Recorded knowledge of "diabetes" dates back to antiquity (Papaspyros, 1952). Diabetes, an Ionic Greek term coined by Greek physician Aretaeus of Cappadakia in the 2nd century A.D., means "to run through a siphon" (Papaspyros, 1952, p. xiii). Initially associated with polyuria, diabetes was also known as "urine of honey" according to "very old Sanscrit texts of Indians" in the 6th century A.D. Symptoms recorded included thirst, muscular weakness, unpleasant odor, somnolency, difficulty breathing, and often problems with digestion (Papaspyros, 1952, p. 1). These Indian doctors also noted that the majority of persons with urine honey were overweight, so they concluded this condition was "a malady of rich and greedy persons, especially of those who consume much rich, starchy food and sugar" (Papaspyros, 1952, p. 2). Japanese and Chinese physicians in the 3rd century A.D, according to Papaspyros, observed and recorded polyuria and "urine to taste so sweet as to attract dogs" (1952, p. 2). Nineteenth-century physicians would introduce changes in the pancreas as the cause of diabetes. It was also during this era that diabetes became known as a metabolic disorder as chemists and physiologists experimented with urine samples of persons with diabetes and conducted rudimentary studies of basal metabolism (Papaspyros, 1952, p. 18). There is a large and growing biomedical literature reporting and further examining the complex pathophysiology of this metabolic disorder. The orientation of clinical medicine and biomedical research that individualizes risk and locates it within the physical sphere of the body

1

perpetuates the idea that risk is individually, not socially and historically, determined.

According to the Centers for Disease Control and Prevention, approximately 24 million children and adults in the U.S., or 8% of the population, have diabetes and nearly one-third are unaware that they have it. The lifetime risk of diabetes among persons born in 2000 in the U.S. is 1 in 3 for men and 2 in 5 for women, with a higher risk being estimated among minority populations throughout their lifespan. While the burden of diabetes in the U.S. is well documented, how the socio-ecological context acts on the body and population groups to increase risk for type 2 diabetes is not well understood. Increasingly, researchers are addressing the broader environmental factors that tend toward a higher prevalence of diabetes in communities of color, but much work remains to be done.

In part I of *Diabetes and Health Disparities: Community-Based Approaches for Racial and Ethnic Populations,* we provide an overview and epidemiology of diabetes in the United States, and argue for approaching the prevention and control of diabetes in racial and ethnic populations from a socio-ecological perspective. Simply put, a socio-ecological approach attends to the social conditions that shape the health of the public. We explore (a) epidemiological, place, and cultural relationships between diabetes and obesity in communities of color; (b) constructs of community from the standpoints of the professional and the persons presumably tied to a particular community as they relate to the development of strategies to eliminate diabetes disparities; and (c) the influence of institutionalized racism and residential segregation in the social construction of diabetes in communities of color, then posit broader evaluation paradigms to document the impact of community-based approaches.

REFERENCE

Papaspyros, N.S. (1952). *The history of diabetes mellitus.* London: Robert Stockwell.

Diabetes and Health Disparities: Community-Based Approaches for Racial and Ethnic Populations[1]

LEANDRIS C. LIBURD

INTRODUCTION

According to the World Health Organization, "diabetes is a global epidemic threatening to overwhelm global healthcare services, wipe out some indigenous populations and undermine economies worldwide, especially in developing countries" (2009). Worldwide, about 194 million adults have diabetes and this number is projected to increase to 333 million by 2025 (International Diabetes Federation, 2008). Emerging rates of type 2 diabetes around the world presage a pandemic of this debilitating and costly chronic disease (Green, Hirsch, and Pramming 2003). Type 2 diabetes, the principal focus of this text, accounts for 90–95% of all diagnosed cases of diabetes in the U.S. (Centers for Disease Control and Prevention, 2008). *Diabetes and Health Disparities: Community-Based Approaches for Racial and Ethnic Populations* seeks to add promising community-based approaches to the fight to eliminate disparities in type 2 diabetes.

The disproportionate and rising burden of diabetes in racial and ethnic communities in the United States is well documented but not

---

[1] The findings and conclusions in this chapter are those of the author and do not necessarily represent the views of the Centers for Disease Control and Prevention.

3

well understood. Despite decades of a national emphasis on improving health among racial and ethnic minority groups (U.S. Department of Health and Human Services, 1986)—including African Americans, American Indians or Alaska Natives, Hispanic/Latino Americans, Asian Americans, and Pacific Islanders—the current diabetes incidence and prevalence and the associated complications of diabetes in these groups are sobering and predicted to increase in the years ahead.

In the past 60 years, we have benefited from an extensive literature on the pathogenesis and clinical management of diabetes. A cross-section of diabetes researchers also posits competing hypotheses about the causes of diabetes. While genes matter, changes in genetic structures likely do not account for the epidemic of diabetes that has occurred over the last 20–25 years (Braun, 2002; Permutt, Wasson, & Cox, 2005). It is generally accepted among diabetes researchers that the different types of diabetes are caused by a complex interaction of genetic and environmental factors. The exact pathways of these mechanisms are not well understood. Yet, any population-based approach to improving diabetes outcomes must acknowledge an interconnectedness of biological, behavioral, physical, and socio-ecological determinants of the disease and develop intervention models specific to one or more of these determinants.

In this text we take a socio-ecological approach to understanding and responding to the disproportionate burden of type 2 diabetes among racial and ethnic populations in the U.S. Simply put, a socio-ecological approach attends to the social conditions that shape the health of the public. A social-ecology orientation to health and disease (a) assumes a population perspective on health determinants, (b) recognizes the complex interactions among multiple levels of influence, (c) examines the social context that shapes behavior, (d) adopts a life course and developmental perspective, and (e) identifies biological mechanisms (Berkman & Lochner, 2002).

More explicitly, a socio-ecological approach argues that we must move beyond clinical interventions in high-risk populations if we want to advance the population's health; identify the central role of socioeconomic conditions, social networks and cohesion, and work conditions in shaping population health; study the impact of "cumulative disadvantage" and exposure to risks for illness across the lifespan; and understand more fully how social and psychological conditions (e.g., chronic stress) interact with biological mechanisms to cause disease (Berkman & Lochner, 2002). A full discussion of the social ecology of health is beyond the scope of this text. However, if we are to reverse current trends in the incidence of diabetes, additional work framed from the socio-ecological perspective is needed.

ORGANIZATION OF THE TEXT

In *Diabetes and Health Disparities*, we argue for a critical re-examination of the core assumptions inherent in traditional explanations of, and interventions for, diabetes in communities of color.[2] Using a framework that favors the social determinants of health, we draw on epidemiological data (chapters 2 and 3); anthropological research (chapter 4); literature from the public health, social science, community interventions, and evaluation literature (chapters 5–7); and case studies from the field (chapters 8–16) to forge a broader public health agenda to address the social conditions that construct risks for type 2 diabetes and its associated risk factors and complications. We acknowledge that although the associations between the social determinants of health and disparities in diabetes prevalence between communities of color and the general population are strong and compelling, there is a paucity of evidence that improvements in the social environment are directly associated with decreases in the incidence of type 2 diabetes.

In fact, this text will raise as many questions as are potentially answered, for example:

- In what instances are cultural, socioeconomic, and political forces more predictive of health behaviors than individual choice (Holmes, et al., 1998; Kumanyika, 1998; Ren, et al., 1999; Tull & Chambers, 2001; Williams, 1996)?
- What are feasible public health interventions and policies in light of the location and inherently political nature of public health (Adler & Newman, 2002; Lurie, 2002)?
- How can we actively engage interdisciplinary social science perspectives in contextualizing the gender, class, and racial distribution of

---

[2] Terms including *communities of color, people of color,* and *racial and ethnic minority groups* are used interchangeably throughout this text to respectfully and collectively capture the following population groups: American Indian or Alaska Native, Asian, Black or African American, Hispanic/Latino, and Native Hawaiian or Other Pacific Islander.

diabetes (Inhorn & Whittle, 2001; LaVeist, 1996; Whittle & Inhorn, 2001)?

■ How well have our community-based public health strategies kept pace with the changing demographics and destabilization of many urban communities?

■ Are we regularly and systematically challenging and refining the assumptions that drive our program planning to ensure these assumptions remain relevant and effective in communities that are rapidly changing racially, ethnically, and economically?

■ What are feasible options for health reform that will eliminate disparities in health care for persons of color with diabetes?

The centrality of access to affordable and quality health care in eliminating diabetes disparities, although a key factor in the fight to reduce the preventable burden of diabetes and its associated complications, is only minimally addressed in this text by Navarro in chapter 6. Although not a prominent aspect of this text, we acknowledge and applaud the multitude of studies, commentaries, and model health services advocating for a more equitable and accessible health care system.

LEARNING OBJECTIVES

The content of *Diabetes and Health Disparities* is guided by the following learning objectives:

■ Increase the reader's understanding of the epidemiology of diabetes in communities of color in the U.S. and its associated risk factors. We pay particular attention to obesity as a risk factor for the development of type 2 diabetes.

■ Support the continued development, implementation, and evaluation of community-based diabetes prevention and control programs grounded in the framework of the social determinants of health. Toward this end, we examine (a) how we understand communities and the framing of community models for diabetes programs, (b) structural influences such as residential segregation that bear on the development of health disparities including diabetes, (c) cultural influences such as obesity on risk factors for the development of diabetes, and (d) biases in our use of the terms *racial and ethnic minority groups* that potentially limit the effectiveness of public health programs intended to improve health outcomes in populations that bear a disproportionate burden of chronic diseases.

■ Provide case studies of community-based diabetes programs that are moving in the direction of social determinants of health framework through greater attention to policy and environmental change in community sectors such as schools, work sites, the food environment, and places of worship. The reader is asked to consider a group of questions that will hopefully inspire additional strategies that address social determinants of health, such as insuring access to affordable and high-quality fresh fruits and vegetables in urban, low-income communities.

■ Advance the evaluation of public health programs addressing diabetes prevention and control in communities of color by assessing a community's ability to develop and leverage its capacity through inter-organizational relationships with new and nontraditional partners within and outside the community; establish measures that reflect this emphasis on shared capacity and outcomes that result from complex clusters of organizational resources and efforts across levels of a community; design evaluations that reflect the time needed to address social determinants of health and that focus primarily on contribution rather than attribution, due to the typically indirect path between programmatic and policy interventions addressing health outcomes through social determinants of health; and consider milestones that help ensure that the longer-term social determinants of health outcomes are realized.

■ Challenge the next generation of public health workers to forge a more robust community-based diabetes prevention and control research and practice agenda, than has been accomplished to date, using theories, community models, and strategies that provide direction toward the elimination of health disparities and achievement of health equity.

THE SOCIAL DETERMINANTS OF HEALTH AND HEALTH EQUITY

According to the World Health Organization's Commission on Social Determinants of Health, "the poor health of the poor, the social gradient in health within countries, and the marked health inequities between countries are caused by the unequal distribution of power, income, goods, and services, globally and nationally, the consequent unfairness in the immediate, visible circumstances of peoples' lives—their access to health care, schools, and education, their conditions of work and leisure, their homes, communities, towns, or cities—and their chances of leading a flourishing life" constitute the social determinants of health (World Health Organization, 2008). Root factors like discrimination, poverty, and other forms of oppression play out at the community level, which affects the community environment (Giles & Liburd, 2007).

The terms *health disparities* and *health equity* are fairly common to health practitioners, program managers, policy makers, and researchers (Braveman, 2006). The terms *health disparities* or *health inequities* are generally used in the U.S., whereas health equity is more common in Europe. In the early 1990s Margaret Whitehead developed a widely accepted definition of health disparities: "differences in health that are not only avoidable and unnecessary but in addition unjust and unfair" (Braveman, 2006, p. 167). Health equity is defined as "providing all people with fair opportunities to attain their full health potential to the extent possible" (Braveman, 2006, p. 167). Inherent in our understanding of health equity is the recognition of the role of social privilege, or what Inhorn and Whittle term "social hierarchies" (2001). According to Braveman, Krieger, and Lynch, "Disparities are not merely differences in health between groups but differences between groups with varying levels of social privilege. Social privilege can be defined as one's relative position in a hierarchy determined by prestige, power, or wealth" (2000, p. 232).

"The most fundamental causes of health disparities are socioeconomic disparities," according to Adler and Newman (2002, p. 61). Socioeconomic status in public health has traditionally been defined by education, income, and occupation (Krieger & Moss 1996; Winkleby, Jatulis, Frank, and Fortmann 1992). Commonly believed, for example, education shapes future occupational opportunities and earning potential and "provides knowledge and life skills that allow better-educated persons to gain more ready access to information and resources to promote health" (Adler & Newman, 2002, p. 61). Similarly, income provides the means to access and purchases housing, schools, nutrition, and recreation. Higher incomes afford better housing and access to goods and services that tend toward health. However, the pathway between socioeconomic status and health is not a direct one, but likely serves as "proxies for other determinants," that is, "differential exposure to conditions that have more immediate effects on health" (Adler & Newman, 2002, p. 67).

In the United States, for example, residential neighborhoods in urban and suburban communities continue to demonstrate historical patterns of segregation by race (Williams & Collins, 2001; Wilson, 1991; Wilson, 2009). Theoretically, racial segregation that appears to be equal in its housing quality and access to services, as may be observed in middle- and upper-middle-class Black communities, might portend a positive health benefit for these residents, but additional research is needed to confirm if this is so. More generally, as has been observed by several scholars, the degree of residential segregation is indicative of the quality of the public schools, the quality of and access to services like shopping and healthcare, property values and the investments of the local government in creating a "livable community," and police protection, among others (Brown et al., 2003).

Persons who live in these communities are intimately aware of the impact of residential segregation and other social determinants of health on daily life and the opportunities to promote health and prevent disease. In 1999 the Centers for Disease Control and Prevention (CDC) launched the REACH (Racial and Ethnic Approaches to Community Health) 2010 program to address avoidable and unfair disparities in six health conditions: breast and cervical cancer screening, cardiovascular disease, diabetes, HIV/AIDS, immunizations, and infant mortality (Giles & Liburd, 2006). Using community-based participatory approaches, REACH was built on a premise described by Inhorn and Whittle as the "new epidemiologies" that "listen to and engage with people articulating their experiences of health and illness within the social, political, economic, as well as biological context of their lives" (2001, p. 558).

In 2007, south Los Angeles's Community Health Councils (CHCs) was awarded a REACH grant to address cardiovascular disease in a largely African American section of the community. Lark Galloway-Gilliam, Executive Director of CHCs, described the root causes of the cardiovascular disease burden in these terms: "The disparities are not simply a result of individual behavior but rather an outgrowth of racial segregation and public and private policies and systems that concentrate poverty." Social justice is fundamental to public health, even though we are still defining and refining strategies to effectively bridge the social context of communities at high risk for diabetes with clinical and other requirements for preventing and managing diabetes. Throughout this text there will be frequent mention of how structural influences expressed through policies and other practices where people live, work, worship, and play help shape diabetes disparities. To effectively eliminate disparities in the conditions that promote diabetes, public health workers involved in diabetes prevention and control in racial and ethnic communities must support and partner with community institutions whose mission supports achieving health equity.

"RACIAL AND ETHNIC POPULATIONS" IN THE UNITED STATES

race: a recent idea created by western Europeans following exploration across the world to account for differences among people and justify colonization, conquest, enslavement, and social hierarchy among humans. The term is used to refer to groupings of people according to common origin or background and associated with perceived biological markers. Among humans there are no races except the human race. In biology, the term has limited use, usually associated with organisms or populations that are able to interbreed. Ideas about race are culturally and socially transmitted and form the basis of racism, racial classification and often complex racial identities.

racial classification: the practice of classifying people into distinct racial groups based on certain characteristics such as skin color or geographic region, often for the purpose of ranking them based on believed innate differences between the groups.

racial identity: this concept operates at two levels: (1) self identity or conceptualization based upon perceptions of one's race and (2) society's perception and definition of a person's race.

racialization: the process by which individuals and groups of people are viewed through a racial lens, through a culturally invented racial framework. Racialization is often referred to as racialism.

racial stratification: a system of stratification and inequality in which access to resources (political, economic, social) depends largely upon one's racial classification.   *(continued)*

racism: the use of race to establish and justify a social hierarchy and system of power that privileges, preferences or advances certain individuals or groups of people usually at the expense of others. Racism is perpetuated through both interpersonal and institutional practices.

ethnicity: an idea similar to race that groups people according to common origin or background. The term usually refers to social, cultural, religious, linguistic and other affiliations although, like race, it is sometimes linked to perceived biological markers. Ethnicity is often characterized by cultural features, such as dress, language, religion, and social organization.

Excerpts from the glossary of American Anthropological Association (2007).

The primary populations of interest for *Diabetes and Health Disparities* are based on the race categories established by the Office of Management and Budget (2000): "The five minimum race categories are American Indian or Alaska Native, Asian, Black or African American, Native Hawaiian or Other Pacific Islander, and White." Hispanic origin (Hispanic/Latino) is indicated separately from race and considered an ethnicity. Persons of Hispanic origin include those of Mexican, Mexican-American, Central American, South American, Chicano or Puerto Rican, Cuban, or other Spanish-Caribbean ancestry. We do not address diabetes in White populations in this text, but recognize that there are largely White communities, such as those found in Appalachia, that suffer a disproportionate burden of diabetes akin to that found in communities of color (CDC, 2005).

We are keenly aware that these race categories and the ethnicity tag-on have little meaning in terms of reflecting the histories, diversity within and among groups within a single category (e.g., Hispanic/Latino), or unique cultural identities embraced across the rich heterogeneity of each racial and ethnic category. In our attention to American Indian or Alaska Native, Asian, Black or African American, and Native Hawaiian or Other Pacific Islander, we argue that race is a social construct and lived experience, not a genetic endowment that tends toward health disparities in populations characterized in this text as racial and ethnic minority groups. According to the American Anthropological Association (1998),

> With the vast expansion of scientific knowledge in this century, however, it has become clear that human populations are not unambiguous, clearly demarcated, biologically distinct groups. Evidence from the analysis of genetics (e.g., DNA) indicates that most physical variation, about 94%, lies *within* so-called racial groups. Conventional geographic "racial" groupings differ from one another only in about 6% of their genes. This means that there is greater variation within "racial" groups than between them. . . . Throughout history whenever different groups have come into contact, they have interbred. The continued sharing of genetic materials has maintained all of humankind as a single species. . . . Historical research has shown that the idea of "race" has always carried more meanings than mere physical differences; indeed, physical variations in the human species have no meaning except the social ones that humans put on them.

A social construct then is "a social mechanism, phenomenon, or category created and developed by society; a perception of an individual, group, or idea that is 'constructed' through cultural or social practice" (*Webster's Dictionary*, 2009). In working with racial and ethnic communities to eliminate disparities in diabetes, it is critical to learn from the community its history, experiences of oppression, meanings ascribed to diabetes and other chronic diseases, and how they construct their own racial and ethnic identity. It is beyond the scope of this book and the expertise of the authors to speak with authority to the diversities of social, political, and cultural experience of these racial and ethnic minority groups, but we are hopeful that what we have included can be used as a beginning from which more authentic local reflection can emerge.

Our concern with race in health then is more appropriately represented as a concern with racism and its impact on the health of people of color in the U.S. According to sociologist William Julius Wilson, racism is "an ideology of racial domination with two key features: (1) beliefs that one race is either biologically or culturally inferior to another and (2) the use of such beliefs to rationalize or prescribe the way the 'inferior' race should be treated in this society, as well as to explain its social position as a group and its collective accomplishments" (2009, p. 15). He argues that racism is expressed through structural forces described as social acts and social processes.

Social acts refer to "the behaviors of individuals within society," such as "stereotyping; stigmatization; discrimination in hiring, job promotions, housing, and admission to educational institutions—as well as exclusion from unions, employers' associations, and clubs—when any of these are the act of an individual or group exercising power over others" (Wilson, 2009, p. 5).

Social processes, on the other hand, refer to "the 'machinery' of society that exists to promote ongoing relations among members of the larger group. Examples of social processes that contribute directly to racial group outcomes include laws, policies, and institutional practices that exclude people on the basis of race or ethnicity" (Wilson, 2009, p. 5). The cumulative impact of the internalization and lived experience of racism is argued to contribute to the excess mortality and morbidity experienced by racial and ethnic groups in the U.S. (Geronimus, Bound, Waidmann, Hillemeier, & Burns, 1996; Geronimus, Hicken, Keene, & Bound, 2006; Williams, 1999; Williams & Mohammed, 2009).

There is a large and growing literature on the impact of racism on health. Health disparities between African Americans and Whites in the U.S., for example, are well documented and can be traced back to the 15th and 16th centuries' slave trade of Africans in North America, continuing through different historical landmarks of the antebellum period of slavery in the South, the post-Civil War and Reconstruction eras, and post-Reconstruction and the span of "Jim Crow," persisting through the Civil Rights era and more recent Black Liberation and Black Power movements of the late 1960s and early 1970s (Byrd & Clayton, 2000; Dubois, 1899; Savitt, 1978; Semmes, 1996). However, as in analyses of the contribution of socioeconomic status to health, the pathways and structural mechanisms through which racism impacts health are not well established.

For example, Jones and colleagues found in their study of "socially assigned race" that "being socially assigned as *White* is associated with large and statistically significant advantages in health status, even for those who self-identify with a non-*white* group" (2008, p. 501). Racism is defined by Jones as "a system of structuring opportunity and assigning value based on the social interpretation of how one looks" (2003, p. 9). According to Jones and her colleagues, the significance of socially assigned race is that "it measures the *ad hoc* racial classification upon which racism operates" (2008, p. 496). In other words, they posit that "perhaps racial health disparities are not due just to disadvantages experienced by members of non-*White* groups, but also to the advantages experienced by *White* people" (Jones et al., 2008, p. 501). A full and compelling discussion of racism and diabetes disparities is beyond the scope of this text. In chapter 6 Navarro discusses the role of institutionalized racism in residential segregation.

New Millennium Communities

Among the strengths of CDC's community-based programs are that they engage members of the affected community in the design and implementation of the program, are grounded in indigenous community structures and practices, and address health care policies and practice as related to diabetes. Although we have considerable experience mobilizing communities around diabetes prevention and control, our models are challenged to keep pace with the changing landscape and dynamics of contemporary racial and ethnic communities.

Over the past 40 years, the demographics of an inner city in many urban areas has been modified by gentrification and the influx of diverse migrant groups from neighboring borders and around the world. For example, according to the U.S. Census Bureau, the Hispanic or Latino population of the United States increased by 57.9%, from 22.4 million in 1990 to 35.3 million in 2000, representing persons of Mexican, Central and South American, Cuban, Puerto Rican, and other Hispanic descent (U.S. Census Bureau, 2000). In 2000 approximately half of the Hispanic/ Latino population in the United States resided in metropolitan areas. Compared with non-Hispanic Whites, low levels of formal education and high levels of unemployment characterize Hispanic/Latino communities and Hispanic/Latino families are more likely to live in poverty. The growing burden of diabetes among Hispanic/Latino residents of the United States, their diverse cultural and linguistic traditions, and the challenges associated with settling in a new country create new opportunities for public health workers to establish meaningful and effective interventions.

Community in the new millennium is often a moving, heterogeneous, hard to conceptualize, often hidden (from formal governmental institutions) target. Community models that once assumed a relatively stable, connected, and demographically and culturally similar population living in a traceable geopolitical location may no longer reflect the reality of many urban residents who are at high risk for the development of diabetes (Wilson & Taub, 2006). Public health workers are called to define community and align our programs based on the actuality of community and not Western, romanticized models. In chapter 5 Liburd and Bowie elaborate on the meanings of community in public health practice and how our framing of racial and ethnic communities informs community models for diabetes prevention and control.

FORGING NEW EVALUATION APPROACHES

Integral to community-based approaches for racial and ethnic populations is the active engagement, leadership, and ownership of the affected community in all aspects of the program. This holds true for the evaluation component of community-based programs as well. In this text community-based participatory approaches to evaluation refer to those where participation by community members who are affected by that which is being evaluated is central throughout the evaluation process. These approaches are designed to build community capacity and have social betterment as a driving force. In other words, the unit of assessment for the evaluation is the community as the social context in which change is sought, rather than individual community members in which health behaviors occur. Chapter 7 explores how community change is achieved and assessed within complex clusters of organizations and their resources and efforts across levels of a community. The chapter also underscores the need for evaluations to reflect the time needed to address social determinants and the often indirect path between programmatic and policy interventions addressing health outcomes through social determinants of health.

Four Generations of Evaluation

As has happened in other disciplines, evaluation has undergone a variety of paradigm shifts. To better contextualize the evaluative stance of this text, we provide a brief historical overview of earlier and more established evaluation models. Guba and Lincoln (1989) summarized four generations of evaluation that provide a context for community-based participatory evaluation (CBPE) and its key tenets. First-generation evaluation was primarily rooted in empiricism or measurement. Second-generation evaluators saw a lack of program description as a key limitation of the measurement approach. That is, evaluators knew what the end result was but we did not know what characteristics of the program itself might have most contributed to this end state, as we had very little understanding of the context. Third-generation evaluators came to believe that although measurement and description were both important, the evaluator, as an objective third party, was in a unique position to judge a program's merit or worth.

While the first three approaches were each seen as key advancements to the field of evaluation, Guba and Lincoln (1989) also noted that each approach had key shortcomings. Each approach fell prey to managerialism whereby, typically, the funder of the evaluation controlled the questions, how information was collected and used, and so on. This can foster disenfranchising conditions in which the funder is in collusion with the evaluator and is able to shape the evaluation to meet the funder's needs. The first three generations of evaluation were also seen as over-reliant on a scientific paradigm whereby an a priori understanding, that is the understanding of the principle investigator, is tested. The a priori understanding in turn reflects biases of the investigator that unduly compromise notions of objectivity. Finally, the first three generations of evaluation tended to assess programs in a way that assumed a single set of values that underlie and drive a given program, for example, the ability of a program to achieve and sustain individual behavior change. These values are often embodied in external standards (e.g., priorities of the funders) and other points of reference by which a program's merit or worth may be judged (e.g., other scientists or practitioners with similar interests). Rather than follow this standard, the fourth-generation evaluator helps to identify information that addresses questions and concerns raised about the program by its stakeholders, particularly those who stand to reap a health benefit from the program's success.

The evaluator in fourth-generation evaluation has several responsibilities. In addition to being an expert in measurement, the evaluator must also be capable of effectively describing programs and making judgments of merit and worth about the programs. In assessing the programs, the evaluator must also reflect the program's history and the contextual factors influencing its success and facilitate creating conditions whereby stakeholders are empowered to learn and take action to improve their program. Fourth-generation evaluations frame the evaluation design on the basis of the claims, concerns, and issues of a broad pool of stakeholders. Claims are what stakeholders identify as the true benefits and goals of a program. For these the evaluation may help to identify evidence that supports or refutes each claim. Concerns are weaknesses, barriers, and challenges associated with the program. Again, the evaluation may help to verify these concerns or identify their causes and possible ways they may be addressed in the future. Evaluations may also be designed to gather information to better understand both sides of an issue (e.g., competing claims or concerns) or any area where stakeholders have a key difference of opinion regarding the program.

Fourth-generation evaluation is a constructivist approach meaning that it largely dispenses with attempts to draw cause-and-effect relationships predicated on building a program's generalizability. Rather than focus on validating a program for wider translation and dissemination, fourth-generation evaluation has as its primary focus the understanding of a program in its current context and in the interest of its stakeholders. The fourth-generation evaluation approach acknowledges that a program's political context can reshape resources, priorities, target population, and so on. The fourth-generation evaluation approach is responsive to this reality and considers these fluctuations an important part of the program itself. These factors are regularly considered, rather than controlled, by maximizing the involvement of stakeholders.

In fourth-generation evaluation the evaluator is the mediator rather than the judge. The evaluator helps to enable the stakeholders, operating from a jointly determined process of negotiation, to reach key recommendations and decisions. The evaluator moves out from controller to collaborator regardless of whether this threatens technical adequacy. The evaluator solicits and incorporates stakeholder input, including the development of the content of the evaluation and the methods chosen. The evaluator is learner and teacher rather than investigator, setting the stage for stakeholders to learn. The evaluator takes responsibility for the implications of the work as much as the other stakeholders. In other words, the evaluator is equally accountable and serves as a change agent rather than passive observer. As a change agent the evaluator helps use the evaluation to frame action rather than simply imparting knowledge.

Community-Based Participatory Evaluation

CBPE is consistent with fourth-generation evaluation in many respects. It begins with the tenet that those within the community who are affected by the program under study are equal participants in framing the evaluation questions and approaches, determining how program success will be defined, identifying intended users and uses of evaluation findings, and so on. An underlying value of this approach is self-determination. Within this framework, self-determination advocates that historically disenfranchised groups should have greater control over the programs and studies that affect the groups. The endpoint is often program improvement rather than a judgment of a program's merit or worth. It may be directed toward improving decision-making and planning, enhancing self-reflection and process learning, or ensuring good use of resources where the priority of each potential purpose can differ depending on the stakeholder group.

These aspects of CBPE help ensure the use of evaluation findings by increasing their relevance within a community's cultural context and resource limitations. The evaluation benefits from expertise and other resources residing in the community and, in the process, engenders community buy-in and enhances the ability of community members to implement proposed changes based on evaluation findings. Not only does including the community throughout the evaluation process help ensure changes to the program but also other implications or uses of the evaluation are driven by the needs and concerns of those most affected (KU Work Group for Community Health and Development, 2007). This level of community involvement in the evaluation of the program helps ensure the sustainability of programmatic changes. In addition, participatory evaluation can build community relationships and infrastructure to support future evaluation and research efforts (Brown & Tandon, 1983; Fetterman, Kaftarian, & Wandersman, 1996; Pinto, Schmidt, Rodriguez, & Solano, 2007). These are especially important considerations when evaluating programs in communities with racial/ethnic health disparities. (For a comprehensive list of strengths and weaknesses of community-based participatory research, the reader is referred to the KU Work Group for Community Health and Development [2007].)

SUMMARY

Overall, in preparing this text we included findings and perspectives from the CDC's program and prevention research experience, along with publications from the epidemiological, social science, community intervention, and evaluation literature. The depth and breadth of the literature are promising and provocative, stimulating questions that help frame the formation of next steps in reducing, and ultimately eliminating, the burden of diabetes in disproportionately affected populations. It is our aim that *Diabetes and Health Disparities* will challenge and inform the vision and work of public health practitioners and researchers, policy makers, community organizers, and community institutions involved in health promotion and chronic disease prevention. In addition, we are hopeful that those charged with training the next generation of public health workers will continue to reach more broadly into the social, economic and political environments in their efforts to eliminate disparities in diabetes prevalence.

REFERENCES

Adler, N. E., & Newman, K. (2002). Socioeconomic disparities in health: Pathways and policies. *Health Affairs, 21(2),* 60–76.

American Anthropological Association. (May 17, 1998). Statement on "race." Retrieved February 2, 2009, from http://www.aaanet.org/stmts/racepp.htm

American Anthropological Association, (2007). *Race: Are we so different? A project of the American Anthropological Association.* Retrieved from http://www.understandingrace.org/resources/glossary.html

Berkman, L. F., & Lochner, A. (2002). Social determinants of health: Meeting at the crossroads. *Health Affairs, 21(2),* 291–293.

Braun, L. (2002). Race, ethnicity, and health: Can genetics explain disparities? *Perspectives in Biology and Medicine, 45(2),* 159–174.

Braveman, P. A. (2006). Health disparities and health equity: Concepts and measurement. *Annual Review of Public Health, 27,* 167–194.

Braveman, P. A., Krieger, N., & Lynch, J. (2000). Health inequities and social inequalities in health. *Bulletin of the World Health Organization, 78,* 232–233.

Brown, L. D., & Tandon, R. (1983). Ideology and political economy in inquiry: Action research and participatory research. *Journal of Applied Behavioural Science, 19,* 277–285.

Brown, M. K., Carnoy, M., Currie, E., Duster, T., Oppenheimer, D. B., Shultz, M. M., & Wellman, D. (2003). *White-washing race: The myth of a color-blind society.* Berkeley, CA: The University of California Press.

Byrd, W. M., & Clayton, L. A. (2000). *An American health dilemma: A medical history of African Americans and the problem of race.* New York: Routledge.

Centers for Disease Control and Prevention. (2008). *National diabetes fact sheet: General information and national estimates on diabetes in the United States, 2007.* Atlanta, GA: U.S. Department of Health and Human Services, Centers for Disease Control and Prevention.

Centers for Disease Control and Prevention. (2007). *National Diabetes Fact Sheet: General Information and National Estimates on Diabetes in the United States.* Retrieved from www.cdc.gov/diabetes/pubs/factsheet07.htm

DuBois, W. E. B. (1899). *The Philadelphia Negro.* Philadelphia: University of Pennsylvania.

Fetterman, D. M., Kaftarian, S., & Wandersman, A. (Eds.) (1996). *Empowerment evaluation: Knowledge and tools for self-assessment and accountability.* Thousand Oaks, CA: Sage.

Geronimus, A. T., Bound, J., Waidmann, T. A., Hillemeier, M. M., & Burns, P. B. (1996). Excess mortality among Blacks and Whites in the United States. *New England Journal of Medicine, 335(21),* 1552–1558.

Geronimus, A. T., Hicken, M., Keene, D., & Bound, J. (2006). "Weathering" and age patterns of allostatic load scores among Blacks and Whites in the United States. *American Journal of Public Health, 96(5)*, 826–833.

Giles, W. H., & Liburd, L. C. (2007). Reflections on the past, reaching for the future: REACH 2010—the first seven years. *Health Promotion Practice, 7*, S179–S180.

Giles, W. H., & Liburd, L. C. (2007). Achieving health equity and social justice. In L. Cohen, V. Chavez, & S. Chehimi (Eds.), *Prevention is primary* (pp. 25–40). San Francisco, CA: Jossey-Bass.

Green, A., Hirsch N. C., & Pramming, S. K. (2003). The changing world demography of type 2 diabetes. *Diabetes Metabolism Research and Review, 19*, 3–7.

Guba, E., & Lincoln, Y. (1989). *Fourth generation evaluation.* London: Sage.

Holmes, M. D., Stampfer M. J., Wolf A. M., Jones C. P., Spiegelman D., Manson J. E., & Colditz G. A. (1998). Can behavioral risk factors explain the difference in body mass index between African American and European American women? *Ethnicity & Disease, 8*, 331–339.

Inhorn, M., & Whittle, K. L. (2001). Feminism meets the "new "epidemiologies": Toward an appraisal of antifeminist biases in epidemiological research on women's health. *Social Science & Medicine, 53*, 553–567.

International Diabetes Federation. (2008). *Diabetes atlas* (3rd ed.). Retrieved April 2008 from http://www.eatlas.idf.org/media/

Jones, C. P. (2003). Confronting institutionalized racism. *Phylon 50(1–2)*, 7–22.

Jones, C. P., Truman, B., Elam-Evans, L.D., Jones C. A., Jones C. Y., Jiles R., Rumisha. S.F., & Perry G.S. (2008). Using "socially assigned race" to probe White advantages in health status. *Ethnicity & Disease, 18*, 496–504.

Krieger, N. and Moss, N. (1996) Accounting for the public's health: an introduction to selected papers from a U.S. conference on "measuring social inequalities in health". *Int J Health Serv 26(3):383–90.*

KU Work Group for Community Health and Development. (2007). Conducting concerns surveys. Lawrence, KS: University of Kansas. Retrieved September 12, 2007, from http://ctb.ku.edu/en/tablecontents/section_1045.htm

Kumanyika, S. K. (1998). Obesity in African Americans: Biobehavioral consequences of culture. *Ethnicity & Disease, 8*, 93–96.

LaVeist, T. A. (1996). Why we should continue to study race . . . but do a better job: An essay on race, racism and health. *Ethnicity & Disease, 6*, 21–29.

Lurie, N. (2002). What the federal government can do about the nonmedical determinants of health. *Health Affairs, 21(2)*, 94–106.

Office of Management and Budget. (March 9, 2000). Bulletin No. 00-02.

Permutt, M. A., Wasson, J., & Cox, N. (2005). Genetic epidemiology of diabetes. *Journal of Clinical Investigation, 115(6)*, 1431–1439.

Pinto, R. M., Schmidt, C. N. T., Rodriguez, P. S. O., & Solano, R. (2007). Using principles of community participatory research: Groundwork for a collaboration in Brazil. *International Social Work, 50*, 53.

Ren, X. S., Amick B. C., Williams D. R. (1999). Racial/ethnic disparities in health: The interplay between discrimination and socioeconomic status. *Ethnicity & Disease. 9*, 151–165.

Savitt, T. L. (1978). *Medicine and slavery: The diseases and health care of Blacks in antebellum Virginia.* Urbana, IL: University of Illinois Press.

Semmes, C. E. (1996). *Racism, health, and post-industrialism: A theory of African-American health.* Westport, CT: Praeger.

Tull, E. S., & Chambers, E. C. (2001). Internalized racism is associated with glucose intolerance among Black Americans in the U.S. Virgin Islands. *Diabetes Care, 24(8),* 1498.

U.S. Census Bureau. (2000). www.census.gov/main/www/cen2000.html

U.S. Department of Health and Human Services. (1986). *Report of the secretary's task force on Black & minority health.* Washington, DC: Government Printing Office.

Webster's Dictionary. (2009) www.websters-online-dictionary.org/

Whittle, K., & Inhorn, M. (2001). Rethinking difference: A feminist reframing of gender/race/class for improvement of women's health research. *International Journal of Health Services, 31(1),* 147–165.

Williams, D. R. (1996). Racism and health: A research agenda. *Ethnicity & Disease, 6,* 1–6.

Williams, D. R. (1999). Race, socioeconomic status, and health: The added effects of racism and discrimination. *Annals of the New York Academy of Sciences, 896,* 173–188.

Williams, D. R., & Collins, C. (2001). Racial residential segregation: A fundamental cause of racial disparities in health. *Public Health Reports, 116(5),* 404–416.

Williams, D. R., & Mohammed, S. A. (2009). Discrimination and racial disparities in health: Evidence and needed research. *Journal of Behavioral Medicine, 32(1),* 20–47.

Wilson, W. J. (1991). Studying inner-city social dislocation: The challenge of public agenda research. *American Sociological Review, 56,* 1–14.

Wilson, W. J. (2009). *More than just race: Being Black and poor in the inner city.* New York: W. W. Norton & Company.

Wilson, W. J., & Taub R. P. (2006). *There goes the neighborhood.* New York: Alfred A. Knopf.

Winkleby, M. A., Jatulis, D.E., Frank, E., Fortmann, S.P. (1992). "Socioeconomic Status and Health: How Education, Income, and occupation contribute to Risk factors for cardiovascular disease." *American Journal of Public Health 82(6):* 816-820.

World Diabetes Day. (2009). *Why Diabetes?: Diabetes is a silent killer that kills one person every 10 seconds.* http://www.worlddiabetesday.org/node/2415

World Health Organization. (2008). Commission on Social Determinants of Health's Final Report, Executive Summary.

Overview and Epidemiology of Diabetes in Racial/Ethnic Minorities in the United States[1]

2

MEDA E. PAVKOV, LINDA S. GEISS, GLORIA L. BECKLES, AND DESMOND E. WILLIAMS

INTRODUCTION

About 194 million adults worldwide have diabetes. This figure is projected to increase to 333 million by 2025 (International Diabetes Federation, 2008). The largest increase is predicted in developing countries, those transitioning from an agricultural to an established market economy. In developed countries, the largest increase is predicted to be among the elderly and in racial and ethnic minorities (see Figure 2.1) (International Diabetes Federation, 2008).

The projected increase in diabetes prevalence is based on current age and gender-specific prevalence of diabetes. The projection takes account of improving life expectancy, population growth, and progressive urbanization. Most prediction models do not assume an increase in the age- and sex-specific incidence rates of diabetes and do not account for the increasing frequency and magnitude of obesity and other major risk factors for diabetes. Since incidence is likely to increase, as is the prevalence of obesity, the true future burden of diabetes is likely to exceed current estimates.

---

[1] The findings and conclusions in this report are those of the authors and do not necessarily represent the official position of the Centers for Disease Control and Prevention (CDC) or the Agency for Toxic Substances and Disease Registry.

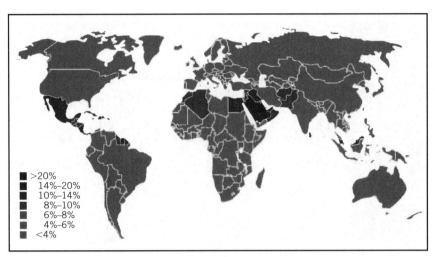

Figure 2.1 Prevalence estimates of diabetes, 2007.

Type 2 diabetes accounts for 90–95% of all diagnosed cases in the U.S. (CDC, 2008). Racial and ethnic minorities, including African Americans, Hispanics, Native Americans, Asians, and Pacific Islanders, are disproportionately affected by diabetes and are at higher risk than the general population of developing complications of diabetes. Possible reasons for this include genetic susceptibility, inadequate access to health care, suboptimal diabetes-related preventive care, and environmental exposures. In 1998 the Department of Health and Human Services established the elimination of racial and ethnic disparities in health outcomes among U.S. residents as a national priority (President's Advisory Commission on Consumer Protection and Quality in the Health Care Industry, 1998; Satcher, 1999). To identify disparities and monitor progress toward achieving this objective, high-quality surveillance data on diabetes-related morbidity and mortality and data on quality of diabetes care among minority populations are required.

TYPES OF DIABETES

Diabetes is a group of metabolic disorders that share the phenotype of hyperglycemia. Several distinct types of diabetes, caused by a complex interaction of genetics and environmental factors, have been described.

Type 1 Diabetes

Type 1 diabetes is an autoimmune process likely triggered by environmental factors in genetically susceptible individuals. This leads to the destruction of the pancreatic beta cells by autoreactive T cells and subsequent deficiency in insulin, the hormone that regulates blood glucose (Barnett, Eff, Leslie, & Pyke, 1981; Eisenbarth, 1986). The rate of decline in beta cell mass varies among individuals and clinical diabetes becomes evident when approximately 80% of beta cells are destroyed (Skyler, 1998). Consequently, persons with type 1 diabetes require lifelong treatment with insulin. The risk of developing type 1 diabetes in relatives of individuals with the disease is relatively low (3–4% if a parent has type 1 diabetes and 5–15% if a sibling does). Hence, most individuals with type 1 diabetes do not have a first-degree relative with this disease. This form of diabetes typically occurs in children and young adults. Type 1 diabetes accounts for 5–10% of all diagnosed cases of diabetes in North America. There exists no consensus on strategies for preventing type 1 diabetes. However, several clinical trials aimed at the prevention of type 1 diabetes are currently in progress.

Type 2 Diabetes

Type 2 diabetes is characterized by insulin resistance, with abnormal insulin secretion and reduced glucose utilization by fat cells, skeletal muscle, and liver. The disease is polygenic and multifactorial, with a strong genetic component. The risk of having the disease is significantly higher in first-degree relatives of those with type 2 diabetes and approaches 40% in offspring with both parents having type 2 diabetes; the concordance of type 2 diabetes in identical twins is 70–90% (Powers, 2008). Type 2 diabetes is associated with older age, obesity, family history of diabetes, history of gestational diabetes, impaired glucose metabolism, physical inactivity, and race/ethnicity. Clinically based reports and population studies suggest that type 2 diabetes in children and adolescents, although still rare, is being diagnosed with increasing frequency, particularly in minority and transitional populations.

Gestational Diabetes

Gestational diabetes is defined as glucose intolerance of variable severity that occurs during pregnancy but resolves on delivery. Gestational diabetes occurs in about 4% of pregnancies in the U.S. and is more frequent among African Americans, Hispanic/Latino Americans, and American Indians (Coustan, 1995). It is also more common among obese women and those with a family history of diabetes. During pregnancy gestational diabetes requires treatment to normalize maternal blood glucose levels and avoid complications in the infant. Women who have had gestational diabetes have a 30–60% chance of developing diabetes in the next 5–10 years (CDC, 2008).

Monogenic Types

Monogenic types of diabetes, such as maturity-onset diabetes of youth types (MODY), result from specific genetic conditions affecting islet cell development or the expression of genes important in insulin secretion. MODY 1, MODY 3, and MODY 5 patients can be successfully managed with a sulfonylurea when insulin is discontinued. Individuals with MODY 2, the result of mutations in the glucokinase gene, have mild-to-moderate stable hyperglycemia that does not respond to oral hypoglycemic agents. MODY 4 is a rare variant caused by mutations in a transcription factor that regulates pancreatic development and insulin gene transcription. Homozygous inactivating mutations cause pancreatic agenesis, whereas heterozygous mutations result in diabetes. Mutations in MODY-associated genes are rare causes of diabetes (<5%).

Neonatal Diabetes

Neonatal diabetes, with onset at <6 months of age, is caused by several genetic mutations. It can be transient or permanent and requires treatment with insulin. Mutations in subunits of the ATP-sensitive potassium channel subunits (Kir6.2 and ABCC8) are the major causes of permanent neonatal diabetes. Although these activating mutations impair glucose-stimulated insulin secretion, sulfonylureas may improve glycemic control. Homozygous glucokinase mutations can cause a particularly severe form of neonatal diabetes.

Secondary Diabetes

Secondary diabetes occurs as a result of another disease or factor and can be transitory. Potential causes of secondary diabetes are other endocrine disorders, such as hyperthyroidism, Cushing's syndrome, and acromegaly; pancreatic disorders, such as pancreatitis; hemochromatosis; hepatitis C; autoimmune diseases; and carcinoid tumors in the lungs, stomach, or intestines. Drugs, chemical agents, and toxins, including common consumer plastics and plastics ingredients (e.g., phthalates and bisphenol A), have been linked to insulin resistance. Medical treatments (e.g., pancreatectomy, orchyectomy, and radiation therapy) and genetic conditions (e.g., cystic fibrosis, Huntington's disease, Down syndrome, Klinefelter syndrome, and Turner syndrome) may disrupt the normal use of insulin and glucose. Treating secondary diabetes involves treating its cause. Treatment addresses the diabetes itself when the underlying cause cannot be resolved, the benefits of medications outweigh the side effects, or the cause remains unidentified. The frequency of secondary diabetes is estimated 1–5% of all diabetes cases.

This chapter will focus on the epidemiology of type 2 diabetes in racial and ethnic minorities in the U.S. We describe the incidence rates and prevalence of diabetes and risk factors disproportionately affecting these populations. We also review complications of diabetes that disproportionately affect racial/ethnic minorities and disparities in health outcomes.

BURDEN OF DIABETES

Approximately 24 million children and adults in the U.S., or 8% of the population, have diabetes. Nearly one-third are unaware that they have the disease (CDC, 2008). Ethnicity-specific age-adjusted prevalence estimates for 2004–2006 indicate that 6.6% of non-Hispanic Whites, 7.5% of Asian Americans, 10.4% of Hispanics, and 11.8% of non-Hispanic Blacks had diagnosed diabetes (see Figure 2.2). Among Hispanics rates were 8.2% for Cubans, 11.9% for Mexican Americans, and 12.6% for Puerto Ricans (CDC, 2008).

Among American Indians and Alaska Natives (AI/ANs) aged 20 years or older receiving care from the Indian Health Service (IHS), 14.2% had diagnosed diabetes, with rates varying from 6.0% among ANs to 29.3% among AIs in southern Arizona (CDC, 2008). In Hawaii the prevalence of diabetes among adult Asians, Native Hawaiians, and other Pacific Islanders is more than two times that in Whites after age adjustment to the 2002 U.S. adult population (CDC, 2003). Similarly, in California Asians are 1.5 times as likely to have diagnosed diabetes as non-Hispanic Whites. Generally, diabetes is diagnosed more often in women than in men, its

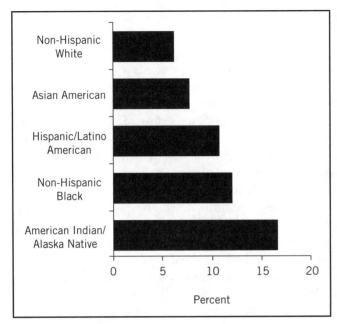

Figure 2.2 Age-adjusted prevalence of diabetes for persons aged 20 years or older by race/ethnicity in the U.S. in 2007

frequency increases with age, and levels off in those aged 80 years and older. The mean age at diagnosis of diabetes is 56 years for non-Hispanic Blacks, 57 years for Hispanics, 58 years for non-Hispanic Whites, and 59 years for other races/ethnicities (Narayan, Boyle, Thompson, Sorensen, & Williamson, 2003).

The lifetime risk of diabetes among persons born in 2000 in the U.S. is 1 in 3 for men and 2 in 5 for women, with a higher risk being estimated among minority populations throughout their lifespan (Narayan et al., 2003) (see Figure 2.3). Among men the lifetime risk at birth was estimated at 45% for Hispanics and 27% for non-Hispanic Whites. Among women the lifetime risk was estimated at 53% for Hispanics and 31% for non-Hispanic Whites. Unlike the general population, the residual risk for developing diabetes remains high for minority groups even at older ages, ranging at age 60 years from 17% in non-Hispanic White men to 32% in Hispanic men and from 20% in non-Hispanic White women to 36% in Hispanic women.

The number of persons with diagnosed diabetes is projected to increase in the U.S. by 198% between 2005 (16.2 million) and 2050 (48.3 million) (Narayan, Boyle, Geiss, Saaddine, & Thompson, 2006),

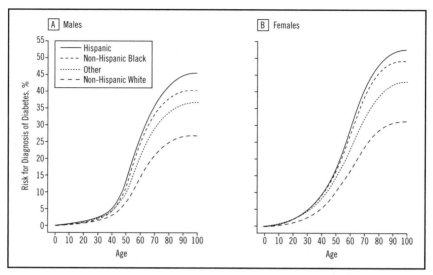

Figure 2.3 Cumulative lifetime risk for diagnosis of diabetes by age, sex, and race/ethnicity

with the largest increase being projected among minority groups. Over the same time, diabetes prevalence is projected to increase by 99% among non-Hispanic Whites (from 5.3% to 10.6%), by 107% among non-Hispanic Blacks (from 7.4% to 15.3%), by 127% among Hispanics (from 5.5% to 12.4%), and by 158% among other races (from 5.4% to 14.0%). In keeping with these figures, the number of individuals with diabetes is projected to increase 481% among Hispanics, 208% among non-Hispanic Blacks, and 113% among non-Hispanic Whites. The largest increase is projected among non-Hispanic Blacks aged ≥75 years old (606%) (Narayan et al., 2006).

Economic Burden of Diabetes

The total cost of diabetes in year 2007 dollars was estimated at $174 billion, including $116 billion in excess medical expenditures and $58 billion in reduced national productivity (American Diabetes Association [ADA], 2008b). Persons with diabetes have medical expenditures that are on average 2.3 times higher than in those without diabetes. Moreover, the annual attributed health care cost per person with diabetes increases with age. This is primarily the result of associated comorbidity with longer duration of diabetes, leading to increased use of hospital and nursing facility resources, physician office visits, non-diabetes related medications, and home care. Of all health care expenditures attributed to diabetes, 56% are incurred by people aged 65 years and older, 35% by those aged 45–64 years, and 9% by those aged 45 years or younger. Although racial and ethnic minorities have a higher prevalence of diabetes within each age group, health resource usage and cost patterns are currently unavailable for these groups, largely because currently available data sources do not support such analyses.

Quality adjusted life years (QALYs), representing the life expectancy and quality of life affected by interventions and treatments, are commonly used in economic analyses of the impact of disease and interventions. Each life year is given a value between 1.0 and 0, with the highest value assigned for perfect health and the lowest assigned for death. Among patients with diabetes the loss of life years and QALYs is projected to be highest for non-Hispanic Blacks. Non-Hispanic Black men diagnosed with diabetes at age 10 years lose 22 life years and 33 QALYs, whereas non-Hispanic Black women diagnosed at the same age lose 2 additional life years and 2 additional QALYs (Narayan et al., 2003).

The burden of diabetes and its complications on the individual and the health care system is significant. However, diabetes is largely preventable through a healthier diet and increased exercise, and diabetes complications are largely preventable through improved care for people with diabetes. Therefore, the cost of diabetes and its complications are also largely preventable.

EPIDEMIOLOGY OF DIABETES

The incidence rate of diabetes is the number of new cases of diabetes that occur during a defined period of time, divided by the number of persons exposed to the risk of experiencing diabetes during this period. If the time period is 1 year, then the estimate represents the annual incidence rate. The denominator is sometimes expressed as person-time (or person-years), representing the time each person contributes to the population at risk being observed. The prevalence of diabetes is defined by the number of persons in a given population who have the disease at a specified point in time. These definitions apply to any other disease or condition. The incidence rate of diabetes and the death rate among people without or with diabetes (rate of people being removed from the population) are major determinants of diabetes prevalence.

Incidence of Diabetes

Hispanic/Latino Americans

The Hispanic/Latino population represents about 15% of the U.S. population, with a growth rate of 24.3%, which is four times the growth rate of the total U.S. population (6.1%) between 2000 and 2006 (U.S. Census Bureau, 2004). Almost 40% of Mexican Americans, the largest Hispanic/Latino subgroup in the U.S., are foreign born, and 59% migrated to the U.S. after 1990 (U.S. Census Bureau, 2004). Hispanic/Latinos with low acculturation frequently lack routine health care, health insurance, and education. Those with low language acculturation have nearly twice the risk of developing diabetes than those with high language acculturation [odds ratio (OR) = 1.90, 95% CI 1.02–3.54] (Pérez-Escamilla & Putnik, 2007).

In 2005 the age-adjusted incidence of diabetes in the overall Hispanic/Latino population in the U.S. was 10.2 per 1000 people, increasing from 7.4 per 1000 in 1997 (CDC, 2008). The 2000 U.S. population was used as the standard for the age adjustment. Specifically, among Mexican Americans in the San Antonio Heart Study, the incidence of type 2 diabetes increased from 5.7% to 15.7% over an 8-year time period ($p = 0.001$), whereas in Whites it increased from 2.6% to 9.4% ($p = 0.07$) (Burke et al., 1999). Although trends were increasing for both ethnic groups, the lack of a significant change among non-Hispanic Whites is likely due to the smaller number of cases ($n = 68$ cases) than among Mexican Americans ($n = 225$). In this study age, sex, body mass index (BMI), ethnicity, and neighborhood were the strongest predictors for diabetes in a stepwise logistic regression analysis. Since mortality declined less in diabetic than in nondiabetic subjects, the increasing incidence rate of diabetes may have contributed largely to the increase in the prevalence of diabetes in this population.

African Americans

African Americans represent 12% of the U.S. population (U.S. Census Bureau, 2001). The age-adjusted incidence of diabetes in 2005 was 10.4 per 1000, increasing from 9.2 per 1000 in 1997; age adjustments were made to the 2000 U.S. population (CDC, 2008). The risk of diabetes is higher for African American men and women than for their White counterparts. In the Atherosclerosis Risk in Communities study (Brancati,

Kao, Folsom, Watson, & Szklo, 2000), the incidence rate of diabetes during 9 years of follow-up was 25.1 per 1000 person years (95% CI 22.4–28.1) in African American women, 2.4 times greater than in White women (10.4 per 1000 person years, 95% CI 9.4–11.4); in African American men diabetes incidence was 23.4 per 1000 person years (95% CI 19.9–27.2) and about 1.5 times greater than in their White counterparts (15.9 per 1000 person years, 95% CI 14.6–17.2) (p < 0.001). In this study new cases were defined by self-report of physician-diagnosed type 2 diabetes, use of hypoglycemic medicines, or fasting glucose level ≥126 mg/dL (7.0 mmol/L). The higher prevalence of potentially modifiable risk factors, particularly a higher adiposity, accounted for almost half of the excess risk in African American women (to a lesser extent in African American men) in a proportional hazards regression analysis (Brancati et al., 2000).

Differences in known risk factors only partially explain racial/ethnic differences in diabetes risk. However, other risk factors for diabetes, such as family history, education, and exercise, are rarely considered. These sometimes unmeasured risk factors could have significant implications on the observed difference and the magnitude of the association between obesity and diabetes, particularly in ethnic minorities.

American Indians and Alaska Natives

Approximately 3.2 million people in the U.S. identify themselves as AI/AN (Indian Health Service, 2008). Most are members of the more than 560 federally recognized tribes. The AN population includes Eskimos, Aleuts, and Indians (Athabascan, Haida, Tlingit, and Tsimsian). In addition to their tribal affiliations, AI/ANs are often distinguished by language and/or cultural groups, some of which extend across the U.S., Canada, and Mexico (Ghodes, 1995). They often live on reservations and in rural communities, mostly in the western U.S. and Alaska, and face pervasive economic and educa-tional disadvantages (U.S. Census Bureau, 1992). Diabetes was either rare or unrecognized among AI/ANs until the middle part of the 20th century. Since then diabetes has become one of the most common serious diseases among AI/ANs.

Population-based incidence rates of diabetes have been reported in few Native American groups in the U.S. (Lee et al., 2002). The lowest incidence of type 2 diabetes has been reported in Eskimos; between 1964 and 1967, the reported incidence among Greenland, Canadian and Alaska Eskimos was less than 1.0% (Schaefer, 1968). Among tribal members aged 45–74 years from Arizona, Oklahoma, South Dakota, and North Dakota, the overall 4-year incidence of diabetes was 19.7%. The annual average incidence of diabetes among persons with normal glucose tolerance was 2.8%. Higher BMI and triglycerides in men and higher fasting insulin in women were significant predictors of diabetes. Those with impaired glucose tolerance progressed to diabetes at an average annual rate of 9.3%, much higher than the 1.5% found in Whites and 7.0% found in both Mexican Americans and Japanese Americans (Harris, 1996).

The incidence rate of diabetes among the Pima Indians of Arizona, who participated in a comprehensive longitudinal study of diabetes, obesity, and diabetes complica-tions since 1965, is among the highest recorded in the world (Knowler, Bennett, Hamman, & Miller, 1978). Although the overall incidence rate of diabetes remained stable over the past 4 decades [age- and sex-adjusted incidence rates of diabetes were 25.3 cases/1,000 person years (95% CI 22.5–28.0) for 1965–1977, 22.9 cases/1,000 person years (95% CI 20.0–25.8) for 1978–1990, and 23.5 cases/1,000 person years (95% CI 20.5–26.5) for 1991–2003 ($p = 0.3$)] (Pavkov et al., 2007), the increasing prevalence of obesity and increasing prevalence of pregnant women with diabetes observed over the last decades have shifted the onset of diabetes to younger ages (Hillier & Pedula, 2003).

Asian Americans

Asian American populations comprise 13.5 million people (4.42% of the total population) and are among the fastest growing segments of the U.S. population. Nearly 75% of Asian Americans are foreign-born (Association of Asian Pacific Community Health Organizations , 2008) and include, according to country of origin, Chinese (24%), Filipino (18%), Asian Indian (16%), Vietnamese (11%), Korean (11%), Japanese (8%), and other Asians (13%) (U.S. Census Bureau, 2001), with great diversity in language, culture, and beliefs.

In general, Asian Americans are at greater risk of type 2 diabetes than Whites, although they are less likely to be obese. The annual incidence of diabetes in Asian Americans enrolled in the Medicare program was 49 cases per 1,000 in 2001, 48% higher than in Whites (McNeely & Fujimoto, 2008). The cumulative incidence of diabetes in Japanese Americans 40–60 years old is estimated at 18.0% over 10 years of follow-up (McNeely & Fujimoto, 2008). These figures were similar in second- and third-generation Japanese Americans of similar age. In Japanese American men living in Hawaii, the incidence of "possible" diabetes, as defined by self-reported disease, medication, or hospital diagnosis, was 12.8%, and the incidence was 5.7% when assessed by hypoglycemic medication usage over a 6-year time period (Burchfiel et al., 1995). Men who developed diabetes had significantly higher age-adjusted mean BMI, weight gain since age 25 years, subscapular skin fold thickness, subscapular/triceps skin fold ratio, glucose, cholesterol, triglyceride, uric acid, hematocrit, systolic and diastolic blood pressure, and heart rate, and significantly lower levels of physical activity than men who did not develop diabetes (Burchfiel et al., 1995).

In the Nurses' Health Study, a 20-year prospective study including White (i.e., of Southern European/Mediterranean, Scandinavian, and other Caucasian origin), African American, Hispanic, and Asian women, the BMI-adjusted risk of diabetes was significantly higher among Asian than White women [risk ratio (RR) = 2.26, 95% CI 1.70–2.99]. Asian women were leaner at baseline but more sedentary, had a lower prevalence of smoking, consumed less alcohol, and ate a healthier diet than the White women (Shai et al., 2006). BMI increased in all racial/ethnic groups, as did diabetes incidence. However, after adjusting for BMI, the risk of diabetes was lowest among Asian women and highest among African American women. Diet measurements suggested that the negative association between diabetes and intake high in fiber and polyunsaturated fat and low in transfat and glucose could be stronger among ethnic minorities than among Whites.

Pacific Islander Americans

Pacific Islanders represent less than 1% of the U.S. population and comprise 19 ethnic groups, the vast majority being of Native Hawaiian, Guamanian/Chamarro, or Samoan ancestry (U.S. Census Bureau, 2001). Colonization and rapid modernization disrupted the islands' traditional lifestyle based on agriculture and fishing. The transition from subsistence to a cash economy was associated with a more sedentary lifestyle and increased consumption of processed foods (McNeely & Fujimoto, 2008). Currently, Pacific Islanders are more likely to be obese and have diabetes than Whites of similar age (Fujimoto, 1995).

Little data concerning the incidence of diabetes in Pacific Islander American populations are available. A 1997–2000 cross-sectional study in the North Kohala region of Hawaii, including White, Filipino, Native

Hawaiian, and Japanese adults, indicated a significantly higher adjusted risk for diabetes among Filipinos (OR = 2.2, 95% CI 1.4–3.5) and Hawaiians (OR = 2.8, 95% CI 1.9–4.2) than among Whites (Kim, Park, Grandinetti, Holck, & Waslien, 2008). The differences persisted after additional adjustment for dietary factors (OR = 1.9, 95% CI 1.1–3.2 and OR = 1.8, 95% CI 1.1–3.0, respectively). In an earlier population survey conducted between 1978 and 1992 in Papua New Guinea, Western Samoa, Mauritius, and Nauru, the incidence rates varied largely among these populations, ranging from 1.2 cases/1,000 person years in periurban and rural Papua New Guinea Highlanders to 22.5 cases/1,000 person years in Micronesian Nauruans and 24.0 cases/1,000 person years in the rural Wanigelas (Dowse, 1996). After adjusting for BMI, within the age range of 25–45 years, the Wanigela people in rural Papua New Guinea were found to have the highest susceptibility to diabetes yet documented for any population in the world, and the incidence rate of diabetes could be even higher for those in urban areas, in whom prevalence of diabetes was nearly three times higher than in rural areas.

Prevalence of Diabetes

Hispanic/Latino Americans

Hispanic/Latino Americans are 1.6 times as likely to have diabetes as non-Hispanic Whites after adjusting for age differences, with Puerto Ricans and Mexican Americans having the highest prevalence (*vide supra*) (CDC, 2008). In the U.S.–Mexico border region, where the population is predominantly of Mexican descent, the prevalence of diabetes was estimated at 15.7%, somewhat higher than the U.S. national prevalence among Mexican Americans of 11.9% (Mier, Medina, & Ory, 2007).

Residents of Puerto Rico are 1.9 times as likely to have diagnosed diabetes as non-Hispanic Whites in the U.S. Results from the Massachusetts Hispanic Elders survey showed significantly higher diabetes prevalence for Puerto Ricans over 60 years of age than Dominican Americans, other Hispanics, and non-Hispanic Whites (Tucker, Bermudez, & Castaneda, 2000).

By contrast, Cuban Americans living in Miami, FL, were found less likely to have diabetes than either Mexican Americans or Puerto Ricans (Flegal et al., 1991). This discrepancy is attributed, at least in part, to Cuban Americans typically having a higher socioeconomic status than other

Hispanic/Latino groups included in the Hispanic Health and Nutrition Examination Survey. On the other hand, it has been suggested that the low American Indian admixture of Cuban Americans may have a protective effect against diabetes. Although functional variants in candidate genes for type 2 diabetes have been identified in Pima Indians, it is yet to be determined whether these genes also influence the occurrence of diabetes in other populations (Baier & Hanson, 2004). Estimates of diabetes prevalence for other Hispanic/Latino subgroups are not reported due to lower precision.

African Americans

African Americans are 1.8 times as likely to have diabetes as non-Hispanic Whites after adjustment to the 2000 U.S. population age (CDC, 2008). Twenty-five percent of African Americans aged 65–74 years have diabetes. Among African American men 25–70 years old, the prevalence of diabetes was 5.7% in the National Health and Nutrition Examination Survey (NHANES) III for 1988–1994 and 8.4% in NHANES IV for 1999–2002, 1.2 and 1.3 as high as in non-Hispanic Whites, respectively. The prevalence of obesity and mean age were similar in African American and non-Hispanic White men, whereas the latter were more likely to have a higher level of education (beyond high school) in both samples (Smith, 2007). Over the last 2 decades, the 2000 U.S. age-adjusted annual prevalence of diabetes was consistently higher in African American women than in African American men, and highest when compared with non-Hispanic White and Hispanic American men and women (CDC, 2008).

Unique susceptibility genes were sought that might explain the higher predisposition for diabetes than in White or Hispanic Americans. However, family-based linkage studies among African American and African populations failed to identify such genes. Recent studies comparing diabetes prevalence in African Americans and Whites of similar socioeconomic status suggest that disparities in diabetes prevalence are more likely to reflect differences in the distribution of risk factors for diabetes than race per se (Signorello et al., 2007).

African Americans have become more heterogeneous by country of immediate origin and degree of admixture. However, national surveillance and other available epidemiologic studies do not identify African Americans by their ethnic and cultural background. Therefore, we can not compare the risk of diabetes among African Americans of different ancestries.

American Indians and Alaska Natives

Data from the population served by the IHS in 2005 indicate that 16.5% of AI/ANs aged 20 years and older had diagnosed diabetes, representing a 1.43-fold increase from 1994 (CDC, 2003, 2008). AI/AN women are generally more likely to be diagnosed with diabetes than men, probably due to women's greater awareness of the disease and greater tendency to seek health care than to true differences in risk for diabetes (IHS, 1997). These estimates only reflect the approximately 60% of AI/ANs who receive care from the IHS or tribal health facilities. For the remaining approximately 40%, the prevalence of diabetes and its risk factors are largely unknown (Burrows, Geiss, Engelgau, & Acton, 2000). Thus, these estimates could be substantially biased.

Although the prevalence of diabetes is lower among ANs than AIs, the largest increase in diabetes prevalence between 1990 and 2001 was found among Eskimos (110%) and Aleuts (81%) (Hall, Sberna, & Utermohle, 2001). In 2002 approximately 30% of AI/ANs aged ≥55 years had diabetes, but the prevalence varied among tribes. Although the prevalence was lowest among youth, AI/ANs aged 20–34 years experienced the largest relative increase during the same time span (74%). Similarly, AI/ANs <35 years old experienced an almost 8% annual increase in diabetes prevalence between 1994 and 2004 (IHS, 2000).

In the Pima Indians the age- and sex-adjusted prevalence of diabetes was 12.7 times as high as in the predominantly White population of Rochester, MN (Knowler et al., 1978). Conversely, the prevalence of diabetes in the Pima Indians from the Sierra Madre Mountains in Mexico is low (Ravussin, Valencia, Esparza, Bennett, & Schulz, 1994). Living in a remote area that only recently became accessible by road, the Mexican Pima have experienced relatively little recent change in environmental conditions. Although estimated genetic distance between these people and the Pima Indians of Arizona is low, the Mexican Pimas' traditional lifestyle may protect them from the development of obesity and diabetes, supporting the notion that type 2 diabetes results from a genetic predisposition/lifestyle interaction.

Asian Americans

Among participants aged ≥30 years old in the 2001 Behavioral Risk Factor Surveillance System (BRFSS) survey, the age-, sex-, and BMI-adjusted odds of diabetes in Asian Americans was 1.6 (95% CI 1.1–2.2), compared with non-Hispanic Whites (McNeely & Boyko, 2004). In second-generation Japanese Americans 45–74 years old, the prevalence of diabetes was approximately 40% higher than in Caucasians of similar age. In Japanese American men at least 70 years old, the prevalence of diabetes was 40% (Rodriguez et al., 1996), twice that of non-Hispanic White men of the same age (Harris et al., 1998). Diabetes prevalence among Filipino women 40–79 years old residing in San Diego and Hawaii did not significantly differ (31.6% in San Diego, 24.9% in Hawaii, $p = 0.79$) (Araneta et al., 2006). Comparatively, a population survey at several sites in the Philippines showed that diabetes prevalence among Filipinas 20–65 years old was 5.3% (95% CI 3.7–6.9) after age-standardizing to the total eligible population in the Philippines (Baltazar, Ancheta, Abanb, Fernando, & Baquilod, 2004). The age- and sex-adjusted prevalence of diabetes in the Philippines was 4.8% (95% CI 3.6–6.0). Age, female sex, central obesity, family history of diabetes, BMI, and physical inactivity were positively and significantly associated with diabetes in this population. Several other regional studies including different Asian subgroups in the U.S. consistently found higher prevalence of diabetes in Asian women than in men, in Asians than in Caucasians, and in Asian groups living in the U.S. than in their countries of origin (McNeely & Fujimoto, 2008).

Pacific Islander Americans

Type 2 diabetes, virtually unknown among Pacific Islanders before World War II, is now increasingly frequent among Pacific Islander Americans. Age-, sex-, and BMI-adjusted odds of diabetes are three times higher (95% CI 1.4–6.7) in Pacific Islanders than in Whites, but are not significantly higher in Asian Americans (OR = 1.6, 95% CI 0.7–3.9) (McNeely & Boyko, 2004). A review of outpatient medical records in the Marshall Islands (Ebeye, the most populous island of Kwajalein Atoll) revealed a prevalence of diabetes of 20% in patients aged 30 years and older and 46% in patients aged 50 years and older (Yamada & Palafox, 2001). Diabetes prevalence among urbanized Western Samoans is twice that of Samoans in the rural communities (7.8% and 3.4%, respectively), even after adjusting for body weight. This difference was attributed largely to rural residents having a higher level of physical activity than their urban counterparts (Zimmet, Ainuu, DeBoer, Faaiuso, & Whitehouse, 1981). In the time period 1996–2000, Native Hawaiians were 2.5 times more likely to have diabetes than non-Hispanic

White residents of Hawaii of similar age (National Diabetes Information Clearinghouse, 2002).

Diabetes in Youth

Type 2 diabetes in youth is characterized by absent or low levels of islet cell and glutamic acid decarboxylase antibodies, and absence of linkage or association with MODY loci. Many children with type 2 diabetes are obese at diagnosis and have a strong family history of type 2 diabetes and diabetes-related comorbidities, and some are the offspring of mothers who had gestational diabetes. Typically, youth diagnosed with type 2 diabetes are pubertal or post-pubertal, are less likely to be significantly ill at presentation than those with type 1 diabetes due to normal or increased insulin production, and have a more centralized distribution of body fat. These clinical characteristics suggest that the pathophysiology of type 2 diabetes in children and adolescents is the same as in adults.

The greatest increase in the prevalence of obesity in the U.S. in the past 10 years has occurred in the young adult population across all ethnic groups (Mokdad et al., 1999). In 2004 data from the NHANES indicate that 37.2% of children aged 6–11 years and 34.3% of adolescents aged 12–19 years were overweight (Hale & Rupert, 2006). More than 17% of youth were classified as obese, with minority youth disproportionately affected; 19.2% of Mexican Americans and 20% of African Americans were classified as obese, compared with 16.3% of White youth. African American girls are particularly affected by obesity, with 23.8% of girls between the ages of 2 and 19 years being considered obese. Studies indicate that racial/ethnic differences in overweight and obesity typically arise during puberty. Because obesity is a strong predictor of diabetes, the disproportion in the prevalence of type 2 diabetes occurring in racial/ethnic minority youth and young adulthood may be attributed in part to these differences.

In 2002–2003 the annual incidence rate of type 2 diabetes in people younger than 20 years in the U.S. was 5.3 per 100,000, more frequently diagnosed in racial/ethnic minorities than non-Hispanic Whites, often during the teens. Among non-Hispanic White youth aged 10–19 years, incident cases were more frequently type 1 diabetes than type 2. Among Hispanic and African American youth aged 10–19 years, the rates of new cases of type 1 and type 2 diabetes were similar (CDC, 2008). For Asian/Pacific Islander and AI youth aged 10–19 years, the incidence rate of type 2 diabetes was higher than of type 1.

Approximately 0.2% of people younger than 20 years in the U.S. have diabetes (CDC, 2008). The prevalence is lower in children 0–9 years old (0.08%) than in those 10–19 years old (0.3%). Among teenagers prevalence was 0.3% in non-Hispanic Blacks and non-Hispanic Whites, 0.2% in American Indians and Hispanics, and 0.1% in Asian/Pacific Islanders. Type 1 diabetes was the predominant form of diabetes in those younger than 20 years, accounting for 80% of diabetes in this population. Among teenage youth the proportion of type 2 diabetes ranged between 6% and 76%, with a higher proportion in minority youth (SEARCH for Diabetes in Youth Study Group, 2006). Nevertheless, the distinction between type1 and type 2 diabetes in youth is often difficult and additional testing for IA-2 antibodies, considered the best indicator of type 1 diabetes at onset, is required to conclusively distinguish the difference (Lipton, 2007).

In Pima Indian children and adolescents, diabetes was first reported in the 1970s and is entirely type 2 diabetes (Dabelea, Palmer, Bennett, Pettitt, & Knowler, 1999; Hanson, 1997; Janssen, Bogardus, Takeda, Knowler, & Thompson, 1994; Knowler, Bennett, Bottazzo, & Doniach, 1979; Knowler, Pettitt, Saad, & Bennett, 1990). Between 1965 and 2003, the average BMI in nondiabetic Pima Indians increased in all age groups including children. However, during the same period the incidence rate of type 2 diabetes increased among Pima Indians aged 5–14 years, decreased in those aged 25–34 years, and did not change significantly in other ages (Pavkov et al., 2007) (see Figure 2.4).

These findings suggest that the increasing obesity in youth, combined with a nearly fourfold increase in the frequency of exposure to diabetes in utero, shifted the onset of diabetes to younger ages (Dabelea et al., 1998; Knowler et al., 1990; Pavkov et al., 2006). The age-specific prevalence of diabetes increased over the same time in subjects <25 years old, but did not show a similar trend in the older ages. Since mortality in young persons remained stable during this period, the increasing prevalence of diabetes in youth is believed to be largely attributable to the increasing incidence of diabetes in this age group. The onset of diabetes in Pima Indians younger than 20 years of age is associated with a nearly 5-fold increase in the incidence of end-stage kidney disease and a 3-fold increase in mortality between 25 and 54 years of age than in adult-onset disease (Pavkov et al., 2006).

Diabetes prevention and treatment programs should target youth at high risk for developing type 2 diabetes. These programs, ideally involving family, school, and community, can help prevent or delay the disease, assisting youth in progressing through adulthood without

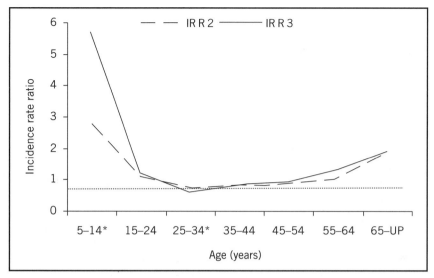

Figure 2.4 Age-specific, sex-adjusted incidence rate ratio of type 2 diabetes in Pima Indians, computed for three time periods between 1965 and 2003. The incidence rate in subjects aged 5–14 years was 5.7 (95%CI = 1.9–17.4) times as high in the last as in the first period, but the rate declined in those 25–34 years old (incidence rate ratio = 0.6, 95%CI = 0.4–0.8). IRR2 = incidence rate ratios in 1978–1990 relative to 1965–1977, IRR3 = incidence rate ratios in 1991–2003 relative to 1965–1977.*P_{trend} <0.05 [26].
Source: From Pavkov et al., *Diabetes Care* 2007.

diabetes-related complications. Establishing community advocacy may prove extremely useful in obtaining legislative support and developing both primary and secondary prevention programs.

RISK FACTORS FOR DIABETES

Factors predicting the occurrence of type 2 diabetes include the presence of certain genetic markers, the prenatal diabetic environment, and postnatal environmental factors (see Table 2.1) (ADA, 2007).

Intrauterine Environment

Offspring of diabetic mothers are at a much higher risk of obesity and diabetes during childhood and as young adults than offspring of non-diabetic mothers. Thus, female offspring of women with diabetes often

Table 2.1

RISK FACTORS FOR TYPE 2 DIABETES

Family History of Diabetes (i.e., parent or sibling with type 2 diabetes)
Obesity (BMI ≥25 kg/m²)
Habitual Physical Inactivity
Race/Ethnicity (e.g., African American, Latino, Native American, Asian American, Pacific Islander)
Previously Identified Impaired Fasting Glucose or Impaired Glucose Tolerance
History of Gestational Diabetes Mellitus or Delivery of Baby >4 kg (>9 lb)
Hypertension (blood pressure ≥140/90 mmHg)
High-Density Lipoprotein Cholesterol Level <35 mg/dL (0.90 mmol/L) and/or a Triglyceride Level >250 mg/dL (2.82 mmol/L)
Polycystic Ovary Syndrome or Acanthosis Nigricans
History of Vascular Disease

Source: Adapted from American Diabetes Association. (2007). Clinical practice recommendations 2007. *Diabetes Care, 30(Suppl 1)*, S1–S103.

have diabetic pregnancies themselves. In addition to susceptibility genes transmitted to the next generation, intrauterine exposure to diabetes can lead to increased risk for long-term diabetes complications. Most of the information about the magnitude of this risk comes from studies in Pima Indians, in whom the proportion of children exposed to diabetes in utero increased nearly four times between 1967 and 1996 and was associated with a doubling of the number of cases of diabetes attributable to this exposure (Dabelea et al., 1998).

Obesity

Obesity is a major risk factor for type 2 diabetes among all races and ethnic groups. The World Health Organization defines overweight as BMI between 25 and 30 kg/m², and obesity as BMI ≥30 kg/m² (World Health Organization, 2000). Derived in predominantly White populations, these cut points are associated with increased risk for diabetes or cardiovascular disease. Mounting evidence suggests that different cut points for overweight and obesity may apply to non-White populations (Huxley, Omari, & Caterson, 2008). Alternatively, such differences may reflect the limitations of using relative body weight as a metabolic risk marker and the importance of accounting for the site of accumulation of the excess adipose tissue. In keeping with these observations, for a BMI <25 kg/m², African Americans have a similarly low risk of diabetes as Whites; by contrast, obesity is associated with a higher risk of diabetes in African Americans than in Whites (McNeely & Fujimoto, 2008). Similarly, for a given BMI Asians have a higher risk of diabetes (McNeely & Fujimoto, 2008). Adjusted weight gain since age 18 years was a stronger predictor for diabetes in Asian women than in other ethnicities; for a 5 kg increment in weight, the adjusted RR of diabetes was 1.84 (95% CI 1.58–2.14) for Asians, 1.44 (95% CI 1.26–1.63) for Hispanics, 1.38 (95% CI 1.28–1.49) for African Americans, and 1.37 (95% CI 1.35–1.38) for Whites (Shai et al., 2006). Compared with non-Hispanic Whites with BMI 30 kg/m^2 in the BRFSS (McNeely & Boyko, 2004), age- and sex-adjusted OR for diabetes was 1.7 (95% CI 0.7–4.5) for Asians with BMI 30 kg/m^2, 1.0 (95% CI 0.5–2.2) for Asians with BMI 29 kg/m^2, 0.9 (95% CI 0.4–1.7) for Asians with BMI 28 kg/m^2, and 0.6 (95% CI 0.3–1.1) for Asians with BMI 27 kg/m^2. The age-, sex-, and BMI-adjusted odds of diabetes were 1.8 (95% CI 1.3– 2.5) when compared with non-Hispanic Whites. A higher percentage of body fat than in Caucasians, greater propensity for intra-abdominal fat deposition (Fujimoto et al., 1995; Park, Allison, Heymsfield, & Gallagher, 2001), or impaired beta cell function (Shin et al., 1997) in Asian Americans compared with other ethnicities are mechanisms believed to be involved in the higher risk of diabetes at any given BMI in Asians.

Overweight and obesity may be components of the pathway between socioeconomic disadvantage and diabetes incidence, as shown in a community sample of 6,147 nondiabetic adults from Alameda County, CA, followed between 1965 and 1999. Socioeconomic position (defined by factors including household income, level of education, marital status, social support, access to medical care, health behaviors, BMI, hypertension, and number of medicines used) significantly predicted the incidence of type 2 diabetes over a 34-year period (Maty, Everson-Rose, Haan, Raghunathan, & Kaplan, 2005). This effect was attenuated in baseline and time-dependent analyses adjusted for body composition and BMI.

Diet and Physical Inactivity

As a result of migration, urbanization, and acculturation, the food choices and activities of members of many racial/ethnic groups have changed dramatically and rapidly. These populations have abandoned their traditional diets and are choosing foods with more animal protein, animal fats, and processed carbohydrates. In many cases urbanization has changed a lifestyle characterized by regular physical activity to a more sedentary one, which predisposes people to overweight and obesity and adoption of other practices like smoking (McNeely & Fujimoto, 2008). Overproduction and heavy advertising of energy-dense foods strongly influenced individual dietary choices during recent decades and could be the prime causes of the recent increase in average BMI in the U.S. and elsewhere (Putnam, Allshouse, & Kantor, L. S., 2002; Silventoinen, 2004).

Among Hispanic high school students, mean consumption of fruits and vegetables was lower than for non-Hispanic Whites but slightly higher than for non-Hispanic African Americans (Crawford, Story, Wang, Ritchie, & Sabry, 2001). Data from NHANES III indicate a higher than recommended consumption of fat among Mexican American women 6–24 years old (Crawford et al., 2001).

In a Chicago inner city study, only 26% of African American adolescents engaged in more than 20 minutes of moderate-to-vigorous daily physical activity, whereas 71% spent at least 4 hours each day in sedentary activities, such as watching television, using the computer, or playing video games (Wang et al., 2006). In addition to the relatively sedentary lifestyle, up to 70% of African American adolescents drank soda more than twice a day and 55% consumed fried foods at the same frequency. Data from large-scale epidemiologic studies showed that African American girls are more likely to consume calorie-dense foods than White girls and eat while watching television or doing homework, even after adjusting for socioeconomic status (McNutt et al., 1997).

Similar changes have also occurred in the diet of other immigrant populations. The dietary intake of Japanese men living in Seattle, WA, was higher in calories, protein, fat, and carbohydrates and lower in fibers than that of similarly aged Japanese men living in Japan (Fujimoto, 1995). The average daily fat intake in Japanese American men was 32.4 grams, compared with 16.7 grams of fat for those living in Japan. Other studies showed that the Japanese Americans' diet has a lower protein/sugar ratio than that of native Japanese, with more animal protein, 1.5–2.0 times more simple carbohydrates, and less complex carbohydrates (Nakanishi et al., 2004). Additionally, Japanese Americans were more likely to report very light or light levels of physical activity than native Japanese people (Kawate et al., 1979).

The Pima Indians in Arizona maintained much of their traditional diet and lifestyle through the end of the 19th century. Increasing settlement of their area by people of European derivation, however, led to diversion of the Pimas' water supply and disruption of agriculture, lead-ing to fundamental changes in their way of life. To survive poverty and malnutrition, the Pima Indians accepted lard, sugar, white flour, and oth-er commodity foods supplied by the U.S. government. Thus, subsistence farming activities of the Pima population in Arizona were replaced by government assistance programs and a cash economy. In the late 1930s, a review of medical records from the two hospitals serving the popu-lation concluded that the prevalence of diabetes was similar to that in the U.S. population (Joslin, 1940). By the 1950s many more Pima were overweight and diagnosed with diabetes (Cohen, 1954), suggesting an increase in the frequency of diabetes in this population coinciding with the rapid transition to a nontraditional lifestyle following increasing con-tact with European Americans (Pavkov et al., 2007).

The Pima Indians now consume a diet that is nutritionally similar to most other Americans, rich in sugar and animal-derived fat and low in fiber and starch. Children are exposed to television commercials that almost exclusively encourage the consumption of highly palatable foods that are high in fat, soft drinks, and snacks with large amounts of excess calories and low cost.

DISPARITIES IN DIABETES COMPLICATIONS

Diabetes is associated with an increased risk for a number of serious, often life-threatening complications, and racial/ethnic minority popula-tions experience an even greater risk of developing these complications. In addition to a higher prevalence of diabetes, other causes of disparities in diabetes complications include enrollment in poorer quality health care plans; ethnic differences in self-care behavior, such as nutritional habits or physical activity; adherence to medication use; biologic varia-tion in blood pressure, hemoglobin A1c, and lipid levels; and psycho-social factors, such as differing levels of trust in providers or the health care system (Brown et al., 2005).

Social and cultural factors, such as body image, educational level, fears, general family integration and support, health literacy, language, myths, and nutritional preferences, may affect the success of the physi-cian-patient relationship and influence patients' adherence to treatment. These factors need to be considered in the day-to-day management of patients from culturally diverse populations and when implementing educational activities. Ascertainment of racial/ethnic-specific behaviors, how family ties may affect diabetes prevention or care, and awareness of the patients' educational level may help improve the quality of care provided to minority groups through improved patient-provider trust and communication.

Heart Disease and Stroke

Heart disease accounts for about 68% and stroke for about 16% of deaths in people aged 65 years and older with diabetes (CDC, 2008). Adults with diabetes have 2–4 times higher risk of fatal heart disease than those without diabetes and the risk for stroke is 2–4 times higher. This is not surprising, since 75% of adults with diabetes have elevated blood pressure ($\geq$130/80 mm Hg) or use prescription medicines for hypertension (CDC, 2008). Nevertheless, the proportion of diabetic persons developing cardiovascular disease varies by ethnicity and may be declining in some groups.

Between 1997 and 2005, the age-adjusted cardiovascular disease (CVD) prevalence was higher among non-Hispanic Whites than Hispanic Americans or African Americans (CDC, 2007). The age-adjusted prevalence of self-reported CVD decreased by 25.3% among African Americans, with rates ranging from 36.3% (95% CI 32.3–40.4) in 1997 to 27.1% (95% CI 23.5–30.7) in 2005 ($p = 0.03$). Among non-Hispanics of any race, the rate decreased by 12%, from 37.9% (95% CI 35.7–40.1) in 1997 to 33.3% (95% CI 31.5–35.0) in 2005 ($p = 0.02$). No decline was found in non-Hispanic Whites and no clear trend was detected among Hispanics during this time period. Better prevention and more effective treatments for CVD risk factors largely contributed to the decrease in self-reported CVD prevalence in persons with diagnosed diabetes.

A study within a nonprofit prepaid health care organization examining disparities in the occurrence of diabetes complications across racial/ethnic groups found persistent racial/ethnic disparities. Disparities remained even after adjustment for a wide range of demographic, socioeconomic, behavioral, and clinical factors (Karter et al., 2002). Relative to non-Hispanic Whites, adjusted hazard ratios for myocardial infarction were 0.56 for African Americans, 0.68 for Asians, and 0.68 for Latinos, respectively ($p < 0.001$); adjusted hazard ratios for stroke were 0.76 for Asians and 0.72 for Latinos, respectively ($p < 0.01$); adjusted hazard

ratios for congestive heart failure were 0.70 for Asians and 0.61 for Latinos, respectively ($p < 0.01$); adjusted hazard ratios for lower extremity
amputations were 0.40 for Asians ($p < 0.001$); and adjusted hazard ratios
for end-stage kidney disease were 2.03 for African Americans, 1.85 for
Asians, and 1.46 for Latinos, respectively ($p < 0.01$). African Americans
had similar risk for stroke, congestive heart failure, or lower extremity
amputations as non-Hispanic Whites, and Latinos had similar risk for
lower extremity amputations as non-Hispanic Whites. Genetic predisposition or other unmeasured environmental factors, or both, may have
accounted for these differences in diabetes complications.

IHS data indicate that the incidence of CVD has increased among
AI/ANs; CVD is now the leading cause of death in those with diabetes
(Galloway, 2005). Among 13 AI tribes in Arizona, Oklahoma, North Dakota, and South Dakota, death rates due to CVD differ substantially by
tribe (Lee et al., 1990). Although the prevalence of diabetes is highest
among AIs in Arizona, fatal coronary heart disease (CHD) is lower than
in other AIs. This difference may be related in part to lower cigarette
smoking and lower levels of total and low-density lipoprotein cholesterol
than in other tribal groups. Although diabetes has a major impact on
CHD and mortality in Pima Indians, the prevalence of CHD, as defined
by major ischemic changes on the electrocardiogram, and death rates
from CHD were significantly higher only in those with ≥ 15 years of
diabetes, relative to subjects with normal glucose tolerance. Impaired
fasting glucose and/or impaired glucose tolerance were not significant
predictors of CHD in a time-dependent analysis, suggesting that the association between CHD and impaired glucose regulation is due primarily to factors other than hyperglycemia per se (Kim et al., 2008).

Diabetic Kidney Disease

Hispanic/Latinos, African Americans, and AI/ANs with diabetes are
at greater risk than Whites for kidney disease as a complication of diabetes. Obesity, increasingly affecting young persons in these ethnic
groups (Ogden et al., 2002), may promote an earlier onset of diabetes and contribute to development of kidney disease earlier in life. A
study in youth who were diagnosed with diabetes for less than 3 years
found that 40% of the predominantly Latino and African American
participants aged 10–18 years had microalbuminuria, compared with
none of the obese nondiabetic control subjects (Ogden et al., 2002).

Those with microalbuminuria had a higher average daytime systolic blood pressure than diabetic individuals without microalbuminuria or the control group.

The incidence of diabetic end-stage kidney disease declined after 1994 in non-Hispanic Whites younger than 40 years of age, but it continued to rise in African Americans of similar age and remained unchanged in Hispanics (National Institutes of Health, 2006). The incidence rate of diabetic end-stage kidney disease among Asian Americans is less than in Whites, but since 1992 Asian Americans experienced the greatest increase in end-stage kidney disease incidence due to diabetes among the various ethnic groups tracked by the U.S. Renal Data System (National Institutes of Health, 2006). Likewise, in Hawaii diabetes is the most common cause of end-stage kidney disease among people of Japanese and Filipino ancestry (Mau et al., 2003).

Between 1999 and 2004, the incidence of diabetic end-stage kidney disease, age-adjusted to the 2000 U.S. standard population, declined among AI/ANs (CDC, 2005), despite an increasing prevalence of diabetes in these populations, suggesting that current diabetes and kidney disease management practices effectively slow disease progression. Although susceptibility to kidney disease differs by ethnicity, if the rise in childhood type 2 diabetes continues, the increasing number of those with longer duration of diabetes will likely increase the frequency of diabetic kidney disease in the affected populations and even reverse the recent decline in diabetic end-stage kidney disease (Nelson, Pavkov, Hanson, & Knowler, 2008).

Diabetic Retinopathy

Diabetic retinopathy is the major cause of blindness among adults with diabetes. However, data from the National Health Interview Survey showed no significant difference in the prevalence of diabetic retinopathy in Whites ≥50 years old (9.4%, 95% CI 7.5–11.2) and other race/ethnicities (12.0%, 95% CI 8.8–15.2) (CDC, 2004). Projected estimates indicate that the number of Americans ≥40 with diabetic retinopathy will increase to 16 million by 2050, up from 5.5 million in 2005 (Saaddine et al., 2008). Moreover, 3.4 million of these will have vision-threatening diabetic retinopathy. The forecasted increase in those with diabetic retinopathy is higher for Hispanic/Latinos than for Whites and African Americans across all age groups, reflecting in part the population growth pattern and its impact on the number of people with diabetes.

Periodontal Disease

A chronic infection of the tissue surrounding the teeth, periodontal disease is a frequent complication of diabetes (Löe, 1993). Data from NHANES III show that prevalence of periodontal disease in Hispanic Americans ≥18 years old with diabetes was 28.5%, similar to that in African Americans (31.3%) and 1.4 times higher than in non-Hispanic Whites (Borrell, Burt, & Taylor, 2005). Comparatively, in NHANES IV the frequency of periodontal disease declined in these three racial/ethnic groups and particularly in African Americans, regardless of diabetes status. The declining trend was attributed, at least in part, to increasing awareness and the lower prevalence of current smoking among all racial/ethnic groups.

Observational studies indicate that periodontal disease has an adverse effect on glycemic control, increasing the risk for diabetes complications. In Pima Indian adults with diabetes, periodontitis predicted macroalbuminuria and end-stage kidney disease in a dose-dependent manner (Shultis et al., 2007). Moreover, periodontal disease was a strong predictor for mortality from coronary heart disease and diabetic nephropathy. Although experimental and epidemiologic studies suggest a link between periodontal disease and cardiovascular and chronic kidney disease, the mechanism by which periodontitis impacts these diseases remains unclear.

Infections and Infection-Related Mortality

Persons with diabetes are more susceptible to certain infections, are more difficult to treat once they acquire these infections, and often have worse prognosis than those without diabetes. Mortality due to infectious diseases in the U.S. ranges between 4% and 14.5% of diabetes-related deaths, most of these being ascribed to pneumonia and septicemia (Bertoni, Saydah, & Brancati, 2001). Decubitus ulcers and cellulitis associated with diabetes are frequently reported as the source of septicemia. Age-adjusted RR for death due to infections is 2.4 (95% CI 1.2–4.7) in women with diabetes compared with those without diabetes; in men with diabetes, the RR is 1.7 (95% CI 0.8–4.7) compared with those without diabetes. Results from a nationally representative cohort suggested that the excess risk of death from infections may be mediated in part by CVD (Bertoni et al., 2001). Available data on the frequency of infections among different racial/ethnic groups with diabetes are sparse, making inferences about disparities unfeasible.

MANAGEMENT OF DIABETES

Prevention

Many observation studies have found that BMI is strongly predictive of diabetes incidence. A number of randomized clinical trials have tested whether intervention on specific dietary components or physical activity will reduce the incidence of diabetes. One such clinical trial, the Diabetes Prevention Program, showed that at-risk individuals can sharply reduce the chance of developing type 2 diabetes through intensive weight loss with the goals of reducing weight, reducing total calories and calories from fat, and increasing moderate physical activity. Lifestyle intervention significantly reduced the development of diabetes by 58%, and in people aged 60 years and older, by 71% (Diabetes Prevention Program Research Group, 2002). The benefits of lifestyle interventions exceeded those of treatment with the oral diabetes drug metformin (31%) and were uniform for men and women across race/ethnic groups, including non-Hispanic Whites, Hispanics, African Americans, Asians, and AIs (see Figure 2.5). Similar healthy behaviors can improve insulin sensitivity, decrease insulin and fasting glucose, and reduce intra-abdominal fat among adolescents, thus preventing the onset and manifestation of diabetes. Whether these interventions also reduce cardiovascular disease and atherosclerosis, major causes of death in people with diabetes, remains to be determined.

Treatment

The ADA treatment guidelines recommend maintaining fasting plasma glucose values within an optimal range of 90–130 mg/dl (5.0–7.2 mmol/L) and an overall A1c goal of less than 7% for persons with diabetes (2008a). Intensive treatment of hyperglycemia prevents microvascular complications of diabetes, but has no significant effect on macrovascular complications. The best way to reduce CVD events in patients with diabetes is to target all cardiovascular risk factors. The largest diabetes trial, enrolling 11,140 patients with type 2 diabetes in 20 countries, confirmed that achieving a mean A1c of 6.5% significantly reduces the risk of diabetic nephropathy, although it did not affect the risk for cardiovascular disease (The ADVANCE Collaborative Group, 2008). Intensive glucose control, defined as the use of gliclazide plus other drugs as required to

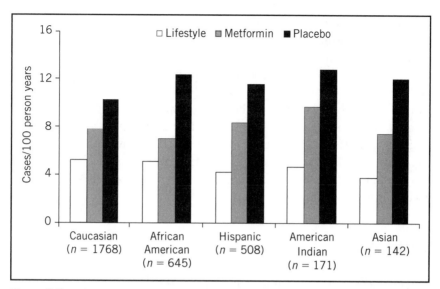

Figure 2.5 Incidence of diabetes by treatment group and ethnicity in the Diabetes Prevention Program. Treatment with metformin and modification of lifestyle were highly effective means of delaying or preventing type 2 diabetes across racial/ethnic groups (Diabetes Prevention Program Research Group, 2002).

achieve an A1c value of 6.5% or less, reduced the incidence of combined major macrovascular and microvascular events, largely by reduction of new or worsening diabetic nephropathy (i.e., development of macroalbuminuria, doubling of the serum creatinine level, the need for kidney replacement therapy, or death due to kidney disease). There were no significant effects on the incidence of retinopathy, major macrovascular events, death from cardiovascular causes, or death from any cause.

Although the recent availability of continuous glucose monitors permits frequent self-monitoring, achievement of consistent euglycemia in the recommended range and the avoidance of hypoglycemic and hyperglycemic excursions remain elusive for many patients with diabetes. A review of studies including data on glycemic, blood pressure, and low-density lipoprotein cholesterol levels in U.S. racial/ethnic minorities with diabetes, published between 1993 and 2003, revealed that minorities had poorer outcomes of care than non-Hispanic Whites. Disparities were particularly pronounced for glycemic control and blood pressure control (Kirk et al., 2005). Reasons for differences in health outcomes include disparities in health coverage, intensity of treatment, effective self-care, and ethnic differences in hemoglobin glycation or red cell survival (Jovanovic & Harrison, 2004). For example, Puerto Ricans with diabetes in New York State are less likely than Whites to have annual A1c or cholesterol testing and receive treatment for hypertension, despite equal access to health care (Peek, Cargill, & Huang, 2007). Similarly, Whites were more likely to have a lipid profile and an ophthalmologic examination than all other racial/ethnic groups. Hispanic/Latino Americans (Kirk et al., 2008) and African Americans (Kirk et al., 2006) have had consistently higher A1c levels than the White population over the past 15 years. This has substantially contributed to the higher prevalence of diabetes complications in these minorities.

SUMMARY

Diabetes affects racial/ethnic minorities in the U.S. disproportionately and is almost exclusively type 2 diabetes. Because diabetes often develops at a younger age in racial/ethnic minority populations, the major complications of diabetes also appear at a younger age, further exacerbating socioeconomic disparities and leading to increased levels of disability and reduced life expectancy. Even though the proportion of youth developing diabetes among the minority U.S. populations is small, the current epidemic of obesity in this age group has been associated with an increasing incidence of diabetes in childhood and adolescence (Pavkov et al., 2007). Given that many of the risk factors for diabetes are modifiable, efficacious treatments and practices have the potential to reduce health disparities. Future clinical trials of potential therapies and public health intervention programs should include racial/ethnic minority populations to ensure that the efficacy of these therapies and programs is assessed directly in the populations that need them most.

REFERENCES

The ADVANCE Collaborative Group. (2008). Intensive blood glucose control and vascular outcomes in patients with type 2 diabetes. *New England Journal of Medicine, 358,* 2560–2572.

American Diabetes Association. (2007). Clinical practice recommendations 2007. *Diabetes Care, 30(Suppl 1),* S1–S103.

American Diabetes Association. (2008a). Clinical practice recommendations 2008. *Diabetes Care, 31(Suppl 1),* S1–S110.

American Diabetes Association. (2008b). Economic costs of diabetes in the US in 2007. *Diabetes Care, 31,* 596–615.

Araneta, M. R. G., Morton, D. J., Lantion-Ang, L., et al. (2006). Hyperglycemia and type 2 diabetes among Filipino women in the Philippines, Hawaii, and San Diego. *Diabetes Research and Clinical Practice, 71,* 306–312.

Association of Asian Pacific Community Health Organizations. (2008). Summary of Asian Pacific Islander health issues. Retrieved from http://www.aapcho.org

Baier, L. J., & Hanson, R. L. (2004). Genetic studies of the etiology of type 2 diabetes in Pima Indians: Hunting for pieces to a complicated puzzle. *Diabetes, 53,* 1181–1186.

Baltazar, J. C., Ancheta, C. A., Abanb, I. B., Fernando, R. E., & Baquilod, M. M. (2004). Prevalence and correlates of diabetes mellitus and impaired glucose tolerance among adults in Luzon, Philippines. *Diabetes Research and Clinical Practice, 64,* 107–115.

Barnett, A. H., Eff, C., Leslie, R. D. G., & Pyke, D. A. (1981). Diabetes in identical twins: A study of 200 pairs. *Diabetologia, 20,* 87–93.

Bertoni, A. G., Saydah, S., & Brancati, F. L. (2001). Diabetes and the risk of infection-related mortality in the U.S. *Diabetes Care, 24,* 1044–1049.

Borrell, L. N., Burt, B. A., & Taylor, G. W. (2005). Prevalence and trends in periodontitis in the USA: From the NHANES III to the NHANES, 1988 to 2000. *Journal of Dental Research, 84,* 924–930.

Brancati, F. L., Kao, W. H. L., Folsom, A. R., Watson, R. L., & Szklo, M. (2000). Incident type 2 diabetes mellitus in African American and White adults: The Atherosclerosis Risk in Communities Study. *Journal of the American Medical Association, 283,* 2253–2259.

Brown, A. F., Gregg, E. W., Stevens, M. R., Karter, A. J., Weinberger, M., Safford, M. M., Gary, T. L., Caputo, D. A., Waitzfelder, B., Kim, C., Beckles, G. L. (2005). Race, ethnicity, socioeconomic position, and quality of care for adults with diabetes enrolled in managed care: The Translating Research into Action for Diabetes (TRIAD) study. *Diabetes Care, 28,* 2864–2870.

Burchfiel, C. M., Curb, J. D., Rodriguez, B. L., Yano, K., Hwang, L. J., Fong, K. O., & Marcus, E. B. (1995). Incidence and predictors of diabetes in Japanese-American men: The Honolulu Heart Program. *Annals of Epidemiology, 5,* 33–43.

Burke, J. P., Williams, K., Gaskill, S. P., Hazuda, H. P., Haffner, S. M., & Stern, M. P. (1999). Rapid rise in the incidence of type 2 diabetes from 1987 to 1996. *Archives of Internal Medicine, 159,* 1450–1456.

Burrows, N. R., Geiss, L. S., Engelgau, M. M., & Acton, K. J. (2000). Prevalence of diabetes among Native Americans and Alaska Natives, 1990–1997. *Diabetes Care, 23,* 1786–1790.

Centers for Disease Control and Prevention. (2005). *National Diabetes Fact Sheet.* Retrieved December 11, 2008, from http://www.cdc.gov/diabetes/pubs/estimates .htm#prev4

Centers for Disease Control and Prevention. (2003). Diabetes prevalence among American Indians and Alaska Natives and the overall population—United States, 1994–2002. *Morbidity and Mortality Weekly Report, 52,* 702–704.

Centers for Disease Control and Prevention. (2004). Prevalence of visual impairment and selected eye diseases among persons aged >50 years with and without diabetes—United States, 2002. *Morbidity and Mortality Weekly Report, 53,* 1069–1071.

Centers for Disease Control and Prevention. (2005). Incidence of end-stage renal disease among persons with diabetes—United States, 1990–2002. *Morbidity and Mortality Weekly Report, 54,* 1097–1100.

Centers for Disease Control and Prevention. (2007). Prevalence of self-reported cardiovascular disease among persons aged >35 years with diabetes—United States, 1997–2005. *Morbidity and Mortality Weekly Report, 56,* 1129–1132.

Centers for Disease Control and Prevention. (2008). National diabetes fact sheet: General information and national estimates on diabetes in the United States, 2007. Atlanta, GA: U.S. Department of Health and Human Services, Centers for Disease Control and Prevention.

Cohen, B. M. (1954). Diabetes mellitus among Indians of the American Southwest: Its prevalence and clinical characteristics in a hospitalized population. *Annals of Internal Medicine, 40,* 588–599.

Coustan, D. R. (1995). Gestational diabetes. In *Diabetes in America* (2nd ed., pp.703–733). Washington, DC: National Institutes of Health, National Institute of Diabetes and Digestive and Kidney Diseases. NIH Publ. No. 95-1468.

Crawford, P. B., Story, M., Wang, M. C., Ritchie, L. D., & Sabry, S. I. (2001). Ethnic issues in the epidemiology of childhood obesity. *Pediatric Clinics of North America, 48(4).*

Dabelea, D., Hanson, R. L., Bennett, P. H., et al. (1998). Increasing prevalence of type II diabetes in American Indian children. *Diabetologia, 41,* 904–910.

Dabelea, D., Palmer, J. P., Bennett, P. H., Pettitt, D. J., & Knowler, W. C. (1999). Absence of glutamic acid decarboxylase antibodies in Pima Indian children with diabetes mellitus. *Diabetologia, 42,* 1265–1266.

Diabetes Prevention Program Research Group. (2002). Reduction in the incidence of type 2 diabetes with lifestyle intervention or metformin. *New England Journal of Medicine, 346,* 393–403.

Dowse, G. K. (1996). Incidence of NIDDM and the natural history of IGT in Pacific and Indian Ocean populations. Diabetes Research and Clinical Practice, 34, S45–S50.

Eisenbarth, G. S. (1986). Type 1 diabetes mellitus: A chronic autoimmune disease. *New England Journal of Medicine, 314,* 1360–1368.

Flegal, K. M., Ezzati, T. M., Harris, M. I., Haynes, S. G., Juarez, R. Z., Knowler, W. C., Perez-Stable, E. J., & Stern, M. P. (1991). Prevalence of diabetes in Mexican Americans, Cubans, and Puerto Ricans from the Hispanic Health and Nutrition Examination Survey, 1982–84. *Diabetes Care, 14,* 628–638.

Fujimoto, W. Y. (1995). Diabetes in Asian and Pacific Islander Americans. In National Diabetes Data Group, *Diabetes in America* (2nd ed., pp. 661–681). Bethesda, MD: National Institutes of Health, National Institute of Diabetes and Digestive and Kidney Diseases. NIH Publ. No. 95-1468,

Fujimoto, W. Y., Bergstrom, R. W., Boyko, E. J., Leonetti, D. L., Newell, M. L. L., & Wahl, P. W. (1995). Susceptibility to development of central adiposity among populations. *Obesity Research, 3(Suppl 2),* 179S–186S.

Galloway, J. M. (2005). Cardiovascular health among American Indians and Alaska Natives: Successes, challenges and potentials. *American Journal of Preventative Medicine, 29,* S11–S17.

Ghodes, D. (1995). Diabetes in North American Indians and Alaska Natives. In *Diabetes in America* (pp. 683–701). Washington, DC: U.S. Department of Health and Human Services. NIH Publ. No. 95-1468.

Hale, D. E., & Rupert, G. (2006). The changing spectrum of diabetes in Mexican American youth. *Review of Endocrinology and Metabolic Disorders, 7,* 163–170.

Hall, L. D., Sberna, J., & Utermohle, C. J. (2001). Diabetes in Alaska, 1991–2000: Results from the Behavioral Risk Factor Surveillance System. *State of Alaska Epidemiology Bulletin Recommendations and Reports.* Anchorage, Alaska. Department of Health and Human Services, Division of Public Health.

Hanson, R. L. (1997). The Pima Diabetes Genes Group: Genomic scan for markers linked to type II diabetes in Pima Indians. *Diabetes, 46(Suppl 1),* 51.

Harris, M. I. (1996). Impaired glucose tolerance: Prevalence and conversion to NIDDM. *Diabetes Medicine, 13,* S9–S11.

Harris, M. I., Flegal, K. M., Cowie, C. C., Eberhardt, M. S., Goldstein, D. E., Little, R. R., Wiedmeyer, H. M., & Byrd-Holt, D. D. (1998). Prevalence of diabetes, impaired fasting glucose, and impaired glucose tolerance in U.S. adults: The Third National Health and Nutrition Examination Survey, 1988–1994. *Diabetes Care, 21,* 518–524.

Hillier, T. A., & Pedula, K. L. (2003). Complications in young adults with early-onset type 2 diabetes: Losing the relative protection of youth. *Diabetes Care, 26,* 2999–3005.

Huxley, R., Omari, A., & Caterson, I. D. (2008). Obesity and diabetes. In J. M. Ekoe, M. Rewers, R. Williams, & P. Zimmet, *The epidemiology of diabetes mellitus* (2nd ed., pp. 57–70). New York: John Wiley & Sons.

Indian Health Service. (2008). Indian Health Service fact sheet. Retrieved August 11, 2008, from http://www.ihs.gov/PublicInfo/PublicAffairs/Welcome_Info/ThisFacts.asp

Indian Health Service. (1997). *Trends in Indian health, 1997.* Rockville, MD: U.S. Department of Health and Human Services.

Indian Health Service. (2000). *Trends in Indian health, 2000–2001* (pp. 3–9). Rockville, MD: U.S. Department of Health and Human Services. Retrieved from http://www.ihs.gov/nonmedicalprograms/ IHS_stats/trends00.asp

International Diabetes Federation. (2008). *Diabetes atlas* (3rd ed). Retrieved April 2008 from http://www.eatlas.idf.org/media/

Janssen, R. C., Bogardus, C., Takeda, J., Knowler, W. C., & Thompson, D. B. (1994). Linkage analysis of acute insulin secretion with GLUT2 and glucokinase in Pima Indians and the identification of a missense mutation in GLUT2. *Diabetes, 43,* 558–563.

Joslin, E. P. (1940). The universality of diabetes. *Journal of the American Medical Association, 115,* 2033–2038.

Jovanovic, L., & Harrison III, R. W. (2004). Advances in diabetes for the millennium: Diabetes in minorities. *Medscape General Medicine, 6(Suppl 3),* 2.

Karter, A. J., Ferrara, A., Liu, J. Y., Moffet, H. H., Ackerson, L. M., & Selby, J. V. (2002). Ethnic disparities in diabetic complications in an insured population. *Journal of the American Medical Association, 287,* 2519–2527.

Kawate, R., Yamakido, M., Nishimoto, Y., Bennett, P. H., Hamman, R. F., & Knowler, W. C. (1979). Diabetes mellitus and its vascular complications in Japanese migrants on the Island of Hawaii. *Diabetes Care, 2,* 161–170.

Kim, H. S., Park, S. Y., Grandinetti, A., Holck, P. S., & Waslien, C. (2008). Major dietary patterns, ethnicity, and prevalence of type 2 diabetes in rural Hawaii. *Nutrition, 24,* 1065–1072.

Kim, N. H., Pavkov, M. E., Looker, H. C., Nelson, R. G., Bennett, P. H., Hanson, R. L., Curtis, J. M., Sievers, M. L., & Knowler, W. C. (2008). Plasma glucose regulation and mortality in Pima Indians. *Diabetes Care, 31,* 488–492.

Kirk, J. K., Bell, R. A., Bertoni, A. G., et al. (2005). Ethnic disparities: Control of glycemia, blood pressure, and LDL cholesterol among US adults with type 2 diabetes. *The Annals of Pharmacotherapy, 39,* 1489–1501.

Kirk, J. K., D'Agostino, R. B., Bell, R. A., et al. (2006). Disparities in HbA1c levels between African-American and non-Hispanic White adults with diabetes. *Diabetes Care, 29,* 2130–2136.

Kirk, J. K., Passmore, L. V., Bell, R. A., et al. (2008). Disparities in A1C levels between Hispanic and non-Hispanic White adults with diabetes: A meta-analysis. *Diabetes Care, 31,* 240–246.

Knowler, W. C., Bennett, P. H., Bottazzo, G. F., & Doniach, D. (1979). Islet cell antibodies and diabetes mellitus in Pima Indians. *Diabetologia, 17,* 161–164.

Knowler, W. C., Bennett, P. H., Hamman, R. F., & Miller, M. (1978). Diabetes incidence and prevalence in Pima Indians: A 19-fold greater incidence than in Rochester, Minnesota. *American Journal of Epidemiology, 108,* 497–505.

Knowler, W. C., Pettitt, D. J., Saad, M. F., & Bennett, P. H. (1990). Diabetes mellitus in the Pima Indians: Incidence, risk factors and pathogenesis. *Diabetes/Metabolism Reviews, 6,* 1–27.

Lee, E. T., Welty, T. K., Cowan, L. D., Wang, W., Rhoades, D. A., Devereux, R., Go, O., Fabsitz, R., & Howard, B. V. (2002). Incidence of diabetes in American Indians of three geographic areas. *Diabetes Care, 25,* 49–54.

Lee, E. T., Welty, T. K., Fabsitz, R., et al. (1990). The Strong Heart Study: A study of cardiovascular disease in American Indians: design and methods. *American Journal of Epidemiology, 132,* 1141–1155.

Lipton, R. B. (2007). Incidence of diabetes in children and youth—tracking a moving target. *Journal of the American Medical Association, 297,* 2760–2762.

Löe, H. (1993). Periodontal disease: The sixth complication of diabetes mellitus. *Diabetes Care, 16,* 329–334.

Maty, S. C., Everson-Rose, S. A., Haan, M. N., Raghunathan, T. E., & Kaplan, G. A. (2005). Education, income, occupation, and the 34-year incidence (1965–99) of type 2 diabetes in the Alameda County Study. *International Journal of Epidemiology, 34,* 1274–1281.

Mau, M. K., West, M., Sugihara, J., Kamaka, M., Mikami, J., & Cheng, S. F. (2003). Renal disease disparities in Asian and Pacific-based populations in Hawaii. *Journal of the National Medical Association, 95,* 955–963.

McNeely, M. J., & Boyko, E. J. (2004). Type 2 diabetes prevalence in Asian Americans. *Diabetes Care, 27,* 66–69.

McNeely, M. J., & Fujimoto, W. Y. (2008). Epidemiology of diabetes in Asian North Americans. In J. M. Ekoe, M. Rewers, R. Williams, & P. Zimmet (Eds.), *The epidemiology of diabetes mellitus* (2nd ed., pp. 323–337). New York: John Wiley & Sons.

McNutt, S. W., Hu, Y., Schreiber, G. B., et al. (1997). A longitudinal study of the dietary practices of African American and White girls 9 and 10 years old at enrollment: The NHLBI Growth and Health Study. *Journal of Adolescent Health, 20,* 27–37.

Mier, N., Medina, A. A., & Ory, M. G. (2007). Mexican Americans with type 2 diabetes: Perspectives on definitions, motivators, and programs of physical activity. *Prevention of Chronic Disease, 4,* 1–8.

Mokdad, A. H., Serdula, M. K., Dietz, W. H., Bowman, B. A., Marks, J. S., & Koplan, J. P. (1999). The spread of the obesity epidemic in the United States, 1991–1998. *Journal of the American Medical Association, 282,* 1519–1522.

Nakanishi, S., Okubo, M., Yoneda, M., Jitsuiki, K., Yamane, K., & Kohno, N. (2004). A comparison between Japanese-Americans living in Hawaii and Los Angeles and native Japanese: The impact of lifestyle westernization on diabetes mellitus. *Biomedical Pharmacotherapy, 58,* 571–577.

Narayan, K. M. V., Boyle, J. P., Geiss, L. S., Saaddine, J. B., & Thompson, T. J. (2006). Impact of recent increase in incidence on future diabetes burden. *Diabetes Care, 29,* 2114–2116.

Narayan, K. M. V., Boyle, J. P., Thompson, T. J., Sorensen, S. W., & Williamson, D. F. (2003). Lifetime risk of diabetes mellitus in the United States. *Journal of the American Medical Association, 290,* 1884–1890.

National Diabetes Information Clearinghouse. (2002). National diabetes statistics: Fact sheet. NIH Publ. No. 02-3892. Retrieved from http://www.niddk.nih.gov/health/diabetes/pubs/dmstats/dmstats.htm

National Institutes of Health. (2006). U.S. Renal Data System 2006 annual data report. In *Atlas of chronic kidney disease and end-stage renal disease in the United States.* Bethesda, MD: National Institutes of Health, National Institute of Diabetes and Digestive and Kidney Diseases.

Nelson, R. G., Pavkov, M. E., Hanson, R. L., & Knowler, W. C. (2008). Changing course of diabetic nephropathy in the Pima Indians. *Diabetes Research and Clinical Practice, 82(Suppl 1),* S10–S14.

Ogden, C. L., Flegal, K. M., Carroll, M. D., et al. (2002). Prevalence and trends in overweight among US children and adolescents, 1999–2000. *Journal of the American Medical Association, 288,* 1728–1732.

Park, Y. W., Allison, D. B., Heymsfield, S. B., & Gallagher, D. (2001). Larger amounts of visceral adipose tissue in Asian Americans. *Obesity Research, 9,* 381–387.

Pavkov, M. E., Bennett, P. H., Knowler, W. C., Krakoff, J., Sievers, M. L., & Nelson, R. G. (2006). Effect of youth-onset type 2 diabetes mellitus on incidence of end-stage renal disease and mortality in young and middle-aged Pima Indians. *Journal of the American Medical Association, 296,* 421–426.

Pavkov, M. E., Hanson, R. L., Knowler, W. C., Bennett, P. H., Krakoff, J., & Nelson, R. G. (2007). Changing patterns of type 2 diabetes incidence among Pima Indians. *Diabetes Care, 30,* 1758–1763.

Peek, M. E., Cargill, A., & Huang, E. S. (2007). Diabetes health disparities: A systematic review of health care interventions. *Medical Care Research and Review, 64,* 101S–156S.

Pérez-Escamilla, R., & Putnik, P. (2007). The role of acculturation in nutrition, lifestyle, and incidence of type 2 diabetes among Latinos. *Journal of Nutrition, 137,* 860–870.

Powers, A. C. (2008). Diabetes mellitus. Anthony S. Fauci, Eugene Braunwald, Dennis L. Kasper, Stephen L. Hauser, Dan L. Longo, J. Larry Jameson, and Joseph Loscalzo, Eds. *Harrison's principles of internal medicine* (17th ed., pp. 2269–2275). New York: McGraw-Hill.

President's Advisory Commission on Consumer Protection and Quality in the Health Care Industry. (1998). Quality first: Better health care for all Americans. In *Final report of the President's Advisory Commission on Consumer Protection and Quality in the Health Care Industry.* Washington, DC: U.S. Government Printing Office.

Putnam, J., Allshouse, J., & Kantor, L. S. (2002). US per capita food supply trends: More calories, refined carbohydrates, and fats. *Food Review, 25,* 2–15.

Ravussin, E., Valencia, M. E., Esparza, J., Bennett, P. H., & Schulz, L. O. (1994). Effects of a traditional lifestyle on obesity in Pima Indians. *Diabetes Care, 17,* 1067–1074.

Rodriguez, B. L., Curb, J. D., Burchfiel, C. M., Huang, B., Sharp, D. S., Lu, G. Y., Fujimoto, W., & Yano, K. (1996). Impaired glucose tolerance, diabetes, and cardiovascular disease risk factor profiles in the elderly: The Honolulu Heart Program. *Diabetes Care, 19,* 587–590.

Saaddine, J. B., Honeycutt, A. A., Narayan, K. M. V., Zhang, X., Klein, R., & Boyle, J. P. (2008). Projection of diabetic retinopathy and other major eye diseases among people with diabetes mellitus: United States, 2005–2050. *Archives of Ophthalmology, 126,* 1740–1747.

Satcher, D. (1999). The initiative to eliminate racial and ethnic health disparities is moving forward. *Public Health Reports, 114,* 283–287.

Schaefer, O. (1968). Glycosuria and diabetes mellitus in Canadian Eskimos. *Canadian Medical Association Journal, 99,* 201–206.

SEARCH for Diabetes in Youth Study Group. (2006). The burden of diabetes mellitus among US youth: Prevalence estimates from the SEARCH for Diabetes in Youth Study. *Pediatrics, 118,* 1510–1518.

Shai, I., Jiang, R., Manson, J. E., Stampfer, M. J., Willett, W. C., Colditz, G. A., & Hu, F. B. (2006). Ethnicity, obesity, and risk of type 2 diabetes in women: A 20-year follow-up study. *Diabetes Care, 29,* 1585–1590.

Shin, C. S., Lee, H. K., Koh, C. S., Kim, Y. I., Shin, Y. S., Yoo, K. Y., Paik, H. Y., Park, Y. S., & Yang, B. G. (1997). Risk factors for the development of NIDDM in Yonchon County, Korea. *Diabetes Care, 20,* 1842–1846.

Shultis, W. A., Weil, E. J., Looker, H. C., et al. (2007). Effect of periodontitis on overt nephropathy and end-stage renal disease in type 2 diabetes. *Diabetes Care, 30,* 306–311.

Signorello, L. B., Schlundt, D. G., Cohen, S. S., Steinwandel, M. D., Buchowski, M. S., McLaughlin, J. K., Hargreaves, M. K., & Blot, W. J. (2007). Comparing diabetes prevalence between African Americans and Whites of similar socioeconomic status. *American Journal of Public Health, 97,* 2260–2267.

Silventoinen, K., Sans, S., Tolonen, H., Monterde, D., Kuulasmaa, K., Kesteloot, H., et al. (2004). Trends in obesity and energy supply in the WHO MONICA Project. *International Journal of Obesity-Related Metabolic Disorders, 28,* 710–718.

Skyler, J. S. (Ed.). (1998). *Medical management of type 1 diabetes* (3rd ed.). Alexandria, VA: American Diabetes Association.

Smith, J. P. (2007). Nature and causes of trends in male diabetes prevalence, undiagnosed diabetes, and the socioeconomic status health gradient. *Proceedings of the National Academy of Sciences, 104,* 13,225–13,231.

Tucker, K. L., Bermudez, O. L., & Castaneda, C. (2000). Type 2 diabetes is prevalent and poorly controlled among Hispanic elders of Caribbean origin. *American Journal of Public Health, 90,* 1288–1293.

U.S. Census Bureau. (2005). *Hispanic Population Passes 40 Million, Census Bureau Reports.* Retrieved from http://www.census.gov/Press-Release/www/releases/archives/population/005164.html

U.S. Census Bureau. (1992). *Minority Economic Profiles, 24,* and unpublished data.

U.S. Census Bureau. (2001). U.S. Census Bureau Population Estimates Program: Profiles of general demographic characteristics. *National summary: 2000 census of population and housing.* Retrieved May 20, 2008, from http://www.census.gov/main/www/cen2000.html

U.S. Census Bureau. (2004). *Current population survey: Hispanic population of the United States.* Retrieved August 11, 2008, from http://www.census.gov/prod/2004pubs/censr-17.pdf, accessed June 16, 2009

Wang, Y., Tussing, L., Odoms-Young, A., et al. (2006). Obesity prevention in low socioeconomic status urban African-American adolescents: Study design and preliminary findings of the HEALTH-KIDS study. *European Journal of Clinical Nutrition, 60,* 92–103.

World Health Organization International Association for the Study of Obesity, International Obesity Task Force. (2000). The Asia-Pacific perspective: Redefining obesity and its treatment. Sydney, Australia: Health Communications.

Yamada, S., & Palafox, N. (2001). On the biopsychosocial model: The example of political economic causes of diabetes in the Marshall Islands. *Family Medicine, 33,* 702–704.

Zimmet, P., Ainuu, S., DeBoer, W., Faaiuso, J., & Whitehouse, S. (1981). The prevalence of diabetes in the rural and urban Polynesian population of Western Samoa. *Diabetes, 30,* 45–51.

3

The Co-Emergence of the Diabetes and Obesity Epidemics in Racial and Ethnic Populations[1]

LEANDRIS C. LIBURD

INTRODUCTION

The rise in the prevalence of type 2 diabetes coincides with the national and international rise in obesity (Mokdad et al., 1999; Mokdad, Ford, Bowman, Nelson, & Engelgau, 2000; Mokdad et al., 2001a; Valdez & Williamson, 2002). The co-emergence of the type 2 diabetes and obesity epidemics, as well as the complexities of their etiologies, in populations that are arguably socially, economically, and politically vulnerable demand a critical re-examination of how we conduct intervention research and public health practice.

Social scientists, such as sociologists, political scientists, feminist scholars, and anthropologists, can add much knowledge to our understanding of the multiple layers that construct the obesity epidemic. In this chapter contributions from clinical evidence, epidemiology, sociology, and public health are presented in a transdisciplinary format to more fully explain the biocultural relationship between diabetes and obesity. The chapter begins with a critical framing of public health and its orientation to obesity as a public health problem. Biomedical and

---

[1] The findings and conclusions in this chapter are those of the author and do not necessarily represent the views of the Centers for Disease Control and Prevention.

public health perspectives on the definition of obesity, its epidemiological and clinical association with the growing burden of type 2 diabetes, and influences of the broader socioecologic environment on the higher prevalence of obesity in communities of color are described. Particular attention is given to the role of socioeconomic status and its association with obesity trends at the population level.

PUBLIC HEALTH AND OBESITY

Public health research and practice is aimed at improving the health of whole communities and is pursued through the interdisciplinary engagement of easily 20 knowledge domains, including epidemiology and biostatistics, environmental health, social and behavioral sciences, nutrition, maternal and child health, and disaster control and emergency preparedness (see Table 3.1).

Although public health administrators would argue that the mission of public health is accomplished through an organized and integrated approach to community health, the knowledge domains that ground public health practice are highly differentiated and sometimes poorly coordinated in the interest of whole communities. Communities in public health are understood in many discrete and overlapping contexts, such as by geopolitical designation (e.g., census tracts, neighborhoods, cities, and states), collectives of people with shared values and interests (e.g., faith communities and civic groups with diverse social and political agendas), and other communities of identity (e.g., by race and gender, sexual orientation, and region of origin). A fuller elaboration of the nuances of community in public health is discussed in chapter 5. Producing evidence-based approaches for disease prevention and health promotion within these contexts requires an understanding of the complexities of organizational structures, interactions, and myriad other dynamics that shape and influence decision making at the local, state, regional, and national levels wherein public health operates and policies and programs are established.

What Is Obesity?

In the strictest sense, obesity means "excess adipose tissue or excess body fat beyond a threshold for what is considered a norm or a reference

Table 3.1

DISTINCTIONS BETWEEN PUBLIC HEALTH AND MEDICINE

PUBLIC HEALTH	MEDICINE
Primary focus on population	Primary focus on individual
Public service ethic, tempered by concerns for the individual	Personal service ethic, conditioned by awareness of social responsibilities
Emphasis on prevention, health promotion for the whole community	Emphasis on diagnosis and treatment, care for the whole patient
Public health paradigm employs a spectrum of interventions aimed at the environment, human behavior and lifestyle, and medical care	Medical paradigm places predominant emphasis on medical care
Multiple professional identities with diffuse public image	
Variable certification of specialists beyond professional public health degree	Well-established profession with sharp public image
Lines of specialization organized, with examples, by analytical method (epidemiology), setting and population (occupational health), substantive health problem (nutrition), skills in assessment, policy development, and assurance	Uniform system for certifying specialists beyond professional medical degree
Biologic sciences central, stimulated by major threats to health of populations; move between laboratory and field	Lines of specialization organized, with examples, by organ system (cardiology), patient group (pediatrics), etiology, and pathophysiology (oncology)
Numeric sciences an essential feature of analysis and training	
Social sciences an integral part of public health education	
Clinical sciences peripheral to professional training	

Source: From Fineberg. (1990).

value" (Kuczmarski, 2007, p. 25). Obesity in the biomedical context infers an "unhealthy excess of body fat" that increases risk of medical illness and premature mortality (Kuczmarski, 2007). According to the National Institutes of Health (NIH, 1998, p. xi), "Obesity is a complex, multifactorial disease that develops from the interaction between genotype and the environment." For each individual, body weight is the result of a combination of genetic, metabolic, behavioral, environmental, cultural, and socioeconomic influences, but the relative contribution of each of these influences on the expression of obesity is not well understood. Epidemiological and clinical research have found obesity to substantially increase the risk of morbidity from hypertension, dyslipidemia, type 2 diabetes, coronary artery disease, stroke, gallbladder disease, osteoarthritis, and sleep apnea and respiratory problems, as well as cancers of the endometrium, breast, prostate, and colon (NIH, 1998). In addition to increased risk for morbidity, persons categorized as obese are socially stigmatized in some settings and subject to varying forms of discrimination (Campos, 2004; Gard & Wright, 2004; Puhl & Brownell, 2001, 2002).

How Is Obesity Measured?

A variety of criteria have been used in the U.S. to define various levels of weight status (Kuczmarski & Flegal, 2000), but the most common method is the body mass index (BMI), calculated as weight in kilograms divided by height in meters squared (Mokdad et al., 1999). Although widely used since the early 1980s as the standard measure for categorizing persons and populations as underweight, overweight, or obese, BMI is not the best measure of body fatness. BMI cannot take into consideration factors like frame size and muscularity. It does not distinguish between muscle, fat, bone and cartilage, or water weight. Furthermore, the BMI calculation requires that a healthy weight for any person is proportional to the square of his height. This leads to misclassification of above average muscularity.

The following definitions from the *Clinical Guidelines on the Identification, Evaluation, and Treatment of Overweight and Obesity in Adults* are used to classify weight status: underweight BMI is <18.5, healthy BMI is 18.5–24.9, overweight BMI is 25–29, and a BMI of 30 and greater is considered obese (NIH, 1998). Although BMI has been found to be a reliable indicator of total body fat, which is related to the risk of disease and death for population assessment and clinical prescreening, there are limits to the utility of BMI in that it may overestimate body fat in athletes and others who have a muscular build or may underestimate body fat in older persons and others who have lost muscle mass. BMI then is best used as a reference measure to alert the population to pay attention to expanding waistlines and declining physical activity in order to spark action that might slow weight gain and increase levels of regular physical activity.

Whereas total body fat is important, where fat is distributed on the body is also significant in signaling adverse health outcomes. Body fat distribution has been broadly characterized as "fat stored peripherally on the extremities (arms and legs) and fat stored centrally on the torso of the body" (Kuczmarski, 2007, p. 30). Men and women are observed to store fat in different patterns, that is, men tend to have more fat in the abdominal region and women tend to store more fat in the hip/buttocks region (Kuczmarski, 2007). Central or abdominal adiposity has been associated with increased risk for the development of type 2 diabetes (Vazquez, Duval, Jacobs, & Silventoinen, 2007).

Abdominal circumference alone does not fully measure the risk for metabolic disturbances like type 2 diabetes. Fat mass in the central region has been described as visceral or intra-abdominal fat, whereas subcutaneous fat is fat stored beneath the surface of the skin. Visceral fat appears to be more highly associated with metabolic abnormalities (Kuczmarski, 2007). A full discussion of the variety of fats that accumulate in and around the body and the debates about their association with the onset of type 2 diabetes and other morbidities is beyond the scope of this chapter. Additional reading will also reveal that how obesity is defined and measured across racial and ethnic groups is also variable in terms of predicting risk for metabolic disorders like type 2 diabetes (Kuczmarski, 2007). Students are encouraged to read the large and growing literature on the clinical implications of excess body fat.

PREVALENCE OF OBESITY IN THE U.S.

The rise in the prevalence of type 2 diabetes coincides with the national and international rise in obesity and the increases in overweight and obesity across all ages, racial and ethnic groups, and both sexes, but the greatest burden is found among women of color (Mokdad et.al., 1999, 2000, 2001a; Valdez & Williamson, 2002). Between 1980 and

2002, obesity prevalence doubled in adults aged 20 years or older and overweight prevalence tripled in children and adolescents aged 6–19 years (Ogden et al., 2006). Specifically, among children and adolescents aged 2–19 years, 17.1% were overweight in 2003–2004 and 32.2% of adults aged 20 years or older were obese, and the prevalence of extreme obesity (i.e., BMI >40) was 4.8% (Ogden et al., 2006). No differences in BMI distributions were found among adult men in this National Health and Nutrition Examination Survey (NHANES), but Mexican American and non-Hispanic Black women were significantly more likely to be obese than their non-Hispanic White female counterparts (Ogden et al., 2006). Among women almost 58% of non-Hispanic Black women aged 40–59 years were obese in 2003–2004, compared with about 38% of non-Hispanic White women of the same age. Higher prevalence of overweight and obesity among women of color have persisted for decades, but interestingly no increase in overall obesity prevalence among women was observed over the 6-year data analysis period (Ogden et al., 2006). The Centers for Disease Control and Prevention also report that groups where the greatest increase in obesity has been observed recently include persons in the age group 18–29, persons with some college education, and persons living in the southern region of the U.S.

The prevalence of overweight in Mexican American male children and adolescents was significantly greater than non-Hispanic White male children and adolescents, whereas prevalence of overweight among non-Hispanic White male children and adolescents did not differ significantly from non-Hispanic Black male children and adolescents (Ogden et al., 2006). As among adults, the picture changes when we consider the overweight status of females. Mexican American and non-Hispanic Black female children and adolescents were significantly more likely to be overweight than non-Hispanic White female children and adolescents (Ogden et al., 2006). A recent study of obesity rates among Latinos in California found that "compared to other races and ethnic groups in California, Latino males and females of all ages have among the highest rates of obesity, overweight, and one of the most severe consequences of obesity: type 2 diabetes" (Latino Coalition for a Healthy California, 2006). They estimate that nearly 7 out of 10 California Latino adults are overweight or obese, and among U.S.-born adolescents their prevalence or overweight is nearly twice as high as among foreign-born Latino adolescents.

OBESITY AS A KEY RISK FACTOR FOR TYPE 2 DIABETES

The type 2 diabetes epidemic is believed to be partly a by-product of a concomitant increase in population obesity levels, because population increases in diabetes have coincided with increases in obesity (Gregg et al., 2004; Mokdad et.al., 1999, 2000, 2001a, 2001b; Valdez & Williamson, 2002). Between 1960–1962 and 1999–2000, for example, the prevalence of diagnosed diabetes in the U.S. increased from 1.8% to 5.8%, an average increase of one percentage point per decade (Gregg et al., 2004). The rate of increase was greatest for those with BMI ≥ 35 kg/m^2, among whom the prevalence tripled (e.g., from 4.9% to 15.1%, probability >99.9%), and whose per-decade increase was almost twice that of the population overall (Gregg et al., 2004, p. 2808).

Whereas the exact mechanisms through which obesity increases the risk of diabetes are not fully understood, obesity results in insulin resistance, which

> is characterized by a reduction in the number and function of insulin receptors and by a disruption of the postreceptor cascade of events. In addition, obesity is often associated with increased insulin production by pancreatic cells. Perhaps as a function of the duration and magnitude of obesity, further deterioration in glucose homeostatic mechanisms occurs when beta-cells become glucose incompetent and clinical diabetes develops. Also, elevated levels of free fatty acids in obesity may increase hepatic glucose production, and play a role in the insulin resistance of target tissues and decompensation of beta-cells, thus promoting type 2 diabetes. (Ford, Williamson, & Liu, 1997, p. 214)

In addition to obesity and insulin resistance, other factors likely driving the increasing prevalence of type 2 diabetes are "reductions in physical activity, changes in diet composition, environmental factors, or an increase in survival" (Gregg et al., 2004). Within the clinical environment, greater opportunistic screening of obese persons for type 2 diabetes is observed while awareness of the association between obesity and diabetes has increased among providers and the lay public (Gregg et al., 2004).

Vazquez et al. (2007) conducted a meta-analysis of the value of three obesity indicators in predicting incident diabetes. The three indicators were BMI, waist circumference, and waist/hip ratio. Waist circumference has been shown to be a good or better predictor than BMI of the metabolic syndrome, diabetes, cardiovascular disease, and all-cause mortality (Vazquez et al., 2007). They also found that waist/hip ratio is the most common obesity-related predictor of diabetes after BMI, but has a weaker correlation with BMI ($r = 0.4$) than does waist circumference. The ability of these obesity indicators to predict diabetes by ethnicity, age, and sex may also differ according to their research. For example, "among Asian populations, central obesity has been shown to be a more consistent predictor of diabetes than is total obesity, while general obesity has been shown to be a better predictor among White US populations and Europeans" (Vazquez et al., 2007, p. 116). Overall, they found waist circumference to be a slightly better predictor of diabetes than BMI; however, "the statistical reality is that waist circumference and body mass index are very highly correlated and likely to behave similarly in diabetes prediction" (Vazquez et al., 2007, p. 126).

In their study of the influence of long-term patterns of weight change (over a period of about 10 years) in the risk for diabetes in a national cohort of U.S. adults in the NHANES follow-up study, Ford and colleagues (1997) found weight gain to be associated with higher incidence of type 2 diabetes. In addition, "participants who developed diabetes during the follow-up period were older and were more likely to be black, have lower educational attainment, have higher blood pressure, and be overweight at baseline than those who did not develop diabetes. . . . the mean weight gain for participants who developed diabetes was greater than that for participants who did not develop diabetes" (Ford et al., 1997, p. 216). In fact, these data suggested that for every kilogram of increase in weight, the risk of diabetes increased by 4.5% (Ford et al., 1997). For the public health practitioner, consideration of each of these obesity indicators, community trends toward weight gain, co-morbidities, and demographic factors such as level of formal education can be instructive for persons at high risk for developing type 2 diabetes.

SOCIOECOLOGIC INFLUENCES ON OBESITY PREVALENCE

Socioecologic influences on the prevalence of obesity in the U.S. encapsulate variables in the social environment, such as socioeconomic position, race and ethnicity, social networks and social support, and work conditions, along with a focus on place, including neighborhoods, schools, work sites, and even nations (see chapter 6). These multiple and interdependent factors, external to the individual, shape individual choices and behaviors associated with obesity and overweight (Block, Scribner, & DeSalvo, 2004; Institute of Medicine, 2002; Kumanyika, 2007; Powell, Slater, Mirtcheva, Bao, & Chaloupka, 2006; Schulz et al., 2005; Zenk et.al., 2005). Higher status as measured by social class or other indicators of social dominance allow people with more resources, such as money, knowledge, social networks, or power, more opportunities to protect their health relative to those in less favored socioeconomic positions (Mechanic, 2003). One can argue that persons who understand energy balance and its relationship to weight gain, whose history and sociality have nurtured a palate for healthy and disciplined eating, who have the time and needed resources to prioritize and incorporate physical activity, who have access to high quality and affordable foods, and have a social network that shares the value of these choices are in a better position to prevent obesity and maintain a healthy weight.

A socioecological orientation to obesity facilitates our understanding of the growing trends of overweight, obesity, and diabetes and what can be influenced to reverse these trends at the level of the population. Mechanic (2003, pp. 433, 437) describes population health as

> most basically about aggregates and not about individuals. It focuses on the upstream factors that structure how people live and the opportunities and constraints they face. . . . Intervention at the population level seeks to influence the rates at which events occur by altering factors that impact large numbers of individuals. . . . As population health is generally conceived, it depends on a wide range of disciplines and professions that have different theoretical orientations, varying methodological approaches, and diverse standards of proof.

The Institute of Medicine, in its landmark report *The Future of the Public's Health in the 21st Century,* proposes a model of the determinants of health that builds upon the work of Dahlgren and Whitehead, which identifies the

> macro-level conditions and policies (social, economic, cultural, and environmental) as potent forces in shaping midlevel (working conditions, housing) and proximate (behavioral, biological) determinants of health.

Macro-level or upstream determinants (such as sex or the virulence of a disease agent) interact along complex and dynamic pathways to produce health at a population level. (Institute of Medicine, 2003, pp. 52–53)

(See Figure 3.1.)

It is the complex, dynamic, and interactive nature of the socioeco-logic conditions that increase the risk for obesity and overweight in all communities that confounds and undermines most public health inter-ventions that have tended to isolate selected behaviors, namely nutrition and physical activity, and delivered interventions that are often decon-textualized, ahistorical, and overly dependent on theories of individual behavior change. Cultural theories and models, systems theories, and even economic theories are often neglected in intervention research and program planning to combat obesity. A socioecologic or population health approach shifts the attention of the public health practitioner to

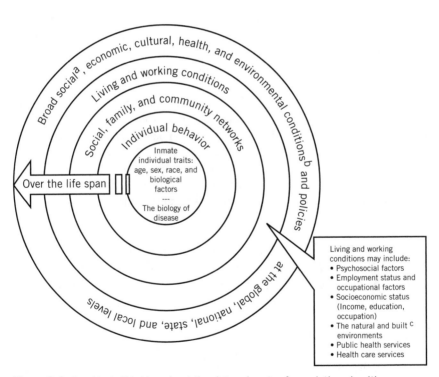

Figure 3.1 A guide to thinking about the determinants of populations health

the macro-level determinants, driving individual choice and behavior in many instances.

In her discussion of ecological models for obesity prevention, Kumanyika (2007) borrows from the work of Booth et al. (2001), which sets forth a framework for determinants of physical activity and eating behavior. In this model they delineate levels or layers of influence that at the center are the "psycho-biological core," and from this center are cultural and social factors that "enable choice" to prevent obesity (Kumanyika, 2007, p. 103). Within the psychobiological core are factors such as genetics and physiology, pleasure, and self-identities, as well as life experience, social roles, socioeconomic status, ethnic identities, and educational attainment (Kumanyika, 2007, p. 103). Within the broader social and cultural circles are factors such as family, religion, community and nongovernmental organizations, architecture and building codes, recreation industry, and the information industry (Kumanyika, 2007, p. 103).

Obesity prevalence from the perspective of this model is shaped by the synergistic and cumulative effect of the interactions of these factors across the lifespan. Population efforts to reverse trends toward growing rates of obesity usually address the most modifiable factors, even though these may not be the primary factors driving the increase in obesity rates. For intervention planning, any one of these factors and the relative importance of each in achieving weight change at the individual and population level is a complex undertaking.

The Food Environment

Medical anthropologists Brown and Krick argue that "cultural and economic factors play critical roles in the etiology of obesity and the increase in obesity prevalence" and that these same cultural and economic factors limit "individual choice and behavior" (Brown & Krick, 2001, p. 111). Specifically, the cultural and economic context in which we live in North America is "*shaped* by powerful socioeconomic forces such as business corporations, [which] constrain individual choices in habitual behaviors... [The economy] establishes an *illusion* of personal choice about work, diet and activity patterns . . . [which creates] *a culturally-constructed 'obesogenic' environment*" (Brown & Krick, 2001, p. 111, italics added). Brown and Krick contend that this obesogenic environment is fueled by the industrial food production system, which "spends a remarkable amount on advertising, particularly on television, for high-calorie, high-profit products" and "shapes both the availability of certain foods (it is hard to find fresh fruits and vegetables in a ghetto market), as well as the manipulative use of advertising to create consumer desire for certain food products" (Brown & Krick, 2001, p. 117).

Specifically, in African American communities there are more fast food restaurants and vendors of alcoholic beverages per capita than in White communities (Williams, 1997), not unrelated to the aggressive marketing of these products to African American consumers. Critser (2000, p. 42) adds,

> it was the poor, and their increasing need for cheap meals consumed outside the home, that fueled the development of what may well be the most important fast-food innovation of the past twenty years, the sales gimmick known as 'supersizing' . . .

Supersizing a typical hamburger, french fries, and soda meal increases the calorie load of that meal from an estimated 680 calories to more than 1,340 calories. According to Critser's observations, the supersize customers in his West Coast urban community are primarily "urban caballeros, drywalleros, and jardineros . . . [and] young black kids traveling between school and home" (Critser, 2000, p. 42). These meals are fast, affordable, highly palatable, and readily available in urban and suburban communities (Schlosser, 2002).

Similarly, studies have found the availability of nutritious foods to be positively correlated with consumption of those foods (Zenk et.al., 2005). A geographic analysis of New Orleans conducted in 2001 found that across 156 census tracts 155 fast food restaurants were identified, with 2.4 fast food restaurants per square mile in predominantly African American neighborhoods, compared to 1.5 restaurants in predominantly White neighborhoods (Block et al., 2004). The Latino Coalition for a Healthy California (2006, p. 1) documents a similar reality:

> Latinos disproportionately live in communities that encourage unhealthy food choices and discourage physical activity, such as places with many fast food outlets, small grocery and convenience stores with limited fresh produce and an ample variety of sweets and other snack items, and few well-equipped and safe areas for children to play and be active.

The frequent absence of major grocery chains, farmers' markets, and whole food markets in these same neighborhoods means that there are fewer affordable sources of fresh fruits and vegetables. This has implications for maintaining a healthy diet, documented by a study in an African American community in North Carolina that found that the availability of grocery stores was directly related to consumption of fresh fruits and vegetables (Morland, Wing, & Roux, 2002). Increasing the ratio of food markets to fast food restaurants and liquor stores in African American communities is a feasible structural change that may improve health benefits for the entire community.

The industrial food production system has changed the culture over the past 25 years in that more meals are eaten outside the home as the number of eating establishments has increased. An economic perspective sees the value of our time is increasing (Phillips, 2002), which contributes to our eating behaviors, whereby eating establishments appeal to American ideals of "getting the most for your money" in the form of large, fat-laden portion sizes and exploit "the appeal of fast food, restaurant food, and convenience food to middle class Americans caught in the 'time squeeze' of frantic daily schedules" (Brown & Krick, 2001, p. 117). Brown and Krick reason that the combined effect of "the cultural and economic contexts predispose individuals to failure" (Brown & Krick, 2001, p. 112) at losing weight and maintaining weight loss, consequently increasing the risk for developing obesity and type 2 diabetes.

Other Living and Working Conditions That Influence Patterns of Obesity

Other factors in the social ecology influencing obesity rates in communities of color include neighborhood safety and time spent outside the home that interferes with the ability to prepare healthy meals at home. Recent research further indicates that perception of neighborhood safety is positively associated with the prevalence of regular physical activity. As time has become more expensive and people are spending more hours at work, more meals are eaten outside the home. This is a phenomenon that cuts across racial, ethnic, and income groups in the United States (Brown & Krick, 2001).

Female-headed households are particularly challenged to purchase and prepare foods at home for their families. A recent study reported higher obesity rates among children whose mothers worked outside the home (Anderson, Butcher, & Levine, 2003). According to this researcher, one factor influencing this finding was the observation that these children did not have the same amount of time for outside play as children with an adult in the home in the afternoons. In the interest of their safety, children without adult supervision were required to remain inside and engage in more sedentary play.

Race, Class, Gender, and Body Size

High socioeconomic status, loosely defined in the public health literature in terms of income, education, and occupation, appears to be protective in the majority population against many of the leading causes of death and disability. Across time and demographic group, high socioeconomic status confers better health except among African Americans as a population group (Lynch & Kaplan, 2001). It is assumed that persons with advanced education, high incomes, and protected white collar occupations minimally have greater access to health insurance, affording optimal use of health care services, adequate housing and nutrition, knowledge of health promotion and disease prevention, and possess the needed resources to purchase a health-promoting and -protective lifestyle.

Meta-analyses of studies of obesity prevalence in the U.S. and internationally, for example, have demonstrated an inverse relationship between high socioeconomic status and obesity among White women (McLaren, 2007; Sobal & Stunkard, 1989). This correlation is not as strikingly unidirectional among African American women (Averett & Korenman, 1999; Kumanyika, 1987). For several decades, epidemiological data reports that high socioeconomic status does not protect African American women as it appears to protect White women (see Figures 3.2–3.7).

The Sobal and Stunkard literature review published in 1989 was a seminal analysis in documenting the association between socioeconomic status (SES) and body size. Using 144 published studies from the 1960s to the 1980s on the relationship between SES and obesity in men, women, and children in the developed and developing world, they found "a consistently inverse association for women in developed societies, with a higher likelihood of obesity among women in lower socioeconomic strata" (McLaren, 2007, p. 29). At that time the relationship between obesity, SES, and men and children in developed countries was inconsistent. However, in developing societies "a strong direct relation was observed for women, men, and children, with a higher likelihood of obesity among persons in higher socioeconomic strata" (McLaren, 2007, p. 29).

In 2007 McLaren published an updated and expanded analysis, building upon the earlier work of Sobal and Stunkard. Her analysis

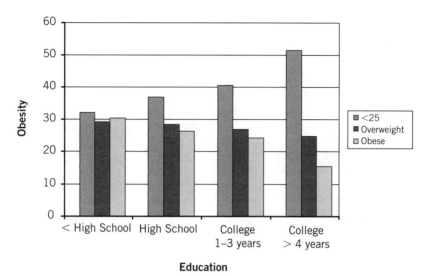

Figure 3.2 Behavioral Risk Factor Surveillance System 2007 BMI for all women with obesity by education.

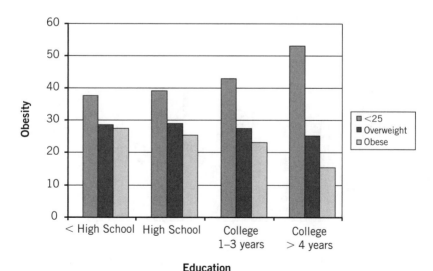

Figure 3.3 Behavioral Risk Factor Surveillance System 2007 BMI for White women with obesity by education.

BRFSS 2007 BMI for Black Women with Obesity by Education

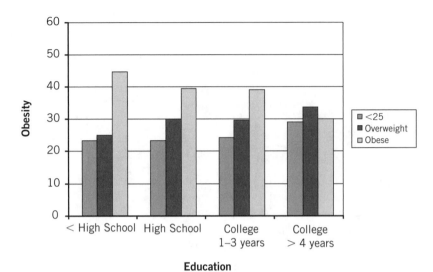

Figure 3.4 Behavioral Risk Factor Surveillance System 2007 BMI for Black women with obesity by education.

BRFSS 2007 BMI for All Women with Obesity by Income

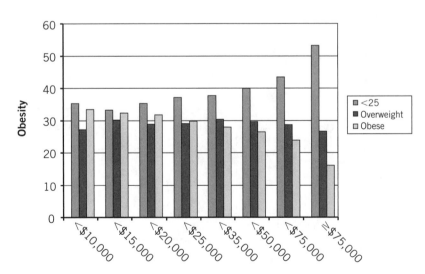

Figure 3.5 Behavioral Risk Factor Surveillance System 2007 BMI for all women with obesity by income.

BRFSS 2007 BMI for White Women with Obesity by Income

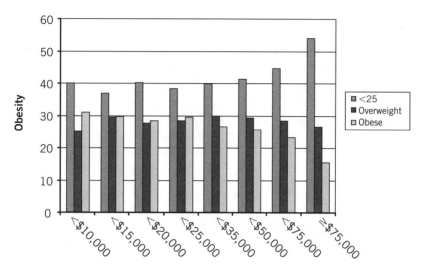

Figure 3.6 Behavioral Risk Factor Surveillance System 2007 BMI for White women with obesity by income.

BRFSS 2007 BMI for Black Women with Obesity by Income

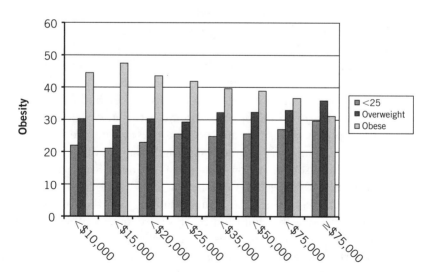

Figure 3.7 Behavioral Risk Factor Surveillance System 2007 BMI for Black women with obesity by income.

focused on patterns of obesity by sex and on countries in different stages of socioeconomic development, and she looked more closely at different indicators of SES. Specifically, McLaren categorized the development status of countries using the human development index (HDI) assigned by the United Nations Development Program. HDI ranks countries based on attributes that include life expectancy at birth, school enrollment and adult literacy, and standard of living based on the gross domestic product. The development of status of countries was characterized as high, medium, or low using these criteria.

Eight categories of SES indicator were established for this review of the literature:

> income and related factors (income, poverty, inability to afford essentials such as food and shelter); education (including schooling and literacy); occupation (occupational prestige or status, employment grade or ordered job type); employment (work status category—e.g., employed versus not employed); a composite indicator (a combination of multiple different indicators of SES); an area-level indicator (e.g., deprivation measured at the neighborhood or regional level rather than the individual level); assets and material belongings (e.g., car ownership, owning versus renting one's dwelling); and other (factors that could not otherwise be classified—e.g., subjective social class). (McLaren, 2007, p. 31)

Race and ethnicity were not examined separately in this analysis. She reviewed 333 articles published between 1988 and 2004.

The outcome of McLaren's analysis was not markedly different from that of Sobal and Stunkard conducted over a decade ago. She found that for women in high HDI countries, the majority of associations (63%) were negative (i.e., lower SES associated with higher body size). This effect was particularly prominent for SES indicators of education, area-level and composite indicators, and occupation. The difference in the Sobal and Stunkard analysis was more striking in that they observed 93% and 75% negative associations for women in the United States and other developed countries, respectively (McLaren, 2007). Among men in high and medium HDI countries, the primary finding was that of "nonsignificance or curvilinearity," followed by "the next most prominent pattern for men in high-HDI countries was negative associations, and this was particularly true for education as an indicator of SES (50 percent negative)" (McLaren, 2007, p. 31). Overall, while the inverse relationship between high SES and obesity still holds in high HDI countries,

McLaren observed "the gradual reversal of the social gradient in weight" as the obesity epidemic becomes more widespread around the world (McLaren, 2007, p. 31).

It is difficult to describe the relationship between SES and obesity because the nuances of SES differ for men and women and also varies across populations, over time within the same population, depending on the SES indicators and categories used, and depending on the type of obesity data used (which cut off points or whether self-reported). Sobal and Stunkard suggest four mediating variables that might help explain the generally observed inverse relationship between SES and obesity among women in developed countries.

The first mediating variable is attitudes toward obesity in developed societies. Specifically, "obesity is a severely stigmatized condition among women" (Sobal & Stunkard, 1989, p. 267). McLaren adds that a certain body shape/size may have prestige that is socially valued and helps to maintain class distinctions for women (McLaren, 2007). Moreover, given the influence of occupation as a SES indicator, McLaren suggests

> it is possible that persons high in the occupational hierarchy may internalize the symbolic value of a thin body and a healthy lifestyle (in line with their class) and at the same time face exposure to a workplace environment that likewise promotes these values. (McLaren, 2007, p. 35)

Dietary restraint is a second mediating variable in that "women of higher SES diet more often than do women of lower SES" (Sobal & Stunkard, 1989, p. 268). An increased level of leisure time physical activity among higher SES women is the third variable that likely explains the lower incidence of obesity in this group. In McLaren's analysis, she finds evidence of a socioeconomic gradient in diet among high HDI countries, "whereby persons in higher socioeconomic groups tend to have a healthier diet, characterized by greater consumption of fruit, vegetables, and lower-fat milk and less consumption of fats" (McLaren, 2007, p. 35). Lastly, inheritance, both genetic and financial, is likely a mediating variable in the expression of obesity among women of higher SES.

Using the mediating variables suggested by Sobal and Stunkard, the literature reports that within the African American community obesity is not stigmatized as one finds in the majority community (Bowen, Tomoyasu, & Cauce, 1991; Kumanyika, Wilson, & Guilford-Davenport, 1993). Kumanyika also cautions that "because blackness is already stigmatized [in American society], the coincidence of obesity and blackness predisposes to double stigmatization," that is, the politics of being Black and overweight "is different from being in any other U.S. racial/ethnic minority group" (Kumanyika, 1998, p. 93). Studies have also documented lower degrees of dietary restraint among African Americans, a greater preference for sweet foods, and greater caloric intake than in Whites (Bowen et al., 1991). When African American women diet, they are reported to lose less weight than their White counterparts (Kumanyika et al., 1993). Additionally, "the culture of weight management may not be well developed within the black community, that is, the day-to-day strategies one might use to maintain weight (e.g., recognizing and compensating for overeating, or returning to pre-partum caloric intake after delivery)" (Kumanyika, 1998, p. 96).

In terms of physical activity and inheritance, Holmes et al. (1998) did not find statistically significant differences in physical activity or weight at age 18 between Black and White women in the Nurses Health Study as explanatory of the higher BMI levels observed in the Black nurses at the time of the survey. The findings in this study suggest the Black women gained more weight in their adult years than the White participants. The specific genetic influence on obesity between these two groups is unknown if Sobal and Stunkard's measures of family and financial inheritance are used. This data was not collected from these women. These studies clearly document the need to question more deeply the usual measures of socioeconomic status and other behavioral variables that have been associated with obesity rates when seeking to understand the disproportionate burden of obesity among African American and other women of color.

Socioeconomic Status as a Category of Social Class

Post-modernists argue that social class has been replaced by "identity politics," "class consciousness," and other iterations of social "difference" (Milner, 1999). By convention, social class reflects the division of society into strata, arranged in a hierarchy of wealth, prestige, and power (Bottomore, 1966). Class, in the sociological sense of a social group "located within a hierarchical order of unequal such groups," is a fairly recent social construction dating from the Industrial Revolution (Milner, 1999, p. 1). Differentials in class status in Western capitalism are achieved through inheritance, occupation, educational attainment, income and investments, and social policies. Individuals within the populace have unequal access to selected occupations, elite educational institutions, and opportunities for higher incomes that leave monies for investments after living expenses are met. Occupations are not equally prestigious or valued. Institutions established to educate students are variable in staff expertise, resources, and facilities, that is, variable in the quality of education that is provided. Overall, the system of social class and its sponsor in the U.S. context, capitalism, is replete with inequalities.

Not surprisingly, when Black race is entered into the equation of social class, there are enduring disparities in wealth,[2] as well as in education and income between Blacks and Whites in the U.S. (Oliver & Shapiro, 1995). According to sociologists Oliver and Shapiro, examination of differences in wealth between Blacks and Whites reveals more than inequality in the sum total of assets and income, but also uncovers a "particular network of social relations and a set of social circumstances that convey a unique constellation of meanings pertinent to race in America" (Oliver & Shapiro, 1995, p. 3). In other words, even when there is perceived equity in income, education, and professional occupation at a given point in time, there is differential access to power that accrues to socioeconomic position. This allows those with wealth to "create opportunities, secure a desired stature and standard of living, or pass class status along to one's children" (Oliver & Shapiro, 1995, p. 2). The historical positioning of African Americans in the U.S. as second-class citizens has structured class divisions that limit African American access to ownership and control of the means of production and to valued occupational niches (Oliver & Shapiro, 1995).

Furthermore, the correlation between SES and health is not as direct when race and gender are considered. The role of SES is also variable across selected health problems (Howard, Anderson, Russell, Howard, & Burke, 2000; Schoenbaum & Waidmann, 1997). In the Nurses Health Study, for example, even though the women were "occupationally homogeneous," the socioeconomic status of the women was not uniform (Holmes et al., 1998, p. 336). Factors that influenced their SES included their husbands' income, personal opportunities for career advancement, and inherited wealth. These factors help explain why studies estimate "middle-income African Americans to have one-third the financial net worth of European Americans with the same income" (Holmes et al., 1998, p. 336).

---

[2] Wealth is defined here as what people own (i.e., financial and material resources that have been accumulated over a lifetime and inherited across generations) (Oliver & Shapiro, 1995).

Class differences are constructed and made material through the social division of privilege. Privilege is further determined in the U.S. by race and income equality between racial groups, but does not eliminate privilege disparity, that is, White privilege or its impact on health. White privilege is likened to class privilege in England, as described by Barbara Wootton: "Ours [class distinctions] is not an official, recognised caste system such as is found, for example, in India. It is something unofficial, unadmitted. One must adapt oneself to it, while at the same time pretending that it does not exist" (Wootton, 1941, p. 10). What do we know about the manifestations of class and privilege among women and African American women that might begin to explain the disparity in obesity rates between the two groups? In chapter 4 an anthropological approach to understanding the meanings of body size among a cohort of professional African American women is presented.

REFERENCES

Anderson, P. M., Butcher, K. F., & Levine, P. B. (2003). Maternal employment and overweight children. *Journal of Health Economics, 22,* 477–504.

Averett, S., & Korenman, S. (1999). Black-White differences in social and economic consequences of obesity. *International Journal of Obesity, 23,* 166–173.

Block, J. P., Scribner, R. A., & DeSalvo, K. B. (2004). Fast food, race/ethnicity, and income. *American Journal of Preventive Medicine, 27(3),* 211–217.

Booth, S. L., Sallis, J. F., Ritenbaugh, C., Hill, J. O., Birch, L. L., Frank, L. D., Glanz, K., Himmelgreen, D. A., Mudd, M., Popkin, B. M., Rickard, K. A., St. Jeor, S., & Hays, N. P. (2001). Environmental and societal factors affect food choice and physical activity: Rationale, influences, and leverage points. *Nutrition Reviews, 59(3, Pt 2),* S21–S39, discussion S57–S65.

Bottomore, T.B. (1966). Classes in Modern Society. New York: Pantheon Books.

Bowen, D., Tomoyasu, N., & Cauce, A. M. (1991). The triple threat: A discussion of gender, class, and race differences in weight. *Women and Health, 17(4),* 123–143.

Brown, P. J., & Krick, S. V. (2001). The etiology of obesity: Diet, television and the illusions of personal choice. In F. E. Johnston & G. D. Foster (Eds.), *Obesity, growth and development* (pp. 111–127). London: Smith-Gordon.

Campos, P. (2004). *The obesity myth.* New York: Gotham Books.

Critser, G. (March 2000). Let them eat fat: The heavy truths about American obesity. *Harper's Magazine,* 41–47.

Fineberg, H. (1990). "Distinction between Public Health and Medicine." Retrieved from http://www.asph.org/files/phvsmed.htm on June 11, 2009.

Ford, E. S., Williamson, D. F., & Liu, S. (1997). Weight change and diabetes incidence: Findings from a national cohort of US adults. *American Journal of Epidemiology, 146(3),* 214–222.

Gard, M., & Wright, J. (2004). *The obesity epidemic: Science, morality and ideology.* New York: Routledge.

Gregg, E. W., Caldwell, B. L., Cheng, Y. J., Cowie, C. C., Williams, D. E., Geiss, L., Engelgau, M. M., & Vinicor, F. (2004). Trends in the prevalence and ration of diagnosed to undiagnosed diabetes according to obesity levels in the U.S. *Diabetes Care, 27*, 2806–2812.

Holmes, M. D., Stampfer, M. J., Wolf, A. M., Jones, C. P., et.al. (1998). Can behavioral risk factors explain the difference in body mass index between African American and European American women? *Ethnicity & Disease, 8*, 331–339.

Howard, G., Anderson, R. T., Russell, G., Howard, V. J., & Burke, G. L. (2000). Race, socioeconomic status, and cause-specific mortality. *Annals of Epidemiology, 10*, 214–223.

Institute of Medicine. (2002). *The future of the public's health in the 21st century.* Washington, DC: The National Academies Press.

Kuczmarski, R. J. (2007). What is obesity? Definitions matter. In S. Kumanyika & R. Brownson (Eds.), *Handbook of obesity prevention* (pp. 25–44). New York: Springer Science & Business Media.

Kuczmarski, R. J., & Flegal, K. M. (2000). Criteria for definition of overweight in transition: Background and recommendations for the United States. *American Journal of Clinical Nutrition, 72*, 1074–1081.

Kumanyika, S. (1987). Obesity in Black women. *Epidemiologic Reviews, 9*, 31–50.

Kumanyika, S. (1998). Obesity in African Americans: Biobehavioral consequences of culture. *Ethnicity & Disease, 8*, 93–96.

Kumanyika, S. (2007). Obesity prevention concepts and frameworks. In S. Kumanyika & R. Brownson (Eds.), *Handbook of obesity prevention* (pp. 85–114). New York: Springer Science & Business Media.

Kumanyika, S., Wilson, J. F., & Guilford-Davenport, M. (1993). Weight-related attitudes and behaviors of Black women. *Journal of the American Dietetic Association, 93*, 416–422.

Latino Coalition for a Healthy California. (2006). Obesity in Latino communities: Prevention, principles, and action. Retrieved from www.LCHC.org

Lynch, J., & Kaplan, G. (2001). Socioeconomic position. In L. F. Berkman & I. Kawachi (Eds.), *Social epidemiology* (pp. 13–35). New York: Oxford University Press.

McLaren, L. (2007). Socioeconomic Status and Obesity. Epidemiol Rev 29:29-48.

Mechanic, D. (2003). Who shall lead: Is there a future for population health? *Journal of Health Politics, Policy and Law, 28(2–3)*, 421–442.

Milner, A. (1999). *Class.* London: Sage Publishers.

Mokdad, A., Bowman, B. A., Ford, E. S., Vinicor, F., Marks, J. S., & Koplan, J. P. (2001a). The continuing epidemics of obesity and diabetes in the United States. *Journal of the American Medical Association, 286(10)*, 1195–1200.

Mokdad, A., Ford, E. S., Bowman, B. A., Nelson, D. E., & Engelgau, M. M. (2000). Diabetes trends in the U.S.: 1990–1998. *Diabetes Care, 23(9)*, 1278–1283.

Mokdad, A., Ford, E. S., Bowman, B. A., Nelson, D. E., Engelgau, M. M., Vinicor, F., & Marks, J. S. (2001b). The continuing increase of diabetes in the U.S. *Diabetes Care, 24(2)*, 412.

Mokdad, A., Serdula, M. K., Dietz, W .H., Bowman, B. A., Marks, J. S., & Koplan, J. P. (1999). The spread of the obesity epidemic in the United States, 1991–1998. *Journal of the American Medical Association, 282(16)*, 1519–1522.

Morland, K., Wing, S., & Roux, A. D. (2002). The contextual effect of the local food environment on residents' diets: The atherosclerosis risk in communities study. *American Journal of Public Health, 92,* 1761–1767.

National Institutes of Health. (1998). Clinical guidelines on the identification, evaluation, and treatment of overweight and obesity in adults. NIH Publ. No. 98-4083.

Ogden, C. L., Carroll, M. D., Curtin, L. R., McDowell, M. A., Tabak, C. J., & Flegal, K. M. (2006). Prevalence of overweight and obesity in the United States, 1999–2004. *Journal of the American Medical Association, 295,* 1549–1555.

Oliver, M. L., & Shapiro, T. M. (1995). *Black wealth/White wealth: A new perspective on racial inequality.* New York: Routledge.

Phillips, P. (2002). "The Rising Cost of Health Care: Can demand be reduced through more effective health promotion?" Journal of Evaluation and Clinical Practice 8: 415–419.

Powell, L. M., Slater, S., Mirtcheva, D., Bao, Y., & Chaloupka, F. J. (2006). Food store availability and neighborhood characteristics in the United States. *Preventive Medicine, 44,* 189–195.

Puhl, R., & Brownell, K. D. (2001). Bias, discrimination, and obesity. *Obesity Research, 9(12),* 788–805.

Puhl, R., & Brownell, K. D. (2002). Confronting and coping with weight stigma: An investigation of overweight and obese adults. *Obesity, 14(10),* 1802–1815.

Schlosser, E. (2002). *Fast food nation.* New York: Perrenial.

Schoenbaum, M., & Waidmann, T. (1997). Race, socioeconomic status, and health: Accounting for race differences in health. *The Journal of Gerontology, 52B(Special Issue),* 61–73.

Schulz, A. J., Zenk, S., Odoms-Young, A., Hollis-Neely, T., Nwankwo, R., Lockett, M., Ridelia, W., & Kannan, S. (2005). Healthy eating and exercising to reduce diabetes: Exploring the potential of social determinants of health frameworks within the context of community-based participatory diabetes prevention. *American Journal of Public Health, 95,* 645–651.

Sobal, J., & Stunkard, A. J. (1989). Socioeconomic status and obesity: A review of the literature. *Psychology Bulletin, 105,* 260–275.

Valdez, R., & Williamson, D. F. (2002). Prevalence and demographics of obesity. In C. G. Fairburn, K. D. Brownell (Eds.), *Eating disorders and obesity* (pp. 417–421). New York: The Guilford Press.

Vazquez, G., Duval, S., Jacobs, D. R., & Silventoinen, K. (2007). Comparison of body mass index, waist circumference, and waist/hip ratio in predicting incident diabetes: A meta-analysis. *Epidemiologic Reviews, 29,* 115–128.

Williams, D. R. (1997). African American health: The role of the social environment. *Journal of Urban Health, 75,* 300–321.

Wootton, B. (1941) End social inequality: a programme for ordinary people. London: K. Paul, Trench, Trubner & Co., Ltd.

Zenk, S. N., Schulz, A. J., Israel, B. A., James, S. A., Bao, S., & Wilson, M. L. (2005). Neighborhood racial composition, neighborhood poverty, and the spatial accessibility of supermarkets in metropolitan Detroit. *American Journal of Public Health, 95(4),* 660–667.

Culture, Meaning, and Obesity Among College-Educated African American Women: An Anthropological Perspective

4

LEANDRIS C. LIBURD

Anthropology seeks to situate obesity and its correlates in the context of culture. In order to develop and implement culturally appropriate public health interventions, we need to have a deeper understanding of the socioecologic environment that influences the disproportionate burden of type 2 diabetes and obesity in racial and ethnic populations in the United States. An anthropological approach to understanding the rise in obesity rates in communities of color is typically more inductive in its epistemology and complements socioecologic models and population health approaches. Qualitative inquiries of this sort do not lend themselves comfortably to traditional survey models and statistical analyses, and the data are not generalizable to the larger population. However, the information can be critical to the formulation of targeted, culturally sensitive community interventions.

In keeping with the primary objectives of this volume, this chapter will elaborate meaning as a determinant of overweight and obesity. Two variables that have been associated with the prevention of obesity in the majority population, specifically among White women, are high socioeconomic status and moral ideologies and cultural meanings attached to body size (Allen, 1998; Sobal and Stunkard 1989). How moral ideologies held by college-educated Black women influence body size and the failure of high socioeconomic status to prevent obesity among Black women has not been a focus of anthropological research.

In this chapter, research examining why high socioeconomic status does not protect African American women from obesity, as it appears to protect White women, is presented. Findings from this research exposes the cultural dissonance and internal struggles of accomplished and talented Black women to possess bodies that "measure up" in a culture where thinness in industrialized and capitalist society is a marker of social distinction and therefore valued by individuals higher on the socioeconomic spectrum (McLaren & Kuh, 2004). Also in the study, using a life history methodology and engaging Black feminist theorists, the influence of intergenerational family norms and ideologies related to body size, the "Black church," higher education, and the professional work environment was examined. To conclude, implications of the perspectives and research presented in this chapter for public health practice are proposed.

CULTURE AND MEANING

Anthropologists have long recognized that body size is not only biologically determined but also culturally constructed (Brown, 1991; Brown & Konner, 1998; Counihan, 1999; Powdermaker, 1960; Scheper-Hughes & Lock, 1998). Culture is a complex concept that has evolved theoretically over the last 100 years, principally through the discipline of anthropology. At its core culture has been described as "a shared, learned, and intergenerationally transmitted pattern of customs, beliefs, values, and behaviors" (Corin, 1995, p. 273). Each individual is born with an innate drive for food, but the ideologies that govern dietary consumption are deeply rooted in the history and material culture of the community in which one is reared (Bordo, 1993; Farb & Armelagos, 1980; Farquhar 2002).

Culture has also been described as a system of meanings and symbols that "define a world view that gives meaning to personal and collective experience, and frames the way people locate themselves within the world, perceive the world, and behave in it" (Corin, 1995, p. 273). Culture defines normalcy and, therefore, the thresholds for "ideal" body proportions and those outside the norm that are obese (Brown, 1992, p. 180). How then are we to examine and understand these complex relationships to obesity? Hortense Powdermaker describes the anthropological approach to understanding obesity this way:

> My basic questions are concerned with the symbolism of fatness and thinness in our society and the relationships of each to other symbols and to

our values. I would be interested in differences in the symbols and in the relative strength of the same symbols in class, ethnic, religious, sex, and age groups, and among individuals. I would assume that there might be conflicting values concerning fatness and thinness, about eating and physical activity, as there are in many other areas of our life, and that some of this conflict might stem from the fact that we live in a rapidly changing society, where traditional values linger beside new ones. I would also be interested in the cultural study of people who are not obese as well as those who are, i.e., some kind of control group in which variables are limited. As an anthropologist, I am naturally interested in a comparative approach, i.e., the symbolism of obesity and thinness in other cultures and the many-sided role of food and eating in them, assuming that this comparative knowledge would illuminate the problem in our society. (Powdermaker, 1960, p. 76)

The anthropological approach is arguably more valid, whereas the epidemiologic approach is more reliable.[1] The epistemology of medical anthropology is not bounded by the need to measure—understood as quantify—the social environment or its cultural antecedents, but embraces as truth the narratives of lived experience.

COLLEGE-EDUCATED AFRICAN AMERICAN WOMEN AND THE OBESITY EPIDEMIC

What is the differential configuration of class and gender experienced by African American women that frames their lives such that in addition to biology the lived experience of being Black and female tends toward overweight and not thinness? If college-educated African American women have comparable incomes, knowledge, and access to health-promoting resources, such as a high-quality diet and opportunities for regular physical activity, why is there a persistent gap in obesity rates between African American and White women? Limited attention has

---

[1] There are several categories of reliability and validity, and specifics of reliability and validity vary when used in quantitative contexts versus qualitative contexts. In this instance, I refer to "simple" validity, that is, how well the social reality being measured through research matches with the constructs researchers use to understand it (Neuman, 2003). In the ethnographic approach the researcher has many more opportunities to clarify with respondents the intent of questions, and to probe with members of the community meanings the researcher might ascribe to certain conditions and practices. Reliability means dependability or consistency, and the structured questionnaires along with the relatively large sample sizes used by epidemiologists help to make this approach more reliable than qualitative approaches.

been given to subjective meanings of body size among African American women in the anthropological and humanities literature (Bordo, 1993; Nichter, 2000). Black feminist scholars in the U.S. and in the Caribbean, on the other hand, have produced scholarship highlighting historic and contemporary negative connotations associated with Black female bodies (Barrow, 1998; Bennett & Dickerson, 2001; hooks, 1995; McClaurin, 2001). bell hooks argues, "Theorizing black experience in the United States is a difficult task" (hooks, 1992). She explains:

> Even those of us righteously committed to black liberation struggle, who feel we have decolonized our minds, often find it hard to 'speak' our experience. . . . Indeed, a fundamental task of black critical thinkers has been the struggle to break with the hegemonic modes of seeing, thinking, and being that block our capacity to see ourselves oppositionally, to imagine, describe, and invent ourselves in ways that are liberatory. (hooks, 1992)

Exploring analyses of Black feminist scholars and other scholars whose work can be used to elaborate social and cultural dimensions of the obesity epidemic will broaden perspectives of public health workers charged with developing culturally sensitive community-based interventions. Critical cultural analyses of selected Black feminist scholars are presented in this chapter to give the reader insight into how the socioecologic influences on eating behavior and physical activity described by Kumanyika (2007) might be interpreted. Perspectives put forth here are those of the scholars and not based on conventional survey research that reflects the opinions of a larger respondent group.

THEORIZING THE BLACK FEMALE BODY

Black race is an identity historically constituted and framed by the larger White society as inferior and marginalized. According to anthropologist Mary Douglas, "the body is a powerful symbolic form, a surface on which the central rules, hierarchies, and even metaphysical commitments of a culture are inscribed and thus reinforced through the concrete language of the body" (Douglas, 1982). The Black body here is a lived body that is symbol and metaphor for hundreds of years of sustained social and political inequality that has culminated in compromised and, in many instances, negative health endowments. Theorizing the Black female body requires the study of the intersections of race and gender that have been largely ignored by theorists in the past (Wallace-Sanders, 2002). Such research would reflect what Wallace-Sanders calls a "collage of Black women's corporeal existence in the United States" (Wallace-Sanders, 2002). In this context, "when Black women stand at the center of the discussion about the female body, their bodies tell a profoundly different story about historic and contemporary American culture" (Wallace-Sanders, 2002). The Black female body defies a uniform or one-dimensional representation. If we are to begin to understand why high socioeconomic status does not protect Black women from obesity as it appears to protect White women, we must consider the historical and institutionalized images of the Black female body in addition to the cultural preferences and family expectations for body size.

Stereotypes about the Black female body in general and the large Black female body in particular abound. Stereotyped representations of Black women include "The Jezebel," "Mammy," "Matriarch," and "bad girls" (Collins, 2000; Douglas, 1999; Newman, 2002). These images have been internalized and acted out in varying degrees within the cultural communities of African American women. These labels are also closely tied to Black women's historical relationships with the White patriarchal power structure (Collins, 2000) and the denuding of Black female bodies (Douglas, 1999). However, in these representations Black female appetite is construed as naturalized, lacking restraint and discipline, and amoral (Witt, 1999).

From childhood African American women learn and internalize that the large Black female body is so-called othered in the Western cultural construction of the female body. The large Black female body is penalized and marginalized from the larger society in pernicious ways. Along with other obese persons, the body size of the large Black woman is leveled against her to restrict her mobility and in other ways deny her humanity. As observed by Kumanyika (1998), being fat and Black can be doubly stigmatizing. This double stigmatization can restrict one's social and professional advancement despite having earned advanced degrees from elite and prestigious institutions. On the other hand, the large Black woman is exploited as a consumer of clothes, food, cosmetics, weight loss programs, gym memberships, and other commodities in attempts to fit more comfortably in the larger society. The impact of these negative representations on Black women's body size has not been widely examined.

TRANSFORMING APPETITES: MORAL INFLUENCES ON THE SHAPING OF BLACK FEMALE BODIES

A qualitative study of professional African American women examining perceptions of body size was conducted in 2005 (Liburd, 2006). The data was analyzed through the lens of the interlocking categories of race, class, and gender. Rooted in Black feminist theory, analyses of race, class, and gender, or intersection theory, recognizes and articulates the simultaneity and interrelatedness of multiple forms of inequality experienced by African Americans and how these experiences have historically shaped the present and future of people of African descent in the U.S. and abroad. Black feminist theorists argue that

> the dynamism of the relationships among race, class, and gender arises from the fact that, while each has its own unique social logic, polarizes different social forces, and generates distinct, characteristic institutional and cultural modalities, each is also, simultaneously, a constituent and formative factor in the development of the others. (Burnham, 2001, p. 2)

This perspective is instructive in analyses of health disparities, particularly if our goal is to understand more fully the root causes of the disparity in diabetes and obesity prevalence.

Research Questions

Using a combination of qualitative and quantitative research methods, I sought to answer the following questions:

1. What are the moral ideologies that a sample of college-educated African American women holds about meanings of body size? What is the impact of these ideologies on preferred body forms among these Black women? What is the impact of these ideologies on this group of Black women's tendencies toward dietary indulgences and/or dietary restraint, sexual indulgences and/or restraint, and regular physical activity and/or sedentariness?

2. In what ways, if at all, do church practices encourage and produce fatness in African American women (e.g., in the

patterning of food habits, the subjective meanings of fatness in women, in religious imagery, and in the social positions of women within the organized church structure)?

3. What is the relationship, if any, between fatness and sexuality as experienced by a sample of African American women involved in a local Black Baptist church (e.g., in terms of attractiveness, body satisfaction, religious perceptions of goodness, sexual repression, and longings for intimacy)?

4. How does the achievement of advanced education (college degree and higher) and professional occupation influence patterns of obesity in this sample of African American women?

Definition of Terms

For the purpose of this study, *Black* and *African American* were used interchangeably to refer to persons of African descent who were born in the United States. Black and African American are understood as a social construction, lived experience, and embraced identity, not as a biological category. This research project does not assume an authentic Black experience, but was designed to capture the diversity of thought among a group of African American women with a shared religiosity and educational and professional background. The designation of Black and African American does not exclude persons of African and Caribbean heritage who represent the first generation to be born in America and who have adopted an African American identity.

Moral influences is defined as a culture's most basic set of shared values, that is, its understandings of good and bad, right and wrong—the basic cultural paradigm in which the people find their sense of personal identity and group solidarity (Paris, 1985). Moral influences include the discourse, behaviors, activities, and other acts that we can observe that reflect a culture's shared values and basic cultural paradigm. *Ideologies* are defined by Neuman (2003) as "fixed, strong and unquestioned assumptions . . . [that] may be founded on faith or rooted in particular social circumstances; and [imply] closed belief systems that change very little." He adds that ideologies "may advance or protect the interests of a particular group" and are "locked into specific moral beliefs." For this study, moral ideologies are the cognitive, mental scripts of the belief systems that characterize the units of analysis in this research project.

Sampling

A purposive sample[2] of 31 professional Black women living in Atlanta, Baltimore, Richmond, and Houston were recruited to participate in this study. Criteria for inclusion in this study were possessing at least a bachelor's degree, identifying as an African American woman, working in a professional (white collar) occupation, and earning >$49,000 per annum (see Tables 4.1– 4.5).

Table 4.1

COLLEGE-EDUCATED AFRICAN AMERICAN WOMEN IN SURVEY: AGE DISTRIBUTION

AGE GROUP	FREQUENCY	PERCENTAGE	BMI MEAN	STD. DEV.
25–35	7	23.33	23.14	5.67
36–45	6	20.00	29.00	6.16
46–55	14	46.67	27.57	4.78
56–65	3	10.00	26.67	3.51

Table 4.2

COLLEGE-EDUCATED AFRICAN AMERICAN WOMEN IN SURVEY: HIGHEST LEVEL EDUCATION STATUS

EDUCATION	FREQUENCY	PERCENTAGE	BMI MEAN	STD. DEV.
BS or BA	6	20.00	28.00	4.86
Master's	15	50.00	26.07	5.71
PhD, MD, or other	9	30.00	27.00	5.52

[2] A purposive sample is a nonprobability sample that seeks cases or respondents that fit particular criteria. Purposive sampling is used when the study population is considered "difficult-to-reach" or a "specialized" population not easily accessed in a random sampling frame. Purposive sampling is also used when a researcher wants to identify particular types of cases for in-depth investigation. The purpose of this type of sample is less to generalize to a larger population than to gain a deeper understanding of types (Neuman, 2003, p. 213).

Table 4.3

COLLEGE-EDUCATED AFRICAN AMERICAN WOMEN IN SURVEY: SELF-REPORTED ANNUAL INCOME

INCOME	FREQUENCY	PERCENTAGE	BMI MEAN	STD. DEV.
49,000	4	13.33	29.00	5.89
49–60k	3	10.00	25.67	4.04
61–75k	5	16.67	22.40	3.44
76–90k	7	23.33	27.29	6.05
91–110k	8	26.67	28.50	5.50
>111,000	3	10.00	26.00	6.08

Table 4.4

COLLEGE-EDUCATED AFRICAN AMERICAN WOMEN IN SURVEY: OCCUPATION

OCCUPATION	FREQUENCY	PERCENTAGE
Health Educator	5	16.67
Health Scientist	2	6.67
Nutritionist	1	3.33
College Faculty	3	10.00
Public Health Analyst	4	13.33
Attorney	1	3.33
Public School Faculty	3	10.00
Statistician	1	3.33
Epidemiologist	2	6.67
Health Communications	3	10.00
Recreation Administrator	1	3.33
Behavioral Scientist	2	6.67
Writer-Editor	1	3.33

Table 4.5

COLLEGE-EDUCATED AFRICAN AMERICAN WOMEN IN SURVEY: BMI DISTRIBUTION

BMI	FREQUENCY	PERCENTAGE
19	2	6.67
20	1	3.33
21	1	3.33
22	4	13.33
23	4	13.33
25	3	10.00
26	2	6.67
27	2	6.67
28	1	3.33
30	2	6.67
33	3	10.00
35	5	16.67

Participants were identified using a modified snowball sampling technique, that is, 10 African American women working at the Centers for Disease Control and Prevention (CDC) were approached by the principal investigator (Liburd) and asked to refer women for the study meeting the above criteria. An initial list of 45 women was generated using this method and every third person on the list was contacted and invited to participate. Additional names were added to the list after the first 15 respondents had been recruited, and a second round of selecting every third person was conducted until a total of 31 women had been recruited. Informed consent was obtained for all life history interviews. The Social, Humanist, Behavioral Institutional Review Board at Emory University approved the study protocols.

Life Histories

Life histories were a key method in the data collection for this research. The method developed by anthropologist John Dollard was used. He defined life histories as

> a deliberate attempt to define the growth of a person in a cultural milieu and to make theoretical sense of it. . . . The material must, in addition, be

worked up and mastered from some systematic viewpoint. . . . from the standpoint of the systematic student of culture . . . the life history is an account of how a new person is added to the group and becomes an adult capable of meeting the traditional expectations of [her] society for a person of [her] sex and age. . . . it may well be argued that without the life history, the transmission of culture forms from one generation to the next cannot be adequately defined. . . . It is possible that detailed studies of the lives of individuals will reveal new perspectives on the culture as a whole which are not accessible when one remains on the formal cross-sectional plane of observation. (Dollard, 1935)

The life history method provides a semistructured opportunity for the respondent to describe the dynamic cultural environment in which she was raised that influenced her ideologies, social interactions, and patterns of behavior. Specifically, early exposures to cultural preferences for food choices and preparation, how leisure time was spent, and typical body sizes of men and women encountered by the respondent can be recalled and documented. This method also maps major life events (e.g., changes in residence, economic status, and childbearing) that bear on the research questions.

Specifically, the life history interview in this study sought to establish an historical framework for the respondent's:

family background, that is, region of birth; 1st-, 2nd-, or 3rd-generation college-educated; occupation of parents; religious upbringing; childhood and current dietary patterns [changes in dietary habits and dietary habits that have been retained over time]; centrality of eating in social interactions; weight and size of female relatives and other women in respondent's social networks observed in childhood and today; and associations made by key women and men in respondent's social networks with size and femininity, womanhood, success, and so on for Black women;

educational background, including universities attended and degrees earned and changes in consciousness about diet, exercise, and weight during college years;

professional background, that is, respondent's occupation and work history, importance of having a particular professional image in this occupation, what the image is, and how it affects the respondent's receptivity and advancement within the workplace;

primacy of weight in respondent's self-image and changes in the valuing of size over time;

weight history, that is, weight at age 18; significant changes in weight over lifetime (may be related to parity, marital status, college-associated weight gain, traumatic life events, etc.); and previous weight loss attempts, weight loss achieved, and weight loss maintained (overall history of weight cycling);

patterns of physical activity (past and present);

self-identified ideal body weight and dress size and efforts taken to achieve or maintain that weight and size;

core values about how Black professional women should be represented (e.g., in terms of work ethic, material professional accomplishments, evidence of advancing the mission and priorities of the respondent's profession, maintaining a professional image as prescribed by the majority culture, and maintaining one's own professional image); and

perceptions of preferred body sizes for women across the life cycle and in different social locations, that is, is there an expectation that Black women will gain weight over time and a cultural acceptance of this pattern, and are there different meanings associated with body size for Black women in the roles of wife, mother, professional, and religious leader? Which roles are primary and a greater determinant of body size? What are some of the positive attributions made within a Black cultural context to large body size among professional Black women? For the women in the study who have children, I explored with them how they were raising their children, male and female, in regard to acceptable body sizes and attitudes and behaviors related to healthy diets and the importance of physical activity.

Limitations of life histories include the cumbersome task of "organizing and conceptualizing the life-history material itself"(Dollard, 1935), the inability to verify the accuracy of the information provided, the risk of reifying culture, and/or overvaluing culture as the explanatory paradigm.

Participant Observation

In addition to the 31 individual in-depth interviews, participant observation was used in this research. Participant observation is a key component of ethnographic and anthropological research. Fieldwork was conducted at the CDC in Atlanta and at a large, suburban church in Dekalb County, GA. Over 12 months of fieldwork, the principal investigator attended weekly worship services and participated in special services offered for women at the church. She also participated in events where food was provided.

Close attention was paid to ideologies expressed about the Christian body; appropriate dietary practices; discourse about body care practices, including the promotion of physical activity; informal conversations about weight, dieting, changes in body and clothing size, and reactions to weight gain and loss in members of the church; symbolism of fatness and thinness; discourse about Christian pleasure and appropriate activities and entertainment; formal and informal systems of support for weight gain and control; typical menus associated with church-sponsored events; and opportunities for group physical activity and competitive sports. The body sizes of women in leadership and other visible positions in the church were included in field notes. This approach was consistent with Powdermaker's theoretical premise of "setting the problem of obesity" in the context of culture (Powdermaker, 1960) given the designation of the church as a moral institution and key social location for the articulation and dissemination of "the Black community's most basic societal values" (Paris, 1985).

The CDC was an ideal site to examine cultural perspectives on obesity in a cohort of highly educated, well paid African American women who, in addition to their educational backgrounds in health and their specific research and work in public health, are inundated daily with messages about obesity, weight control, and physical activity. Yet, the prevalence of overweight and obesity among these women mirrors that observed in national surveys. For some the presence of overweight and obese Black women in key roles at the nation's premier public health agency contradicts the applied premises of public health and biomedicine. In fact, conducting research with Black women immersed in public health research and practice unveiled their own struggles with many assumptions and the institutionalized logic of health promotion and chronic disease prevention as promoted by the CDC.

Participant observation occurred at the CDC during the business day and at professional conferences. Comments heard by the principal investigator about body size expressed by senior managers and African American women were noted. Field notes included messages sent to the workforce about reflecting a healthy lifestyle and any changes made in the workload to accommodate the expectation for healthier body sizes. The body sizes of African Americans in leadership positions in the agency, the amount of time professional Black women spent in sedentary activities, the foods available in the workplace, the participation of African American women in the fitness and exercise programs provided at the CDC, and how women tried to balance the demands of work and family were observed and recorded in the field notes. In conversations the principal investigator inquired about the stresses associated with being Black, female, and a professional working at the CDC and how this impacted the women's ability to pursue a healthy lifestyle.

Data Analysis

All interviews were audiotaped and transcribed by a professional transcription service. The qualitative analysis involved a content analysis of the transcripts by two investigators, Leandris Liburd and Apophia Namageyo-Funa. Text data from all interviews were analyzed manually and independently by the investigators. After completing the independent analyses and initial coding, we then met to confer and agree on the code book and later major themes that emerged in the transcript. The data are reported as aggregated data. Consistent with usual procedures in reporting ethnographic research, direct quotes from the transcribed interviews of respondents are incorporated in the theoretical analysis and interpretation of findings. Names are replaced with pseudonyms to protect confidentiality and anonymity.

Findings

Among the women in this study, cultural messages about preferred body forms for a Black woman were communicated by example, in talk, in commercial fashion, and in music. Black female bodies within the midrange of size (i.e., dress sizes in the range 10–14) best articulate these attributes according to the women in this study (see Figure 4.1).

Nutrition epidemiologist Melinda Green,[3] PhD, MPH, made this observation:

> I think we as middle class Black women, educated Black women, unlike some other cultures or some other racial groups, don't aspire to acculturate

---

[3] This and all other survey respondents' names are pseudonyms.

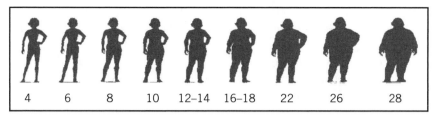

4   6   8   10   12–14   16–18   22   26   28

Figure 4.1 Silhouettes that approximate dress sizes 4–28.

as, you know, some others do. Our concern is more about educating our kids, bringing our community along, and building our career [rather] than worrying about what size we are. I think that most of us do aspire to be a healthy weight, which is why you're hearing so much about size 12 [as an ideal size], but we're not trying to be a size 6 or a size 8, or you know . . . We're not trying to look like a White woman or to acculturate in that way. We have different emphases, different values, and I'm not saying we are not concerned about our health, because I think we are. It's just that we can be healthy, and a lot of data are showing this, without being a size 6 or 8.

Melinda's statement captures the primary themes that emerged about the values that drive the behaviors and priorities of these professional, college-educated Black women. They are deeply committed to higher education and see the achievement of advanced education as the key to economic and social success. In many instances, these women are financially independent and build and sustain middle- and upper-middle-class lifestyles. Expectations are high, and these women work hard to advance their careers and live through high levels of daily stress. The welfare of their families, children, and larger community are extremely important to them and insuring the welfare of so many adds to their overextended days and obligations. Time is very expensive, and discretion over the use of their time is valued.

The passage of women in this study from childhood to womanhood in many instances lacked an explicit focus on body size and weight, but tended to concentrate more on the care (e.g., grooming, personal hygiene, and good nutrition), carriage, and adornment of the body and its shapeliness. What was important is how she carried herself physically, socially, and morally. For example, Linda Jones, PhD, MPH, describes how women's bodies were regarded in her family:

I was born in Virginia in Richmond. My family was made up of a mother, father, and brother and my extended family included a great number of aunts, sisters to my mother. My memorable events related to body size include really not focusing so much on weight in terms of its acceptability but being more focused on image. How you looked in your clothes and whether you ate a balanced meal or not. I don't recall within my own family the issue of being overweight or being underweight as something that was dwelled upon.

Now for me, as a child growing up, what I do remember quite strikingly is that I was considered to be skinny and that I had not a finicky appetite in terms of what I ate but in terms of the amount that I ate. And so I do recall being taken to our community doctor and my mother being very concerned that I needed some kind of—I don't think she went in asking for some type of appetite-enhancing medication, but she was concerned that I needed to have a better appetite than I did. So I do remember being given something by the doctor that at some point in time—maybe it was a placebo, I have no idea, but I do remember being given—maybe it was some kind of liquid vitamin, because thinking back now to kind of what it tasted like, it might have been some kind of multivitamin. I do remember, you know, that maybe it did make me want to eat a little bit more, but I was always a big fruit eater, but I never was a large, large child, so perhaps weight for me was not—it was more being underweight than it was being overweight.

But as far as the other females in my family, I don't remember it, certainly not as a child. And I don't have events until later in adult life where body image and weight became more of an issue. And that was true even for women in my community. I don't remember conversations about so-and-so being so large or so-and-so being so thin.

Among women raised in the segregated South of the 1950s and 1960s, body size norms were considered in the context of the biological diversity found among African-descended people. This is not to say that body size was ignored, but the range of acceptable body sizes was significantly large enough that only persons at culturally determined extremes of either thinness or fatness were anomalous. Thick, big-boned, heavy-set, and shapely were the principal adjectives that characterized the discourse of body size among the women. Interestingly, prior to about 10 years ago, women who were very small or characterized as too skinny were mocked, derided, and deemed in need of some intervention. Carol Simmons, PhD, recalls how her family and friends integrated her particularly small frame into a culture of shapeliness:

I was born in Long Island, NY. That was just where I was born. I didn't stay there long, though, because I was born while my father was transferred to the North for a job because of extreme racism here in the South. There was a lot of racism against African Americans and my father was by trade a plasterer and he was a business owner. So his livelihood was wherever he could get a job doing plastering. So it was not atypical for African Americans if they couldn't find a job here to go either west or north. We came back to Atlanta when I was about 2 years old.

Now as far as memories of women in particular in our family and weight; I think it's always been a struggle for most of the women in my family that I know of personally, especially my mom and my sister. Ironically, I had the opposite weight problem. When I was growing up, I was considered too skinny because I was a very sort of scrawny, little, you know, late bloomer. I didn't really mature until I was in the 12th grade. I didn't have breasts until I was in 11th grade. I mean literally flat-chested. So I was kind of a straggler in terms of developing, you know, body development and weight and I was keenly aware of it because a lot of my cousins, they were already shapely. In fact, I used to be, believe it or not, I don't have this problem now, but I used to be self-conscious because I thought I was too skinny. . . . And I'm not sure that if I were in another culture, and I know it may be specific to African-Americans, but in another culture I would never have had that pressure. I would have in fact been looked upon as just right as opposed to bony. I was called bony, tiny. In fact, that's my nickname, Tiny.

Now my sister, on the other hand, always had the opposite problem. Not really a problem, because when she was growing up, she was considered shapely. She had the big, round, you know, butt, behind, rear end, okay, we'll make it professional, and she had a small waist. She was like the perfect shape. But then as she got older, she began to develop a weight problem, much more than I did. I did in my mid-30s and I was actually more, you know, I had more weight on me in my mid-30s than I ever had, but now that I'm in my 40s, I really try to control it. But yeah, I think as I was growing up, there was not the focus on being too small. You know, people just kind of wanted to just be shapely.

Those women who were taunted as children for being too skinny now experience a greater degree of social inclusion as college-educated professional women interacting closely with the majority culture where size is attached to professional identities, social status, and upward mobility.

While growing up, few of the women recall hearing about any connections made between body size and physical health or risk for disease. There was frequent talk of chronic conditions like diabetes and high blood pressure, but these conditions were not associated with being overweight but rather with diet composition (e.g., high salt and fat intake). This was not the case for Tameka Durand, MPH. Her mother, who was a grade school teacher, taught her as a young girl:

> You could be large, but then there is larger. . . . I would say the threshold is when you are not able to shop in like a regular store, like you have to go to a plus size store to find your clothes. That differentiates you from being large or obese to the point that you stand out because of your weight. . . . Initially when I went to college, I was eating a lot of junk food, eating late at night staying up to study. There was this thing called the Freshman 15. I experienced that. I did get the Freshman 15. I came home and my mother was like, "Oh my goodness, look at how much weight you have put on! I'm going to put you on a diet." I wasn't large. Don't get me wrong. My 15 pounds had me like at a size 9/10, but it was larger than I normally was and my mother felt like I was on the road to bad health and she didn't want me to be unhealthy. Her saying was, "You're too young to be overweight. You're too young to have weight problems. That's something that comes later on in life."

Overall, a healthy body was one that was first of all functional, that is, able to move within and outside of the community with some degree of physical and social ease. A healthy body was also able to fulfill its commitments and accomplish the tasks assigned to it, and the healthy Black body did not dishonor or offend the collective sensibilities of the Black community in terms of values associated with insuring that its members are well nourished, strong, resilient, and sharp physically, mentally, and commercially in dress and presentation. The inability to walk up stairs, experiencing shortness of breath at the least bit of exertion, and in general being easily winded were physical markers that coded a person as obese. According to the women in the study, women characterized as obese wore dress sizes 20 and higher. Regina Jefferson, PhD, MPH, comments,

> I think there are probably some unspoken standards in terms of women outside of the home and church domains that heaviness wouldn't play out, or being way overweight wouldn't cut it, [particularly] to the point where you're huffing and puffing, or that kind of thing.

Therefore, body size was only medicalized (i.e., pathologized) when mobility was hindered, breathing impaired, or one was bedridden as a result of illnesses associated with excess body weight.

Women in this study attended and graduated from the leading universities in the United States. For example, two women in the study are graduates of Stanford Medical School, three earned doctorates in public health from Johns Hopkins University, and several are graduates of Emory University. Other universities represented include the University of Notre Dame, Harvard Law School, Georgia Tech, the University of North Carolina at Chapel Hill, and Wellesley College. A number of the women attended historically Black colleges as undergraduates, including Spelman College, Hampton University, Howard University, Tuskegee University, Fisk University, and Shaw University. Three women earned master's degrees from historically Black colleges: Clark Atlanta University, Morehouse School of Medicine, and Meharry Medical School.

For many young women, entering college is their first experience being away from home, and for those attending majority institutions, it is their first intimate exposure to majority culture. The undergraduate years are a time of great transformation both emotionally and socially for all young women. Students are challenged to critically examine the values and beliefs they grew up with and adopt new ways of thinking that advance them into the knowledge class. Greater attention to body size occurs during the college years.

Carol Simmons attended Emory University as an undergraduate and recalled this about her experience:

> I think I noticed that this whole rail-thin, White female image was very pervasive when I went to school, but there were two effects to that: One was that I became more conscious of not only my weight but [also] the differences in my weight and the majority group's weight. When I thought about other [Black] women I knew, their weight and the majority group's weight was different. [The other effect was] I saw in the White community their struggle as well with anorexia, with bulimia. A lot of eating disorders were very apparent when I went to school at Emory.

We learned earlier that Carol's body was very small in the context of other women in her family and her community. However, in the context of White women, she actually saw even smaller body forms. Carol's exposure to the White female students at Emory introduced her to a radically different orientation to the female body:

> Most of the white women I was exposed to at Emory were always talking about their weight. They were always focusing on it. And that was not my

experience even with the Black students at Emory. I mean, we were doing the teenage thing—dieting, [and] trying to be "in" so we wouldn't be fat—but I don't think we had the obsession that a lot of the White girls that I knew had. So, I saw the downside to endorsing an image that women were trying to live up to that wasn't an image that women in my community had to live up to.

Crystal Peete, a Harvard Law School graduate and the mother of two young sons, had a similar experience during her undergraduate years at a small women's college in California. The college was also known as a "finishing school" for young White women. Crystal is almost 6 ft tall and average build. She runs marathons, but also really loves to eat. Her husband is a physician and was born in the Caribbean. They met while she was attending college. At the time Crystal attended college, there were about 600 students, of whom fewer than 60 were African American. How did this environment affect her body image? Crystal shared:

I started focusing more on "I'm too big, my hips are too big, my thighs are too big!" I was comparing myself to the women around me. I felt like, I'm tall anyway and I'm big-boned, so I'm going to be bigger than many people anyway. I mean, certainly, all of the women in the majority weren't little, but it certainly seemed like more of them were little than more of us. They were smaller than us and then the magazines and, you know, the TV shows showed them being pretty small and even the Blacks on TV were pretty small. So, I started thinking about my hips . . . [and] I took a pretty drastic move. I actually had liposuction and that was after a friend of mine who is White told me she got it. Now this girl was like a size 4, okay, and she got liposuction. I had liposuction out of my hips, and do you know that was the worst mistake, because it's like, it messes up your body in the sense that things get moved around and now I truly have hips. It doesn't work.

Crystal would matriculate at three other majority institutions: the University of Texas's Lyndon B. Johnson School of Public Policy, Columbia Law School, and Harvard Law School. She began a pattern of yo-yo dieting during these years and said at one point that she had "clothes in her closet that ranged from size 2 to size 20-something." Once while working at a law firm, she and another Black female attorney noticed, "there are no overweight people at the law firm. This is a law firm of the *beautiful people*." Crystal and her colleague agonized over this revelation a bit:

What does this mean? Does it mean that overweight people aren't being hired? I mean, I don't know. But, does it mean there's an expectation that they want people to not be overweight? I don't know, I mean, is this just a coincidence? I don't know. In my legal department, I would probably say that nobody is really overweight.

The "finish line" had just moved for Crystal. In addition to her impressive education credentials and her apparent competence as an attorney, she has found that she must also concern herself with achieving and maintaining a body form that fits her professional arena.

As more African American women enter professional environments previously less accessible to them, they find themselves challenged to pursue and achieve a body size that is acceptable within corporate and white collar environments. Failure to achieve the desired or acceptable size can close doors of opportunity to these women. Linda Jones recalled,

> The alienation I have seen experienced by women with whom I have worked involves one woman in particular. While growing up, she attended a prestigious private school up through high school. She graduated and went to a good university and got an undergraduate degree. After that she went to an elite university and got an MBA, but she is now working as a temp. There is no doubt in my mind that the reason she does not get the kind of employment that she is worthy of getting—she is very bright and she gets along very well with people—is because of her size. I worked with her while she was working on her MBA, but she has not been able to get a job and I believe that she is alienated because of her body size. I think about her often because I think that she is discriminated against, and I also believe that this experience impacts Black women more than it impacts White women.

Such negative perceptions eclipse their academic and professional achievements and undermine their character in a majority culture where one's economic status and social position is inscribed in the body.

Across Black communities where the participants were raised, acceptable body sizes were stratified based on life stage and social position. Young women were expected to have bodies that were shapely and sexually appealing to men. The single, most influential variable among participants in this study in determining how young women both adorned and disciplined their bodies was determined by the male gaze and the marriage market. As long as women remained single, even into middle age and beyond, there is an expectation to ignore aging as an inevitable biological process and commit to the body work needed to insure a size that would attract male attention and ideally lead to a serious, committed relationship. After marriage and childbearing, women were expected to gain some weight, but be careful to "not let herself go" (i.e., to abandon all interest in their figure and appearance). Among professional women, there was an expectation that they manage both their weight and how they dressed in order to be taken seriously. Older women, particularly grandmothers, were freer to indulge their appetites and be content with a higher body weight.

Until recently, Linda Jones had never had a weight problem. She had been slender since childhood and was much disciplined in her eating and physical activity. However, at the age of 52, Linda is seeing her body change both in terms of weight and the distribution of body fat. She is going through menopause. For the first time, she has a protruding stomach and she complains that her clothes do not fit. Linda is single and not currently in a relationship. She is also a faculty member at a prestigious university.

> I think part of the formation of our images comes out of our life experiences, and for me I had never been considered overweight. I had never been on a diet. I had always been physically active and as I got older and as I have reached this age of 52, my clothes now don't fit. My dress sizes have changed, and for the first time in a very long time, I'm faced with this issue of being overweight and having to really come to terms with what that means. I think that part of it is that the weight wouldn't be as much of an issue for me if I wasn't in one of those institutions where the expectation is that I should maintain an ideal body weight and be physically active. And that I'm also in a social class where I ought to be able to take advantage of resources for purchasing food, for gaining physical activity, and for eating food in way that would help me maintain—establish and maintain—an ideal body weight. And I think also it has something to do with the fact that I am also not in a relationship, and that I may become less attractive as my weight potentially would stay the same or increase.

Taken together, workplace expectations for smaller body sizes, social expectations of single women to maintain a smaller body size, and the economic consequences of exceeding acceptable body size standards create considerable social and professional pressure for these women to be concerned about their weight.

Body Size and Black Women in Church

Social structures and institutions, kinship systems or social networks, and patterns of authority and power construct culture at the community and individual levels. These same social structures, institutions, and systems influence dietary choices and preferences. There is a growing literature that suggests involvement in a religious community and personal commitment to religious beliefs and practices are positively associated with healthy outcomes (Matthews et al., 1998; Strawbridge, Cohen, Shema, & Kaplan, 2001). Of particular relevance for Black women is a developing discourse pioneered by womanist theologians to advance improvements in health and health care experienced by the Black church and larger Black community (Douglas, 1999; Townes, 1998). It is unclear, however, the extent to which the social and political ideologies of Black church life—namely, influences on dietary practices, physical activity, and body size—support and reinforce attitudes, beliefs, and behaviors that would promote healthy body sizes for Black women.

Despite the recognition of the influence of social networks like faith-based institutions in the socioecologic model of determinants of health, there is limited research on the relationship between religion, religious practice, and body weight. Ferraro found that "obesity is highest in states where religious affiliation is more prevalent and in states with a higher proportion of African American residents" (Ferraro, 1998, p. 238). Black women were described as being more religious, obesity was associated with higher levels of religiosity, and social class was inversely related to both obesity and religiosity. He reports finding no evidence "that religion plays a major role in aiding the management of body weight in the United States," despite biblical admonitions against gluttony and perceptions of fasting and other ascetic behavior as virtuous (Ferraro, 1998, p. 238). Consistent with findings in this research, he reports,

> [T]here are some denominations which may be virtually silent on the issue of body weight. Such denominations typically emphasize the acceptance of people regardless of lifestyle and do not play a strong role as moral entrepreneurs (e.g., Unitarians, Presbyterians). Still other denominations may be oriented to the moral importance of certain health behaviors such as smoking and alcohol consumption, but give little attention to body weight (e.g., fundamentalist denominations). (Ferraro, 1998, p. 225)

Those congregations that foster acceptance of the individual regardless of physical appearance appear "to buffer or reduce any negative effects of obesity on well-being" (Ferraro, 1998, p. 239). Given the consolation and comfort obese people may find in church, Ferraro is skeptical that faith-based institutions will "become a major avenue of intervention in the immediate future" (Ferraro, 1998, p. 239). However, the growing twin burden of diabetes and obesity in congregations with large numbers of African Americans calls for greater participation of these community institutions in health promotion and chronic disease prevention.

When considering the role of the church in promoting healthy body sizes among professional African American women, this research did not find the church a significant influence in promoting weight control or healthier body sizes. More often than not, the church was a place of refuge and a safe space for women of all sizes, particularly large women. Largeness among Black women in the churches attended by the participants in this study was associated in many instances with nurturance. Among many of the women in this study who were in daily contact with the culture of thinness, they found within the church an affirmation and acceptance of their size in the Black church. This acceptance was typically implicit rather than explicit. Body size and weight were simply not discussed.

At the church where this fieldwork was conducted, the women perceived a relaxed "body environment" for women. Alma Mitchell remarked,

> Well, we have a diverse congregation, I think. Other races are represented here, so you see other body structures and types. I do feel that I fit in fine. I don't feel that there is a standard around me that I need to aspire to that I felt as a younger woman in my 20s when I was in church. Now I feel like I set my own precedence. I make my own rules. It's not as important to me what other people think or how other people view me physically as much as it is important to me how I see me. I do, though, rely on my husband to give me input on how I present my weight.

In response to the question regarding what women looked like who were "out front" (i.e., visible and in leadership roles) in the church, easily half of the women reported they observed women of all sizes in the congregation or they stated the women were "large but not obese." Ruth Hill remarked,

> Most of them were heavy. They were stylish but heavy. . . . I never thought about that until I became a lot older and mature after having children. I have come to believe that eating is the indulgence that women allowed themselves when they are trying to come out from certain habits in the world. They might say, "I don't drink alcohol and I don't do drugs. I don't

smoke cigarettes." The one indulgence that women in the church, I feel, give themselves permission to indulge in is eating.

As noted by Ruth, more explicit comment was made about the impropriety of smoking and consuming alcohol than about overeating. In a conversation I had with a female associate pastor of a Black Baptist church in Atlanta, she commented that pastors avoided making statements from the pulpit that would publicly embarrass persons in the congregation. It is possible to maintain one's privacy about smoking or alcohol consumption while in the public space of the church, but it is not possible to hide one's obesity. Even when there was an emphasis in the church about honoring one's body as the temple of the Holy Spirit, it was rarely if ever accompanied by "fat bashing" or attempts to shame or coerce congregants to lose weight.

Large women were particularly visible in the church choir, and music is a central feature of Black worship. Large, talented Black women who sing in the choir are celebrities who are celebrated within the church and little mention is made of their size. Regina Jefferson recalls,

> I remember there was a woman in my husband's choir who had to be at least a size 26 or 28, but she would dress "to the nines" [extremely well]. I mean, she would walk like she was walking on eggshells. The woman was just gorgeous. She was extremely heavy, but somehow she carried it off in that "complete package." In contrast, there was another woman in the choir who was like her same size, but who was less skillful in dressing herself. She got many more [negative] comments about her size than did the woman who knew how to carry it off. I think the issue is to look good, and if you can carry off the looking good, if you can maintain the confidence in your size and carry it off, I don't think those people got the comments. It probably would have been the women who couldn't carry it off who were more subject to it.

Big, booming, and powerful voices seemed rightly housed in big bodies given the perception of largeness being associated with vocal talent as normative. Even beyond the cultural space of the church, well-known opera singers like Leontyne Price and Marian Anderson were also large, buxom women with powerful voices and a mesmerizing stage presence. In general, the ability to sing well and stir the emotions of the congregation toward tears or joy overshadowed and minimized body size in the cultural environment of the church, according to the participants in this study.

About one-third of the women in this study reported explicit expectations of their church for disciplined bodily practices that included weight control, physical activity, and healthy diets in response to the recognition that their bodies were "the temple of the Holy Ghost." From a modern language translation of the Bible, the scripture referenced by several of the women was that recorded in I Corinthians 6:18–20:

> Keep away from the desires of the flesh. Every sin which a man does is outside of the body; but he who goes after the desires of the flesh does evil to his body.
>
> Or are you not conscious that your body is a house for the Holy Spirit which is in you, and which has been given to you by God?
>
> And you are not the owners of yourselves; For a payment has been made for you: let God be honoured in your body.

The scripture above captures expectations of asceticism historically associated with the early Christian church. Derived from the Greek word *askesis*, meaning exercise or training, asceticism typically involves "celibacy, fasting, poverty, seclusion, and, often, a degree of self-mortification in a program of self-discipline and self-denial intended to achieve a spiritual goal" (Newman, 2002).

Linda Jones is a member of a non-denominational church in Baltimore that is very committed to fostering healthy bodies and attention to health and fitness is modeled by both the pastor and his wife. She described how she perceives the emphasis on health in her church:

> The head of my church is very physically active and he has an ideal body weight, as does his wife. So I think there is a little bit of, I guess, a little bit of intimidation that I feel, because when I joined the church in 1996, I was in that ideal body weight. I remember my pastor saying, "Are you still swimming?" Sometimes that's what people will say when they really have noticed that you've gained weight and they think that you have gained it because you are no longer exercising. And so he has asked me on an occasion or two if I'm still swimming. So I think that certainly in terms of the kind of doctrine that operates in my church of the body being the temple of the Holy Spirit, there is an expectation that we are not only responsible for our spiritual health but our physical health as well, and [the implication is] that if we are really people of faith and people of the gospel, then we will take care of our bodies and be responsible for what we ingest and for our lifestyles.

Linda's church was in the process of building a family life center that would house a basketball court and other fitness equipment to encourage physical activity and a healthy lifestyle among the parishioners.

Additionally, food is an important part of church sociality. Women are generally overrepresented on kitchen committees and in other functions of hospitality. When food was served during special events at the church where fieldwork was conducted, the menu was economical and carbohydrate-rich (e.g., spaghetti and meatballs, rolls, and cake). "Dinners" were available for sale each Sunday in the atrium of the church and constituted fried chicken, beans and rice, noodles, a green vegetable, one or two meats, and homemade cakes. For only $5 one could purchase this large, calorie- and fat-laden, midday meal. This service was provided by two members of the church whose business was catering. Therefore, it was a regular source of income for the caterers and the church, in addition to providing a time for members to eat and for fellowship after the church service.

Study Limitations

The findings from this qualitative, ethnographic study cannot be generalized to the larger community of college-educated African American women or to other church congregations. The position of the principal investigator as a college-educated, professional, and obese Black woman may impose unintended biases in observations and interpretations of findings. These same characteristics may have enhanced rapport with respondents and sensitivities to raced, gendered, and cultural practices and social interactions that are important in this research.

Situating the influences on Black female body size within a moral and cultural framework is necessarily a complex undertaking that argues for the inclusion of multiple voices in the articulation of how moral ideologies, practices, and social interactions influence the shaping of Black female bodies. Synthesizing multiple voices, social locations, and intergenerational effects on ideology and practice into a coherent theoretical framework without testing the theoretical assumptions in a larger, random sample study using a survey methodology limits the validity of the findings. Additional research is needed with a larger sample of college-educated Black women to test the validity of the theoretical assumptions underlying these analyses.

This study is further limited by the lack of a comparison group (e.g., a demographically similar group of White, Latino, or American Indian respondents). Without a similar inquiry of White and other racial and ethnic women, we cannot tease out how the experiences of these African American women are culturally distinct from other women. Future research should be designed as a cross-cultural analysis with other racial and ethnic groups of women.

Additionally, participants in this research were subject to multiple and overlapping sociocultural influences on their body size. In addition to the cultural determinants addressed in this study, Black female bodies are also likely shaped by childhood trauma, personal coping strategies, medical history, the overplacement of fast food restaurants and liquor stores, and the paucity of options for fresh fruits, vegetables, and other nutritionally superior food options in communities of color, to name a few. Although this study addresses the cultural production of Black female bodies in a limited context, focused attention to the impact of these other social determinants is beyond the scope of this study.

Discussion

This research discovered again that African American women—even those who are college-educated—define and perceive obesity differently. The 50% of African American women categorized by BMI as overweight would in fact deem themselves as being a healthy and attractive weight (i.e., in dress sizes 10–14). Yet, even though these women view this larger size as ideal, particularly after childbirth and into the middle age years, they still struggle with fitting a larger African-descended body in a majority culture that abhors largeness in women. Black women in their 20s and early 30s were much more focused on preventing weight gain and avoiding the stigma of obesity than earlier generations of Black women. Among the second-generation, upper-middle-class women in the study, restrained eating and close attention to maintaining an ideal weight were already established in their cultural framework.

As professional women working outside the home, these women are in daily contact with the culture of thinness but find some refuge and affirmation in the Black church. All of the women in this study are very health-conscious and desire the benefits of a healthy lifestyle and a healthy weight, but they find it difficult to incorporate this additional body work into their already overcommitted and overextended lives. There is a space for the primary prevention of obesity and overweight that many of the women in the study missed. Specifically, women in their 40s did not generally grow up seeing their mothers and other adult women in their communities engaging in planned physical activity. The health benefits of regular physical activity may be a new expectation and cultural norm that could dramatically impact the lifestyles and health of professional Black women.

IMPLICATIONS FOR PUBLIC HEALTH PRACTICE

This research marks an important beginning for additional intervention research intending to improve chronic disease outcomes for African American women. There are a number of lessons learned that can be integrated into public health interventions. For example, these women valued professional productivity and advancement, family, and quality of life. These priorities were clearly reflected in how they committed their time and resources.

For most of the women, and particularly those with children at home, if opportunities for healthy eating and physical activity were not easily accessible to them in the course of the workday, they would be less likely to engage in either. Any campaign intending to change patterns of food consumption and physical activity must then address and modify the social environments of the workplace, family, and culturally motivated sources of pleasure. For example, employers could grant 2 to 4 paid hours each week for the express purpose of attending to a healthier lifestyle. This might allow women to shop for food, incorporate an hour of physical activity, or provide needed opportunities for physical activity for their children.

Additionally, these programs must affirm the professional Black woman's perception that being Black and female in particular spaces imposes a unique set of challenges in addition to the ones faced by all women. The professional Black women in this study perceived themselves as more vulnerable to job insecurity, because they occupied positions in arenas previously dominated by White men and women. These Black women were competitive and high achievers in the workplace, but more often than not, their competitiveness was tied primarily to insuring their economic survival and secondarily to achieving notoriety in their chosen fields. Their perceptions of vulnerability added to the tendency to overachieve and strive for a level of perfectionism in the workplace that tended toward chronic stress and a lifestyle that was not balanced.

Public health campaigns must also define practical steps that a professional Black woman can take in the course of a week to facilitate health promotion and stress reduction.

Although not much was spoken in the interviews about physical activity, the promotion of greater physical activity within this demographic of women is needed. Even though they possessed the resources to access fitness facilities, this was not highly valued. Purchasing fitness programs and structuring time to work out in the context of an already overcommitted day were not the choices of most of the women in this study. Even though their professional work was sedentary, paying in time and money to "work" more was not part of their indigenous cultural framework. While growing up, many of the women observed their mothers and other women in their communities dieting, but adding physical activity to support their weight loss was a foreign concept. Arguably, these women appeared to have a more working class attitude toward exercise and physical activity, that is, taking care of oneself meant resting after work and attending to one's family in spite of the known health benefits of physical activity.

Programs intended to increase physical activity in this demographic of African American women must not eliminate fitness facilities or other more structured options for physical activity. Programs should include workplace policies that grant time away from work for physical activity, activities that accommodate children, activities that promote sociality and social support like walking with a friend or spouse, and strategies that promote physical activity over weight loss, allowing the woman to feel good about her efforts even when weight loss does not occur.

For example, over the past 10 years, I have observed more and more African American men and women walking to achieve greater fitness at a nearby middle school track. In the middle of the track is a football field. I can imagine a track with a playground in the middle that allows mothers to walk around the track while still being able to keep an eye on their children playing. This track could be made even more appealing by adding a bike lane for older children to ride their bikes or skate, for example, while their mother is walking and still able to keep her eye on the children. In a progressive county or neighborhood, paid staff would be available to assist in monitoring the activities of the children to ensure their safety.

Also, increased physical activity can be achieved through dance. African Americans have a rich heritage of dance that can be directed toward increasing physical activity and is both available and acceptable to middle class Black women and their families. More importantly, dancing is enjoyable, relieves stress, and provides an opportunity to detach from the head and concentrate on the body, a much needed reprieve for the professional Black woman. African dance, salsa, swing, and praise dance are among the forms of dance that appeal to Black women of all body sizes. Among the challenges to the successful implementation of a dance intervention is ensuring that the form of dance accommodates varying levels of skill, talent, and mobility. The dance should not compromise a woman's sense of respectability and decorum, understood to represent her social, occupational, and in some instances religious status. Again, the extent to which children can participate or be cared for during the time of the class will likely increase participation by professional Black women.[4] Public performances by the dancers and dance parties foster recreation and a celebration of African American culture, re-establishing play as a necessary component of Black middle-class life for enjoyment as well as the health of a population disproportionately affected by type 2 diabetes and obesity.

The current and projected burden of type 2 diabetes among all African Americans in the U.S. necessitates new and added attention to the influences of the sociocultural environment, the workplace, and moral ideologies in constructing body size and risks for obesity. It is inadequate and a missed opportunity to achieve the mission of public health if we fail to promote and support an expanded research and practice agenda that addresses these factors.

REFERENCES

Allen, C. (1998). Caribbean bodies: Representation and practices. In C. Barrow (Ed.), *Caribbean portraits: Essays on gender ideologies and identities* (pp. 275–293). Kingston, Jamaica: Ian Randle Publishers.

Barrow, C. (Ed.). (1998). *Caribbean portraits: Essays on gender ideologies and identities.* Kingston, Jamaica: Ian Randle Publishers.

Bennett, M., & Dickerson, V. D. (Eds). (2001). *Recovering the Black female body.* New Brunswick, NJ: Rutgers University Press.

Bordo, S. (1993). *Unbearable weight: Feminism, Western culture, and the body.* Berkeley, CA: University of California Press.

---

[4] I have noticed during my daughter's ballet classes that the African American mothers bring their daughters to class, then sit outside the dance studio for an hour either talking to each other or reading until class is over. This is a missed opportunity for mothers to increase their own physical activity by participating in a dance class while their daughters are doing the same. With some encouragement from the dance studio, this is a highly feasible option for professional Black women.

Brown, P. J. (1991). Culture and the evolution of obesity. *Human Nature, 2(1),* 31–57.

Brown, P. J. (1992). Cultural perspectives on the etiology and treatment of obesity. In A. J. Stunkard & T. A. Wadden (Eds.), *Obesity: Theory and therapy* (pp. 179–193). New York: Raven Press.

Brown, P. J., & Konner, M. (1998). An anthropological perspective on obesity. In P. Brown (Ed.), *Understanding and applying medical anthropology* (pp. 401–413). Mountain View, CA: Mayfield Publishing Co.

Burnham, L. (2001). Working paper series, no. 1: The wellspring of Black feminist theory. In L. Burnham (Ed.), *The wellspring of Black feminist theory.* Oakland, CA: Women of Color Resource Center.

Collins, P. H. (2000). *Black feminist thought.* New York: Routledge.

Corin, E. (1995). The cultural frame: Context and meaning in the construction of health. In B. C. Amick, S. Levine, A. R. Tarlov, & D. C. Walsh (Eds.), *Society and health* (pp. 272–304). New York: Oxford University Press.

Counihan, C. M. (1999). *The anthropology of food and body.* New York: Routledge.

Dollard, J. (1935). *Criteria for the life history.* New Haven, CT: Yale University Press.

Douglas, K. B. (1999). *Sexuality and the Black church.* Maryknoll, NY: Orbis Books.

Douglas, M. (1982). *Natural symbols.* London: Routledge and Kegan Paul.

Farb, P., & Armelagos, G. (1980). *Consuming passions: The anthropology of eating.* Boston: Houghton Mifflin.

Farquhar, J. (2002). *Appetites: Food and sex in post-socialist China.* Durham, NC: Duke University Press.

Ferraro, K. F. (1998). Firm believers? Religion, body weight, and well-being. *Review of Religious Research, 39(3),* 224–244.

hooks, b. (1992). *Black looks: Race and representation.* Boston: South End Press.

hooks, b. (1995). *Art on my mind: Visual politics.* New York: The New Press.

Kumanyika, S. (1998). Obesity in African Americans: biobehavioral consequences of culture. *Ethnicity and Disease.* Winter; 8(1): 93–96.

Kumanyika, S. (2007). Obesity Prevention Concepts and Frameworks. In *Handbook of obesity prevention.* Eds. Kumanyika, S. and Brownson, R.C. New York: Springer.

Liburd, L. C. (2006). *The medical anthropology of type 2 diabetes at the intersection of race, class, and gender.* Emory University. Department of Anthropology. Emory University Dissertations (Ph.D.)

Matthews, D. A., McCullough, M. E., Larson, D. B., Koenig, H. G., Swyers, J. P., & Milano, M. G. (1998). Religious commitment and health status. *Archives of Family Medicine, 7,* 118–124.

McClaurin, I. (Ed.). (2001). *Black feminist anthropology: Theory, politics, praxis, and poetics.* New Brunswick, NJ: Rutgers University Press.

McLaren, L., & Kuh, D. (2004). Women's body dissatisfaction, social class, and social mobility. *Social Science & Medicine.* 58: 1575–1584

Neuman, W. L. (2003). *Social research methods: Qualitative and quantitative approaches.* Boston: Allyn & Bacon.

Newman, S. (2002). *Oh God! A Black woman's guide to sex and spirituality.* New York: One World Ballantine Books.

Nichter, M. (2000). *Fat talk: What girls and their parents say about dieting.* Cambridge, MA: Harvard University Press.

Paris, P. J. (1985). *The social teaching of the black churches.* Philadelphia, Fortress Press.

Powdermaker, H. (1960). An anthropological approach to the problem of obesity. *Bulletin of the New York Academy of Medicine, 36,* 75–83.

Sobal, J., Stunkard, A. J. (1989). Socioeconomic Status and Obesity: A Review of the Literature. *Psychological Bulletin 105(2):* 260–275.

Scheper-Hughes, N., & Lock, M. (1998). The mindful body: A prolegomenon to future work in medical anthropology. In P. J. Brown (Ed.), *Understanding and applying medical anthropology* (pp. 208–225). Mountain View, CA: Mayfield Publishing.

Strawbridge, W. J., Cohen, R. D., Shema, S. J., & Kaplan, G. A. (2001). Religious attendance increases survival by improving and maintaining good health practices, mental health, and stable marriages. *Annals of Behavioral Medicine, 23(1),* 68–74.

Townes, E. M. (1998). *Breaking the fine rain of death: African American health issues and a womanist ethic of care.* New York: The Continuum Publishing Co.

Wallace-Sanders, K. (Ed.). (2002). *Skin deep, spirit strong.* Ann Arbor, MI: The University of Michigan Press.

Witt, D. (1999). *Black hunger: Food and the politics of U.S. identity.* New York: Oxford University Press.

5

The Centrality of Community in Eliminating Diabetes Disparities

LEANDRIS C. LIBURD AND JANICE V. BOWIE

INTRODUCTION

Community is to public health what the body is to biomedicine. That is, the community in its multiple conceptual iterations is the primary focus of public health. The centrality of community in public health is what distinguishes its practice and epistemology from other enterprises concerned with health, illness, and disease in the populace. As the body has been theorized and contemplated across disciplines, so has the concept of community captured the attention and imaginations of theorists across the social sciences, albeit with little consensus.

Constructs of community in public health practice and research encompass a broad array of realities from the standpoints of the professional and the persons presumably tied to a particular community. The multiple dimensions of communities as "organized systems of people in relation to one another" (LaBonte, 1997) who typically share one or more identities, including physical and social spaces, are explored in this chapter. While the exact nature of these systems and the relationships of the people that bind them vary across time and space are not well articulated or integrated uniformly in public health practice, community remains the principle unit of practice in chronic disease prevention and health promotion.

Too often in the history of population-based public health, geography, political units, and demographic characteristics have been the de facto definition of community by virtue of facilitating data collection. Quantitative data collection methods and descriptive epidemiology represent the cornerstone of public health. Indeed, national attention to the disproportionate burden of death and disability in communities of color and the institutionalization of a concern with improving minority health were mobilized in response to compelling epidemiological data (US DHHS, Secretary's Task Force on Black & Minority Health, 1986). However, the apparent inability of public health researchers and practitioners to construct a definition of community that is simultaneously precise and narrow enough to meet the requirements for statistical analyses and descriptive epidemiology, while capturing the intangibles of community that arguably represent the more authentic relational dimensions of this entity, have important implications for people with and at risk for type 2 diabetes.

In this chapter, a snapshot of the literature seeking to define and theorize community and offer some distinctions important for practice in the language of community, such as community-based, community-driven, community-recruited, and community-participatory, is provided. In the arena of health disparities, the word community can be understood in a host of ways, including to delineate who holds power and who does not in public health work and as a euphemism for marginalized groups like the poor, racial and ethnic groups, and other disenfranchised members of our society. Ostensibly, definitions of community (i.e., who's in and who's out) are never value neutral with regard to power (Spears, 2006). As such, community can also be a euphemism for political constituents, that is, special interest groups, the voting public, and others with access to policy makers who wield significant influence over public health practice and research. How then might the interpersonal dimension of community be operationalized to facilitate eliminating diabetes disparities in racial and ethnic populations? In the conclusion of this chapter, we discuss some of the lingering challenges associated with how we define community and the implications of these definitions for subsequent approaches to community-based public health.

WHY CONSIDER COMMUNITY IN PUBLIC HEALTH?

The promotion of a greater good is the hallmark of public health. To achieve improvements in health requires an understanding of the determinants of health and changes in strategies at individual, interpersonal, community, and societal levels (Marmot, 2001). The value of micro- and macro-level approaches in achieving improved health outcomes is essential, given that the goals of community health promotion and chronic disease prevention cannot be accomplished solely through individual-focused initiatives.

The ecological model shown in Figure 5.1 depicts the interplay of factors and levels of influence on health and health outcomes. Illustrating diabetes, the first level, individual, represents biological and personal factors like age, family history of diabetes, obesity, and physical inactivity. At the relationship or interpersonal level, factors include social networks that may influence or undermine positive health behaviors, such as social patterns of eating and cultural beliefs about the disease, and established patterns of diabetes self-management that may or may not be consistent with clinical recommendations. Community in this model, the third level, explores the settings where social relations occur, which from the standpoint of diabetes can include the availability of healthy food systems and other forms of environmental supports for health. The final level is societal, which considers the broader factors that foster or negate health, such as economic policies that dictate foods stocked by bodegas; urban planning that ignores the necessity of sidewalks, bike lanes, and well-routed public transportation; and housing policies that segregate neighborhoods by race and income. (See chapter 6 by Navarro for a detailed discussion of the impact of residential segregation on the social construction of health disparities in communities of color.)

Studies show that community-level factors influence behaviors even when controlling for individual-level factors (Sampson, Raudenbush, &

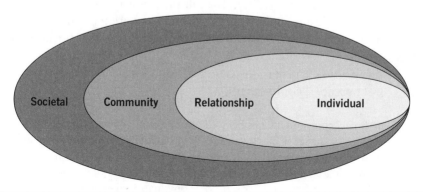

Figure 5.1 The Social Ecological Model

Earls, 1997). It is at the community level that population health is most impacted and vital in aiding our understanding of its value and orientation for planning comprehensive, integrative, and well-balanced approaches for diabetes prevention and control.

WHAT IS A COMMUNITY?

Definitions of community vary according to the discipline of the theorist—sociology, anthropology, health services research, epidemiology, and human or social ecology—and the purpose of the inquiry.
—D. L. Patrick and T. M. Wickizer (1995, p. 47)

Practical problems with defining the community in public health emerge each time practitioners undertake new research or interventions. Historically, the term community figures prominently in early definitions of public health:

> Public health is the science and art of preventing disease, prolonging life, and promoting physical and mental health through organized community efforts for the sanitation of the environment, the control of community infections . . . and the development of the social machinery which will ensure to every individual in the community a standard of living adequate for the maintenance of health. (Winslow, 1920, p. 30)

In 1920 C. E. A.Winslow did not make explicit what he meant by community. This lack of precision in definition remains characteristic today. While the term is richly evocative and easily understood in everyday language (Green & Kreuter, 1999), its multiplicity of meanings can cause problems in the design, implementation, and evaluation of public health interventions intended to improve health outcomes for a particular population group.

There is little or no consensus on what defines a community, a point that has not escaped commentary:

> [T]he term "community" has been defined in so many ways and used in so many contexts, that it has lost much of its meaning. Community may be used to refer to the psychological sense of community, a political entity, a functional spatial unit meeting sustenance needs, a unit of patterned social interaction, or simply an aggregate of individuals in a geographic location. (McLeroy, Bibeau, Steckler, & Glanz, 1988, pp. 362–363)

In recognition of this lack of clarity, scholars have attempted to pin down the meaning. As early as 1931, sociologist C. R. Hoffer identified 43 different definitions of the term, but noted that they had three characteristics in common: (a) they are human groups, (b) they carry out shared activities, and (c) they occupy space (Hoffer, 1931). He conceptualized communities as differing from neighborhoods in that communities encompassed indirect as well as face-to-face contacts and are less tangible than neighborhoods. In 1955 Hilary cited as many as 94 different definitions, all which concerned humanity, but still no universal definition emerged (Amick et al., 1995, p. 47).

Definitions of community vary by theorists, discipline, and the nature of inquiry, and public health practitioners employ a wide array of definitions using their own lens and purposes (Patrick & Wickizer, 1995, p. 47). In a survey carried out by MacQueen (2001) of diverse groups from drug users to vaccine researchers, the following characteristics of community were mentioned by more than half of the respondents surveyed:

1. a common physical location,
2. shared perspective or interests,
3. joint action or activities, and
4. interpersonal relationships.

Another definition used in public health conceptualizes community as containing six elements:

1. membership or sense of identity and belonging,
2. a common symbol system like language,
3. shared values and norms,
4. mutual influence,
5. shared needs and commitment to meeting them, and
6. shared emotional connection (Israel, Checkoway, Schulz, & Zimmerman, 1994).

In this conceptualization, a shared geographic location is possible but not necessary to constitute a community. For example, we observe characteristics associated with community in public health efforts using on-line health education, support groups, and advocacy groups, to name a few. An even more nuanced and multifaceted definition of community in public health is found in Walter's work, which describes it as changing over time and with context, as arising in the context of commitment to shared activities, and as including researchers in addition to those researched (Walter, 1997).

In a recent review, McLeroy, Norton, Kegler, Burdine, and Sumaya (2003) distinguish four implicit conceptualizations of community employed by public health researchers: as setting, as target, as resource, and as agent. They note that the community as setting construct has dominated public health to date, in line with the ongoing focus on individual behavior change, while the least used construct in public health is community as agent, which involves "respecting and reinforcing the natural adaptive, supportive, and developmental capacities of communities" and "carefully work[ing] with these naturally occurring units of solution as our unit of practice" (McLeroy et al., 2003, p. 530). Community as agent best captures a community-driven perspective in public health practice. Beneficiaries of community-driven public health interventions are not passive recipients, but are actively and centrally engaged in defining the content and parameters of the program in ways that fit and bolster the indigenous community structure.

A Synthesis of the Literature[1]

This literature review was conducted by four graduate students at Emory University, capturing three semesters of study of the meaning of community in public health and medicine. The goal of this synthesis of selected literature was to examine current uses of the term community in public health. Toward that end, we performed a systematic search of articles that employed the term in the most influential journals in public health and medicine. We restricted our search to articles from 20 journals, 10 in the public health literature and 10 drawn from medicine. We chose the journals in each field with the highest impact factors, as determined by the ISI Journal Citation Reports for the year 2003 (the most recent year for which impact factors were available).[2] We performed a MEDLINE search

---

[1] The authors would like to acknowledge that this review of the literature was contributed by graduate fellows and faculty of the Center for Health, Culture and Society at the Rollins School of Public Health and the Department of Anthropology of Emory University.

[2] The journals reviewed from public health were: *American Journal of Epidemiology, American Journal of Preventive Medicine, American Journal of Public Health, Annual Review of Public Health, Cancer Epidemiology Biomarkers and Prevention, Environmental Health Perspectives, Epidemiologic Reviews, Epidemiology, International Journal of Epidemiology,* and *Tobacco Control.* The medical journals reviewed were: *American Journal of Medicine, Annals of Internal Medicine, Annual Review of Medicine, Archives of Internal Medicine, BMJ, Canadian Medical Association Journal, Journal of the American Medical Association, Lancet, Medicine,* and *New England Journal of Medicine.*

utilizing the keywords *community health planning* and *community health services*, limiting the results to articles from the 20 journals listed here. The one exception was the *Canadian Medical Association Journal*, which is not included in MEDLINE. For this journal, we searched EMBASE using the keyword *community health*. Those articles not containing the word community in their text were excluded from our analysis.

We coded the remaining 156 articles (99 from public health journals and 57 from medical journals) as to their use of the word community. Three of the students coded each use of the word in each of the articles, using codes developed through a grounded theory process of iterative testing and refinement (Bernard, 1995; Coffey & Atkinson, 1996). Differences of opinion were resolved through discussion and consensus. Data analysis was carried out in Microsoft® Excel® and Epi Info™ (Centers for Disease Control and Prevention, 2005).

This exercise yielded several revealing insights into the operationalization of the word community in the public health and medical literature on the topic. First, very few of the articles examined put forward an explicit definition of community. Only 4 of the 156 articles reviewed (2.6%) actively discussed the intended meanings of the term as used in the article. Second, there were multiple and changing meanings of community in most articles. In 92 of the 156 articles (59%), we observed the term used in more than one sense (e.g., might refer to a neighborhood in one part of the article and a shared characteristic like poverty in another part). On average the term community was used in 2.3 different ways per article. We identified six categories of usage (see Table 5.1), including (a) geographic locale, (b) shared characteristics, (c) level of social organization, (d) a group outside that with whom the researcher usually works, (e) as a synonym for public, and (f) as an adjective.

Identifying Community

Geographic Locale

The most common operationalization of the term community was geographic: 57% of all articles used it to refer to a particular area. Interestingly, articles published in public health journals were significantly more likely to use a geographic definition than articles in medical journals (73% of articles in public health journals vs. 30% of articles in medical journals; $p < 0.0001$). The types of geography used to define community in the articles we reviewed are listed in Table 5.2.

Table 5.1

USES OF THE TERM COMMUNITY IN THE ARTICLES REVIEWED

	NUMBER OF ARTICLES	PERCENTAGE OF ALL ARTICLES
Geographic Locale	89	57
Shared Characteristic	51	33
Level of Social Organization	18	12
Groups outside the Focus of the Research	60	38
Synonym for Public	12	8
Adjective	63	40

Table 5.2

GEOGRAPHIC UNITS REFERRED TO AS A COMMUNITY IN THE ARTICLES REVIEWED

GEOGRAPHIC UNIT USED	NUMBER OF ARTICLES USED
Neighborhood	22
City	21
Governmental District	20
Village or Small Town	18
Service Area of an Organization	14
Other	15

The advantages to defining community geographically are that it is often politically expedient and generally very convenient for public health researchers and professionals. Describing community geographically means that the target population of an intervention is more easily captured for data collection and described. Given that residence in a given geographic area predicts risk for many health problems (Frumkin, 2003; Krieger, Chen, Waterman, Rehkoph, & Subramanian, 2005), it may also provide a valid proxy for risk.

However, the operationalization of community as a geographic entity may raise concerns about construct validity, as it relies on the assumption that the geographic unit in question is residentially segregated, that is, that the people living in an area constitute a community in some meaningful sense. Drawing on MacQueen's definition, use of the word community implies social connections in the local setting, an assertion that may or may not be correct when geographic locale dictates the boundaries of what constitutes the community. In some cases, the question may be one of scale. In the case of rural villages, it may be safe to assert meaningful social connections; however, to refer to an entire city as a community, as 21 articles did, may be imprecise. Similarly, assuming that those living in the service area of an organization constitute a community, as did 14 of the articles we reviewed, may not be accurate. Such definitions become problematic when they result in poorly planned or implemented public health programs. For example, a local diabetes education program that relies simplistically on the expected diffusion of information across community social networks is likely to fail if these social networks do not exist.

Shared Characteristics

Thirty-three percent of the articles reviewed described community as arising from a shared characteristic among a group of people. Shared characteristics used to define communities in the articles reviewed are listed in Table 5.3. Articles about public health interventions in the United States were more likely to define communities in terms of shared characteristics than those describing health projects in poor countries (33% of American articles vs. 14% of international health articles; $p = 0.035$). This may be because community often provides a convenient euphemism for categories of ethnicity or class.

It is interesting to note that international health articles using community as a shared characteristic only used it as a euphemism for class, whereas articles about the United States most commonly used the word as a euphemism for ethnicity. Such usage often seemed to have less to do with the existence of an actual community among the people in question than with the need of a researcher to find an acceptable term for such uncomfortable categories as Black people or poor people. As an example, the Black community is often used to refer to all Black people in a given area, or even in a nation as a whole, whether or not they actually belong to a community characterized by regular interaction, shared

Table 5.3

SHARED CHARACTERISTICS USED TO DEFINE COMMUNITY
IN THE ARTICLES REVIEWED

	NUMBER OF ARTICLES
Ethnicity	30
Class	19
Lifestyle	9
Occupation	5
Church Membership and Faith	4
Disease	2
Other	4

goals, or any of the other characteristics associated with community in MacQueen's definition. Using the term in this way assumes homogeneity and eludes differences within a population, distinctions that may too often be ignored and are medically important.

Frequency of interaction in the communities thus described is rarely, if ever, explored. It appears that community is a "feel good" word that can easily be used by researchers as a gloss for otherwise unacceptable categorizations based on race, class, sexual orientation, or lifestyle. This is likely an unconscious process, such that the use of community to refer to such populations is so common as to have become naturalized. Nonetheless, we must be careful to avoid reinforcing structural inequalities through such usage.

Level of Social Organization

Eighteen articles (12% of the total) used community to refer to a level of social organization that was larger than the family but smaller than, say, a nation. The primary advantage of this usage is community's availability as a term that may flexibly describe a variety of social levels at which individuals experience a sense of group identity and/or may share common needs and goals, such as households, neighborhoods, organizations, and illness communities. Again, as with geography, the question of scale is important. Clearly delineating the scale of the community in research or interventions will make those endeavors better conceptualized and targeted.

Groups outside the Focus of the Research

Thirty-eight percent of the articles reviewed used community to mean all people other than those with whom the researcher usually works. Of the 156 articles reviewed, 43 used community to refer to everyone not in a nursing home or hospital, 9 to describe everyone not affiliated with a university, and 8 in some other, similar sense (e.g., in one article on drug users, community referred to everyone who did not use drugs). Perhaps not surprisingly, the use of community to refer to everyone not in the hospital was especially prevalent among articles in medical journals. Fully 46% of the articles reviewed in medical journals used the term in this sense, as compared to 17% of the articles in public health journals ($p = 0.0001$). The drawbacks to the use of the word in this sense will by now be clear, that is, not everyone outside of the hospital or the university constitutes a homogenous group or one that interacts with one another in the meaningful way evoked by the term.

Community as a Synonym for Public Health

Twelve articles (8% of the total) used community as a synonym for public health in the phrase community health. This usage was primarily limited to British journals.

Community as an Adjective

The use of the term community as an adjective is perhaps the least well-defined. A full 40% of the articles we examined used the term as an adjective in such phrases as community member and community-based organization. A substantial proportion of articles in both medical and public health journals referred to community as an adjective. Use was highest, however, in articles relating to international projects where fully 52% of the articles used community as an adjective, usually in reference to an intervention. Table 5.4 provides a complete listing of adjectives often used to describe community.

Summary of the Literature Review and Recommendations

Although interventions, organizations, and research were repeatedly described as community-based in the articles we reviewed, the nature

Table 5.4

USES OF COMMUNITY AS AN ADJECTIVE IN THE ARTICLES REVIEWED

COMMUNITY USED AS ADJECTIVE TO DESCRIBE:	NUMBER OF ARTICLES
Interventions	39
Members and Representatives	12
Agencies and Organizations	12
Research	9
Capacity	5
Health Workers	4

of the communities in which they were supposedly based was almost never discussed. A candid exploration of the power relationships that determine which individuals or organizations become able to speak for communities was likewise largely absent. Phrases like community participation commonly referred to the participation of anyone other than the researchers. When community is used in such a generalized way, the diversity of voices every community contains is masked. If we are to improve the measurable results of community-based interventions (Merzel & D'Afflitti, 2003; Susser, 1995), we must also attend to the conflicts and alliances that are an unavoidable component of community life (Paul & Demarest, 1984). Speaking more directly to these social realities of community work, and thus endeavoring to learn from them, can only strengthen the ability of public health practitioners to conduct effective research and interventions.

The importance of taking into consideration the multiple facets of community, including ties between people and their shared actions, is a common thread in these definitions. This point was stated strongly in the World Health Organization's 1989 report on community involvement in health (CIH), which stated that "CIH will be quite meaningless in practice if 'community' continues to be used in an undifferentiated way for a geographically defined area" (Oakley, 1989, p. 21). In other words, although collection of statistical information such as ethnic composition and educational attainment of the community may be useful, it does little to elucidate whether the area in question considers itself a community.

In this review of the literature, the vast majority of researchers overlooked precisely those aspects of community that may be most salient. Three of the four aspects of community identified as most important by MacQueen (shared perspective and interests, joint action or activities, and interpersonal relationships) went unexplored in the articles reviewed. The "we feeling" or sense of *communitas* that gives the term community a positive connotation—the very connotation that the papers reviewed are drawing on in employing the term, especially in its use as a euphemism for class or race—was almost totally neglected. Conceptual clarity and agreement regarding the meaning of community, then, has not been reached in the literature on community health.

Regardless of the definition used or discipline of origin, we can agree that community is important to health and well-being. Practitioners and researchers must work together to improve our understanding of the characterizations of community if we are to more fully address the link between community and health.

First, researchers should be explicit in their manuscripts about what they are referring to when they use the term. This helps avoid some of the conceptual muddiness that is brought up by its polyvalence. The polyvalence of community is not bad in and of itself, because the multiple meanings are part of what makes the term so useful. Problems arise for the reader when it is assumed that the term is well-defined. At the level of social networks, reference to MacQueen's attributes (common physical location, shared perspective and interests, joint action or activities, and interpersonal relationships) is a helpful beginning.

Second, we argue that researchers avoid using community as a euphemism for racial and ethnic groups, lower classes, and groups defined by their involvement in so-called risky behaviors. Members of the majority population (e.g., White, middle-class American citizens) are rarely referred to as belonging to communities based on their ethnicity, class, or sexual orientation, but Black, poor, and gay people are placed in communities in a manner that tacitly reinforces the structural inequalities associated with these identities. We would do better to realistically address the heterogeneity and complexity of such identities, including the impact of stigma and marginalization on health and well-being.

Third, with respect to community-level studies, considerable confusion remains about how theories are used or not used. Related to theory construction and testing is the ecological fallacy that threatens the validity of results in community studies. Ecological fallacy is known as error in the interpretation of statistical data in a socioecological study, interpreting general data too particularly or minutely (Last, 1997). The fallacy emerges from projecting to the level of individuals the generalizations that apply to a population or vice versa. It is important for public health professionals to gain more understanding of how to measure and analyze constructs of theories, especially when transforming them into real world settings where theory, research, and practice ought to converge (Glanz, Rimer, & Lewis, 2002; Last, 1997).

Fourth, when using community as an adjective in phrases like community intervention and community-based research, an exploration of what community is being evoked, including a discussion of how that community was defined, who has been chosen as representatives to speak for this community, and in what manner changing community needs and membership will be addressed, should be included in articles describing the research or public health program. A critical distinction is the extent to which community-based research and practice emphasizes conducting interventions in a community as a place or setting (see Table 5.1).

Overall, notions of community can be used to harness and mobilize power, usually through a process of identification in which self-identified community members work to involve others they view as community members. Alternatively, however, definitions of community can also be a way of siphoning off power by excluding unwanted voices from those included in a given community's boundaries. In working with and for communities, researchers must ask: Whose power are we harnessing? To what purpose? On whose authority? And are we doing so in a way that posits real empowerment or just reframes the same old imbalances?

WHY IS COMMUNITY IMPORTANT IN DIABETES PREVENTION AND CONTROL?

Social networks and social support can affect mortality, psychological and physical functioning, and health perceptions, how individuals and families manage disease and illness, and many other intermediate health outcomes.
— *D. L. Patrick and T. M. Wickizer (1995, p. 50)*

At its core, community entails a network of social relations. Community is also a key marker of the quality of human relations and so "resonates with our ideals about the nature of human life" (Norton, McLeroy, Burdine, Felix, & Dorsey, 2002, p. 197). The term refers to something both real and ideal and is replete with both pragmatic and symbolic meanings

(Norton et al., 2002). Cultural anthropologist Victor Turner used the term *communitas* to refer to an acute psychological sense of community that emerges during collective ritual and is characterized by social equality, solidarity, and togetherness (Turner, 1974).

Social cohesion is described as the bonds that link or bring people together by promoting positive norms and facilitative conditions, which leads to collective efficacy. Social cohesion is thought to promote health directly by enabling communities to strengthen their ability to prevent and contain disease at the community level. There is a large, longstanding body of evidence that supports the case that communities, especially neighborhoods, with high social capital—a concept similar to social cohesion—are healthier places. Both social capital and social cohesion have been linked to economic development (Woolcock, 1998), investment in public goods like education (Goldin & Katz, 1998), crime and violence rates in a community (Kennedy, Kawachi, Prothrow-Stith, Lochner, & Gupta, 1998; Sampson et al., 1997), and improved health status (Holtgrave & Crosby, 2003; Kawachi, 1999).

In addition to the traditional correlates of diabetes—demographic characteristics, family history, and access to care—the social determinants of health and social context may more strongly influence individual and collective health behavior, as well as drive beliefs and actions about diabetes prevention, treatment, and control. Understanding social context makes it possible to evaluate a wider range of factors that potentially impact diabetes-related health disparities (Emmons et al., 2008). Although mechanisms of the impact of social cohesion and social relationships on community health need further investigation, there is compelling and persuasive evidence that the lack of social relationships continues to be a major risk factor for disease and death (House, Landis, & Umberson, 1988; Marmot, Friel, Bell, Houweling, & Taylor, 2008; Patrick & Wickizer, 1995; Berkman & Syme, 1979).

Patrick and Wickizer (1995) offer an organizing framework for studying community and health that illuminates pathways by which community operates directly or mediates risk factors and health outcomes. We have customized the framework (see Figure 5.2) to illustrate a few of the characteristics and processes of diabetes that may be relevant for intervening and future study. According to the developers of the organizing framework, social and physical environments are influenced by cultural, political, and economic systems, each respectively reflecting such elements as beliefs and values, health policy and community organizing, and distribution of income, employment, and housing (Patrick & Wickizer, 1995, p. 67).

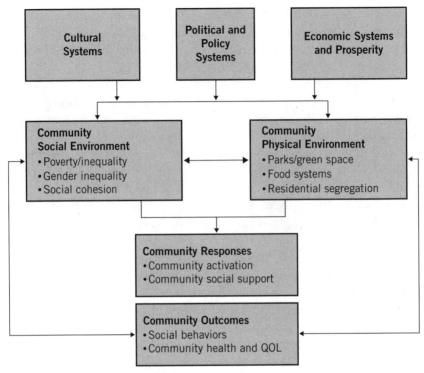

Figure 5.2 A Framework for Studying Community and Health

The next determinants illustrated in the framework are the social and physical environment. In the example of diabetes, as in many chronic diseases, social inequality and poverty are hypothesized to be among the most salient contributors to a health disparity. Physical characteristics of inadequate food systems, the lack of places to engage in physical activity, and residential segregation should also be considered in the model as impacting diabetes control. The final components of the framework include community-level responses needed to support healthy behaviors, community health, and quality of life. The model elucidates both direct and indirect effects of community, noting that the social and physical environment may influence community outcomes directly or indirectly. In addition to its direct effect on community health, poverty might also have an indirect effect through community response. Designing and organizing medical care to low-income, uninsured individuals diagnosed with diabetes is an example of community response.

Finally, the model draws attention to a few of a longer list of determinants operating or having an influence at the community level, largely because communities exist not only as physical structures but also as social and economic ones (Patrick & Wickizer, 1995). Determinants with social and economic consequences, such as deprivation and inequality, systematically influence community life and the life chances of its residents. Most evidence recognizes that behavior does not occur in isolation and that for community-based efforts to yield beneficial outcomes for both place and people, social and cultural influences will need to be supported to advance health and well-being for those experiencing diabetes or any other potentially severe chronic disease.

LINGERING CHALLENGES

After naming a community in the most productive way to influence positive changes in health status, we are challenged to access and engage those affected through respectful and equitable processes and to acknowledge their agency in defining a partnership with us in eliminating an identified burden of disease. This type of approach democratizes science and is bidirectional with the community. It is cooperative and is structured for co-learning. It fundamentally changes the role of the researcher, the researched, the practitioner, and those for whom a program is intended to benefit. Toward this end we have not adequately challenged the assumptions of participation in public health research and practice. There is now a growing body of community-based participatory literature and trade journals to respond to this challenge like the journal *Progress in Community Health Partnerships: Research, Education, and Action,* which is published by Johns Hopkins University Press and funded by the Robert Wood Johnson Foundation.

Participatory research is one strategy and a "first step toward community involvement" (Nichter, 1999, p. 300). Anthropologist Mark Nichter, drawing upon his work in South India, believes participatory research (a) fosters an alliance between professional researchers and lay representatives, affording the latter the opportunity to contribute to the process and direction of enquiry; (b) challenges assumptions made by planners and decision makers, providing a check to the incompleteness and time-bound nature of expert knowledge and placing the opinions of stakeholders center stage; and (c) enables dialogue by translating popular knowledge into a form that planners and decision makers understand, as well as translating expert knowledge into a form the lay population can understand (Nichter, 1999, p. 305). In this context, we have an opportunity to expand our understanding of what it means to be a culturally competent researcher and practitioner.

Another critical issue related to participation is the extent to which community-based research and practice emphasizes community as a place or setting, with or without active engagement of community members, and with them involved in a few or most aspects of the research process or project. Figure 5.3 highlights these distinctions as fundamental to ensuring a definition that accurately represents and guides research and practice with communities. Granted, not all community members desire to be completely immersed in a research study or project; yet, participant voices and perspectives should be made transparent and may require different types of representation, depending on the focus of the research or project. For example, engaging people with diabetes and family members of people with diabetes is essential in the development of community-based interventions.

The demographics of what we have known over the past 40 years as the inner city is steadily being modified by gentrification and the influx of diverse migrant groups from neighboring borders and around the world, among other things. How is gentrification shifting the disease burden among historically segregated communities of color? How is social cohesion and social capital within these displaced communities affected such that poor health status is exacerbated? The answers to these and other questions can inform public health work to eliminate diabetes disparities.

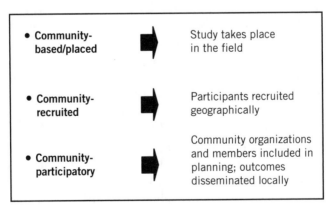

Figure 5.3 Language of Community Public Health Research

Extant community involvement models have not kept pace with the changing demographics, landscape, and dynamics of contemporary urban environments. There is a need for more intervention research, for example, that describes the diversity within racial and ethnic groups and captures aspects of this diversity in strategies to eliminate diabetes disparities (e.g., clarifying historical, geographic, and cultural differences between Hispanic/Latino groups and incorporating this knowledge into diabetes prevention and control programs). Approaching communities disproportionately affected by diabetes as communities of identity allows us to explore the multidimensionality of ethnic and cultural identity and how health-related beliefs, practices, social interactions, and norms are shaped within these communities and in response to external forces (Jones & Liburd, in press).

Public health practitioners have a rich history of seeking out and engaging community leaders in public health interventions. More often than not, we find these leaders juggling numerous social, economic, and political challenges that are ever-changing and reconstructing their environment. There tends to be a limited pool of community volunteers and health advocates in any one community, and their time and talents are desired by many. The household status and day-to-day patterns of contemporary urban communities (e.g., single-parent homes, two-income families, long work hours, long commutes, and absence of the extended family to assist with homemaking and childrearing) suggest urban dwellers may be turning inward. For example, persons with young families appear to be choosing to invest more time after work in their children's activities and other personal interests, and elder residents express concerns about their safety at selected times and places. How can we recruit more community members and institutions into the work of eliminating diabetes disparities?

Today, public health workers and the communities they serve observe the market and other forces of modernity steer and shape their realities, including many of the risks to their health. There is a need to understand the lived experience of race in the U.S. We must work to discourage policies that mitigate community health. There are encouraging signs by more recent public health action that has named key sectors of the political economy as units of practice and communities of identity suitable for public health interventions, such as the fast food industry, local agriculture, and working with systems of education to increase the number of persons graduating from high school. Some examples of these community-based approaches are provided in chapters 8–16. We are inspired by the growing movement of participatory and community-driven approaches to eliminating diabetes disparities in communities of color across the United States.

REFERENCES

Amick, B.B., Levine, S. Tarlov, A.R., & Walsh, D.C. (1995). Society and Health. New York: Oxford University Press.

Berkman, L. F., & Syme, L. (1979). Social networks, host resistance and mortality: A nine-year follow-up study of Alemeda County residents. *American Journal of Epidemiology, 109,* 186–204.

Bernard, H. R. (1995). *Research methods in anthropology: Qualitative and quantitative approaches* (2nd ed.). Walnut Creek, CA: AltaMira Press.

Centers for Disease Control and Prevention. (2005). Epi Info™ 3.3.2. Atlanta, GA: Centers for Disease Control and Prevention.

Coffey, A., & Atkinson, P. (1996). *Making sense of qualitative data: Contemporary research strategies.* Thousand Oaks, CA: Sage Publications.

Emmons, K., Puleo, E., McNeill, L. H., Bennett, G., Chan, S., & Syngal, S. (2008). Colorectal cancer screening awareness and intentions among low income, sociodemographically diverse adults under age 50. *Cancer Causes & Control, 19,* 1031–1041.

Frumkin, H. (2003). Healthy places: Exploring the evidence. *American Journal of Public Health, 93(9),* 1451–1456.

Glanz, K., Rimer, B. K., & Lewis, F. M. (2002). *Health behavior and health education: Theory research and practice* (3rd ed.). San Francisco: Jossey-Bass.

Goldin C., & Katz, L. G. (1998). *Human capital and social capital: The rise of secondary schooling in America, 1910 to 1940: Paper no. 6439.* Cambridge, MA: National Bureau of Economic Research Working.

Green, L. W., & Kreuter, M. W. (1999). *Health promotion planning: An educational and ecological approach.* Mountain View, CA: Mayfield.

Hoffer, C. R. (1931). Understanding the community. *American Journal of Sociology, 36(4),* 616–624.

Holtgrave, D. R., & Crosby, R. A. (2003). Social capital, poverty, and income inequality as predictors of gonorrhea, syphilis, chlamydia and AIDS case rates in the United States. *Sexually Transmitted Infections, 79,* 62–64.

House, J. S., Landis, K. R., & Umberson, D. (1988). Social relationships and health. *Science, 241(4865),* 540–545.

Israel, B., Checkoway, B., Schulz, A., & Zimmerman, M. (1994). Health education and community empowerment: Conceptualizing and measuring perceptions of individual, organizational and community control. *Health Education Quarterly, 21,* 147–170.

Jones, H., & Liburd, L. (in press). Reversing the tide of type 2 diabetes among African Americans through interdisciplinary psychology and medical anthropology research. In *Urban health and society: Interdisciplinary approaches to research and practice.* Eds. Freudenberg, N., Klitzman, S., and Saegert, S. San Francisco: Jossey Bass.

Kawachi, I. (1999). Social capital and community effects on population and individual health. *Annals of the New York Academy of Sciences, 896,* 120–130.

Kennedy, B., Kawachi, I., Prothrow-SmithStith, D., Lochner, K., & Gupta, V. (1998). Social capital, income inequality, and firearm violent crime. *Social Science & Medicine, 47*, 7–17.

Krieger, N., Chen, J. T., Waterman, P. D., Rehkoph, D. H., & Subramanian, S. V. (2005). Painting a truer picture of US socioeconomic and racial/ethnic health inequalities: The Public Health Disparities Geocoding Project. *American Journal of Public Health, 95(2)*, 312–323.

Labonte, R. (1997). Community, community development, and the forming of authentic partnerships: Some critical reflections. In M. Minkler (Ed.), *Community organizing and community building for health.* New Brunswick, NJ: Rutgers University Press, pp. 88–101.

Last, J. M. (1997). *Public health and human ecology* (2nd ed.). Stamford, CT: Appleton and Lange.

MacQueen, K. M. (2001). What is community? An evidence-based definition for participatory public health. *American Journal of Public Health, 91(12)*, 1929–1938.

Marmot, M. (2001). Income inequality, social environment, and inequalities in health. *Journal of Policy Analysis and Management. Winter; 20(1):* 156–159.

Marmot, M., Friel, S., Bell, R., Houweling, T. A., & Taylor, S. (2008). Closing the gap in a generation: Health equity through action on the social determinants of health. *Lancet, 372(9650)*, 1661–1669.

McLeroy, K. R., Bibeau, D., Steckler, A., & Glanz, K. (1988). An ecological perspective on health promotion programs. *Health Education Quarterly, 15(4)*, 351–377.

McLeroy, K. R., Norton, B. L., Kegler, M. C., Burdine, J. N., & Sumaya, C. V. (2003). Community-based interventions. *American Journal of Public Health, 93(4)*, 529–533.

Merzel, C., & D'Afflitti, J. (2003). Reconsidering community-based health promotion: Promise, performance, and potential. *American Journal of Public Health, 93(4)*, 557–574.

Nichter, M. (1999). In R. A. Hahn (Ed.), *Anthropology in public health: Bridging differences in culture and society* (pp. 300–324). New York: Oxford University Press.

Norton, B. L., McLeroy, K. R., Burdine, J. N., Felix, M. R. J., & Dorsey, A. M. (2002). Community capacity: Concept, theory, and methods. In R. J. DiClemente, R. A. Crosby, & M. C. Kegler (Eds.), *Emerging theories in health promotion practice and research: Strategies for improving public health.* San Francisco: Jossey-Bass.

Oakley, P. (1989). *Community involvement in health development: An examination of the critical issues.* Geneva: World Health Organization.

Patrick, D. L., & Wickizer, T. M. (1995). Community and health. In B. C. Amick, S. Levine, A. R. Tarlov, & D. C. Walsh (Eds.), *Society and health* (pp. 46–92). New York: Oxford University Press.

Paul, B., & Demarest, W. J. (1984). Citizen participation overplanned: The case of a health project in the Guatemalan community of San Pedro La Laguna. *Social Science & Medicine, 19(3)*, 185–192.

Robinson, R. G. (2005). Community development model for public health applications: Overview of a model to eliminate population disparities. *Health Promotion Practice, 6(3)*, 338–346.

Sampson, R. J., Raudenbush, S. W., & Earls, F. J. (1997). Neighborhoods and violent crime: A multilevel study of collective efficacy. *Science, 277*, 918–924.

Spears, E. G. (2006). *Toxic knowledge: A social history of environmental health in the New South's model city, Anniston, Alabama, 1872–present.* Atlanta: Emory University.

Susser, M. (1995). The tribulations of trials: Intervention in communities. *American Journal of Public Health, 85(2)*, 156–158.

Taylor, C. (1978). Development and the transition to global health. *Medical Anthropology, 2*, 59–70.

Turner, V. (1974). Passages, margins, and poverty: Religious symbols of communitas. In *Dramas, fields, and metaphors: Symbolic action in human society* (pp. 231–271). Ithaca, NY: Cornell University Press.

U.S. Department of Health and Human Services. *Planned approach to community health: Guide for the local coordinator.* Available at http://www.cdc.gov/nccdphp/patch/. Retrieved June 12, 2009.

U.S. Department of Health and Human Services. (1986). Secretary's Task Force on Black & Minority Health. *Report of the Secretary's Task Force on Black & Minority Health.* Washington, D.C.: U.S. Department of Health and Human Services, Office of Minority Health.

Walter, C. L. (1997). Community building practice: A conceptual framework. In M. Minkler (Ed.), *Community organizing and community building for health* (pp. 68–83). New Brunswick, NJ: Rutgers University Press.

Winslow, C. E. A. (1920). The untilled fields of public health. *Science, 51(1306)*, 23–33.

Woolcock, M. (1998). Social capital and economic development: Toward a theoretical synthesis and policy framework. *Theory and Society, 27*, 151–208.

World Health Organization & United Nation's Children's Fund. Primary health care: Report of the International Conference on primary health care, Alma-Ata, USSR, 6–12 September 1978. Geneva: World Health Organization.

Wright, R. J., & Subramanian, S. V. (2007). Advancing a multilevel framework for epidemiologic research on asthma disparities. *Chest, 32*, 757S–769S.

6

Recontextualizing Place: The Influence of Residential Segregation on Health Disparities in the United States

AMANDA M. NAVARRO

INTRODUCTION

For centuries scholars have demonstrated the relationship between place, health, and well-being (Institute of Medicine, 2002). Place refers to the various environments (e.g., social, economic, physical, and built) and settings (e.g., school, church, workplace, and neighborhood) where people live, work, learn, play, and worship (Institute of Medicine, 2002). Early origins of public health recognized the influence of place on health and the effectiveness of environmental interventions to control and eradicate infectious diseases (e.g., safe water systems, food safety, and reduced crowding). However, as the prevalence of infectious diseases declined in the 20th century, public health interventions were more narrowly directed at the individual's behavior and risk-reduction level to address chronic diseases.

In recent years, the importance of place to health status has once again been brought to our attention as our understanding of how social, economic, and political conditions and resources either promote good or bad health. These life-enhancing conditions and resources, referred to as the social determinants of health, can have a significant influence on health outcomes (Baker, Metzler, & Galea, 2005). The social determinants include employment and education opportunities, transportation, housing, retail provision, recreation facilities, land use, health services, environmental hazards, social networks and social cohesion, and cultural norms and values. These determinants have shown multiple effects on health, including higher rates of death and disease burden, low birth weight, and decreased self-rated health (Macintyre & Ellaway, 2003; White & Borrell, 2006; Williams & Jackson, 2005).

The unequal distribution of life-enhancing conditions and resources across various populations is increasingly recognized as a significant contributor to racial and ethnic health disparities (Schulz et al., 2008). When remedies are available but not used, modifiable inequalities in living conditions become inequities that are morally unacceptable. For example, one critical health-related neighborhood problem is the inadequate supply of affordable housing. Safe and well-maintained housing is associated with health by protecting against communicable diseases, injuries, poisonings, and chronic diseases, as well as reducing psychological and social stresses (Anderson et al., 2003). Excessive housing costs can force household members to limit expenditures on other necessities (e.g., food, transportation, and medical care) and contribute to family instability (e.g., frequent moving and homelessness). These effects of housing insecurity have negative implications for both physical and mental health (Anderson et al., 2003). In addition, unhealthy housing conditions are associated with increased risk of diabetes (Schootman et al., 2007). Recent evidence suggests that affordable housing can help improve physical and mental health outcomes by freeing resources for food and health care expenditures, reducing stress, creating an increased sense of security and control over one's physical environment, and limiting exposures to allergens and toxins (Lubell, Crain, & Cohen, 2007).

In this respect, the concept of place can also be an important construct in understanding the role of social, political, and economic forces that foster increased health risks and poor health outcomes, particularly as it relates to the social and political institutions that create and perpetuate social inequities in health (House & Williams, 2003; Mays, Cochran, & Barnes, 2007). To quote Pompay and colleagues, "The study of the places people inhabit may still allow us to explore the way in which structures work themselves through into the dynamics of everyday life" (Pompay, Williams, Thomas, & Gatrell, 2003, p. 400).

Some argue that these persistent inequities are due to racism, an ideology of inferiority that is used to justify the differential treatment of members of racial and ethnic groups by individuals and societal institutions (House & Williams, 2003). To explain the relationships between deliberate decisions of the powerful and undesirable consequences for the powerless, some researchers have now posited that race-based differences in health are in large part due to racism. As such, racism is increasingly being recognized as a primary driving force that influences decisions made by persons and institutions that control economic and political power to restrict opportunities for communities of color. The construct of racism, translated through institutional policies and practices, can limit access to opportunities and resources that promote health (House & Williams, 2003; Jones, 2000; Schulz, Williams, Israel, & Lempert, 2002; Williams, 1999). Even when controlling for socioeconomic status, racial disparities in health persist as a result of correlated structural factors like segregation, economic disadvantage, and discrimination (Hofrichter, 2003).

The spatial segregation of racial and ethnic populations, that is, the physical expression of institutional racism, is a primary cause of racial differences of socioeconomic status by limiting access to education and employment opportunities and a key mechanism by which racial inequality has been created and reinforced (Williams, 1999; Williams & Collins, 2001). Increasing evidence generated by various academic disciplines, such as social epidemiology, anthropology, psychology, demography, and sociology, have revealed the significant impact that underlying social and economic structures have on communities and their ability to support and promote good health.

Specifically, researchers have argued that race-based residential segregation can have multiple effects on economic and educational opportunities, which can "adversely affect health by creating a broad range of pathogenic residential conditions that can induce adverse effects on health status" (Gee, 2002; Schulz et al., 2002; Williams & Collins, 2001). Several conceptual frameworks that illustrate the structural forces (e.g., macro, social, and public policies) that influence social and economic determinants of health, as well as community-based models that elucidate the pathways by which racial residential segregation produces disparities in diabetes, do exist (Schulz et al., 2005; World Health Organization, 2007). However, the need to explicitly test the multiple pathways and effects of racism on public and institutional policy, residential segregation, and health inequities remains.

This chapter reviews evidence that suggests that racism, manifested through deliberate public policy and institutional decisions, causes the segregation of poor communities and communities of color, which subsequently creates unhealthy living conditions and perpetuates health inequities. This chapter will explicitly explore the role that residential segregation in urban areas plays in limiting access to opportunities and resources essential for promoting health and preventing chronic diseases like diabetes, and in turn, influences health outcomes among racial/ethnic groups. As a growing proportion of the world's population live in urban areas that increasingly become concentrated with economically and socially disadvantaged populations, cities will become the "predominant social context for most of the world's population" (Galea, Freudenberg, & Vlahov, 2005) and a critical focal point to address racial and ethnic health disparities. This chapter will focus on three general issues: (a) the physical, social, and economic disintegration of some parts of urban America; (b) the role of residential segregation (i.e., separation of racial/ethnic groups and concentration of the poor) in creating unhealthy neighborhood living conditions; and (c) the impact of negative neighborhood conditions on health outcomes. In the conclusion, we propose several approaches to address residential segregation as means for eliminating disparities in diabetes as an example.

THE DISINTEGRATION OF SOME PARTS OF CONTEMPORARY URBAN AMERICA

The large migration in the latter half of the 20th century of primarily White middle-class and working-class Americans from cities to the surrounding suburbs led to significant reductions in population size, density, diversity, and resources in the cities (Freudenberg, Galea, & Vlahov, 2006). Referred to as the spatial mismatch hypothesis, the migration of high-wage manufacturing jobs from older urban areas to newer suburban areas in the Northeast and Midwest, coupled with discriminatory institutional policies and practices, has influenced unemployment and higher poverty rates among African Americans in urban communities (Kain, 1992). This mass exodus deprived cities of economic and social opportunities, including jobs and education, and concentrated illness and disease in these areas (Freudenberg, 2000; Galea, Freudenberg, & Vlahov, 2005). The divestment of resources in urban areas has led to the dwindling of essential resources and services to promote health and prevent disease, producing urban pockets of poverty and racially segregated neighborhoods (Vlahov, Gibble, Freudenberg, & Galea, 2004).

While all forms of segregation were declared unconstitutional through a series of U.S. Supreme Court rulings, beginning with *Brown v. Board of Education* (1954), racial and economic segregation is still prevalent in many urban neighborhoods across the nation (Kwate, 2007; Williams & Collins, 2001). Regarded as the "American apartheid," African Americans, and to some extent Hispanics/Latinos, continue to be concentrated in central cities, which are typically the oldest, more dilapidated, and most socioeconomically deprived part of the metropolitan area (Acevedo-Garcia & Lochner, 2003; Zenk et al., 2005). This has resulted in fewer services and resources that are provided in neighborhoods in which more socially disadvantaged people are concentrated. Thus, people who are already poor also live in resource-deprived neighborhoods that lack the adequate infrastructure to lead healthy lives (Macintyre & Ellaway, 2003).

For example, research shows that residential segregation has resulted in segregated public elementary and high schools across the country. For many communities, local government controls funding for public school education; thus, the resources in those communities determines the quality of schools (Williams & Collins, 2001). Therefore, the exodus of businesses and jobs decreases the local tax base, impacting the ability of municipalities to provide adequate funding for education. The concentration of poverty in these communities is considered to be the primary cause of problems experienced by segregated schools. The lack of adequate community resources to provide quality public school education (e.g., limited curricula, deteriorated facilities, and less qualified teachers) due to residential segregation, coupled with higher levels of neighborhood crime, contributes to poor academic performance and high rates of school dropouts (Charles, 2003; Williams & Collins, 2001). Conversely, children residing in more integrated, affluent neighborhoods were significantly more likely to attend high school and enroll in a four-year college (Charles, 2003). Research suggests that education is the strongest predictor of health, showing that less education results in earlier death and higher rates of diabetes-related risk factors like being overweight and physical inactivity (Freudenberg & Ruglis, 2007).

Municipal government policies can significantly influence urban health by providing services, regulating activities that affect health, and setting parameters for urban development (Galea et al., 2005). A variety of government activities, such as those in housing, employment, criminal justice, transportation, employment, and public education, can affect health. Policies promulgated by these various sectors can play a powerful role in reducing or exacerbating health disparities by determining the level of essential services to provide in local communities.

One example of this was the massive housing destruction and en-
suing epidemics that occurred in the Bronx in the 1970s as a result of
planned shrinkage. A term first used by civic leaders in New York City,
planned shrinkage was a process proposed to guide the downsizing of
urban areas by removing essential municipal services like police patrols,
fire departments, garbage removal, public transit, and sanitation services
from communities through a variety of policy mechanisms (Fullilove,
2003). Planned shrinkage was applied to many New York City communities, among them the impoverished area of the South Bronx where they
were subjected to the withdrawal of fire services beginning in 1971. The
reduction in fire services contributed to an enormous increase in fires,
which moved across the neighborhood in a contagious fashion and triggered a fire and housing abandonment epidemic in the area (Fullilove,
2003). This resulted in outmigration, homelessness, and overcrowding,
which ultimately had profound effects on the public's health. Studies
examining the impact of this contagious housing destruction on the
health of local residents showed large numbers of residents displaced
into adjoining neighborhoods, which resulted in marked increase and
subsequent spread of illnesses and a decrease in social conditions (i.e.,
violence and disruption of social networks) in these surrounding areas
(Fullilove, 2003). Referred to as "the synergism of plagues" (Wallace,
1988), "the self-reinforcing, interactive mix of contagious urban decay
and deterioration in both public health and public order" led to marked
increases in tuberculosis, gonorrhea, HIV, homicides, suicides, drug
overdose deaths, infant mortality, and low birth weight (Wallace, & Wallace, 1998). On the basis of this research, it is apparent that the depletion
of municipal services in the Bronx provides a stark illustration of the col-
lapse of public health triggered in large part by government policies.

Contemporary housing and lending practices and city zoning decisions have exacerbated residential segregation of racial and ethnic
groups across urban neighborhoods (Charles, 2003; House & Williams,
2003). For example, redlining—which refers to the practice of denying
or increasing the cost of services, such as banking, insurance, employment, and access to health care and food to particular geographical areas
because of the race or income of its residents—has affected the health of
cities. Redlining has its roots in federal policy, which subsidized home-
ownership by insuring low-interest bank loans for home mortgages (PolicyLink, 2008). This policy has been attributed to the increase of residential segregation by demarcating low-income, minority neighborhoods as

least desirable, further accelerating the deterioration of neighborhoods and increasing the exposure to harmful conditions and diseases.

A recent study found that Chinese Americans residing in nonred-lined areas had poor general and mental health, were more likely to be exposed to negative neighborhood attributes (e.g., toxic waste facilities, fast food restaurants, alcohol, and junk food advertisements), and lacked institutional resources (e.g., shortage of physicians, poorer schools, and lack of supermarkets and adequate public transportation) (Gee, 2002).

Zoning and other land-use decisions are often based on economic and political considerations and have been detrimental to urban poor, racial, and ethnic communities (Klitzman, Matte, & Kass, 2006). This land-use planning tool is used to designate certain areas as appropriate for certain uses (e.g., residential, commercial, and industrial) and can have a significant influence on neighborhood conditions and health outcomes (Maantay, 2001). For example, industrial areas tend to carry higher environmental burden than residential areas, such as poor air quality, noise pollution, storage of hazardous materials, and the proliferation of noxious waste-related facilities (Maantay, 2001). These noxious land uses tend to be concentrated in poor communities and communities of color, having significant implications for health disparities. Zoning policies, although intended to protect the public's health and safety, have often shown to be exclusionary. By delineating between more and less desirable areas, zoning policies can either attract or deter commercial businesses and essential services into these neighborhoods (Maantay, 2001). For example, zoning regulations can prohibit low- and moderate-income housing in certain municipalities, as well as provide little incentive for supermarkets and green spaces to be built.

The subprime lending crisis in 2008 exposed the discriminatory practices by lending corporations in targeting low-income minority communities for high-risk loans. Recent evidence demonstrates that lending practices by major mortgage lending institutions discriminated against residents of low-income communities of color by providing higher-rate mortgages, loans, and closing title fees to African American and Hispanic/Latino borrowers as compared to White borrowers (Bocian, Ernst, & Li, 2006; Campen et al., 2007; Woodward, 2008). Many cities are experiencing significant difficulty funding public services with balanced budgets as a result of the housing market crisis that is a driving force in the economic downturn that started in December 2007. Unlike past downturns when housing was viewed as an area of economic strength to help mitigate fiscal damage, approximately two-thirds of our nation's cities have experienced an increase in foreclosures and a third are facing a drop in revenue (Dorn, Garrett, Holahan, & Williams, 2008). These communities are further burdened by the negative impacts of the subprime crisis—foreclosures, depleting property values, lower tax bases, abandoned homes and increased crime—which is further aggravating health inequities.

IMPACT OF RESIDENTIAL SEGREGATION ON NEIGHBORHOOD LIVING CONDITIONS

Residential segregation continues to persist between racial, ethnic, and poor populations due to social, economic, and political forces that have historically concentrated large numbers of low-income, racial, and ethnic groups in central cities. Despite general declines in residential segregation in the United States from 1980 to 2000, African Americans continue to experience higher rates of segregation than any other racial/ethnic group (Iceland, Weinberg, & Steinmetz, 2002; Wilkes & Iceland, 2004). One study showed that the poorer the neighborhood, the greater the proportion of African American residents, with over eight times as many African Americans in the lowest-wealth neighborhoods compared to the highest-wealth areas (Morland, Wing, Diez Roux, & Poole, 2002). Further, despite improvements in economic integration, African Americans with higher incomes are less able to reside in neighborhoods that are commensurate with their socioeconomic status and tend to live in poorer neighborhoods than do Whites (Kwate, 2007). Other studies reported increasing residential segregation of Hispanics/Latinos and Asians in the many metropolitan areas (Charles, 2003; Iceland et al., 2002; Logan, Stults, & Farley, 2004).

Segregated urban neighborhoods are not designed to promote or facilitate the maintenance of healthy behaviors; therefore, their attributes (e.g., toxic buildings, air pollution, lack of green spaces, and limited access to healthy foods and quality health care services) pose negative health consequences (Perdue, Stone, & Gostin, 2003). This "urban health penalty" constructs the concentration of poor people in urban areas and exposes them to unhealthy physical and social environments, which leads to a disproportionate burden of poor health (Freudenberg, Galea, & Vlahov, 2005). Given the growing evidence that disease burden and resources for health are socially and spatially structured, coupled with increasing proportions of racial and ethnic populations inhabiting impoverished neighborhoods, increased attention has focused on examining how urban neighborhood conditions affect health and contribute to racial and ethnic health disparities. The following discussions will elucidate how residential segregation creates poor neighborhood conditions, particularly as it relates to limited access to health services, green spaces, and healthy foods, which ultimately contributes to disparities as in diabetes.

Access to Health Services

Across our nation's communities, inequities in access to health care services exist for those that are uninsured, Medicaid recipients, many racial and ethnic groups, and other vulnerable populations. Access to quality health care is an important component of diabetes management and the prevention of complications associated with diabetes. Poverty and the lack of insurance have a significant impact on people's ability to obtain care. Persons who lack health insurance are more likely to have unmet needs for health care and lack a usual source of care (National Center for Health Statistics [NCHS], 2007). Not having medical insurance is a major barrier to the receipt of needed health care services (Diamant, Hays, Morales, Ford, Calmes, & Asch, 2004). Adults and children from all racial and ethnic groups are more likely not to have a usual place of care than Whites (NCHS, 2007). Of those having a usual place of care, Whites are more likely to use a doctor's office or HMO, whereas Hispanics/Latinos primarily used a clinic or health center, and African Americans have a greater likelihood of using the hospital emergency room or outpatient department (Lethbridge-Cejku & Vickerie, 2005). Studies have also shown that many low-income individuals do not seek needed medical care due to competing priorities, such as having to pay for food, shelter, or utilities bills (Diamant et al., 2004). Further, rising fuel costs, the home foreclosure crisis, and the nation's economic downtown have led to the increase in delaying or not seeking care because of people's limited family budgets (Cunningham & Felland, 2008).

Residential segregation and the subsequent divestment of services in many urban centers have contributed to inequities in health care. Residents living in segregated communities face greater barriers in accessing health services due to a growing shortage of providers and health services and the greater likelihood of being uninsured (Cunningham & Felland, 2008). Approximately 56 million Americans are medically disenfranchised, that is, with no or inadequate access to primary and preventive care due to local shortages of such physicians (National Association of Community Health Centers & The Robert Graham Center, 2007). According to a recent report released by the National Association of Community Health Centers (NACHC), over 50 million people do not have access to a usual source of care because of a lack or inequitable distribution of primary care physicians (NACHC & The Robert Graham Center, 2007). Exacerbating the problem is the lack of physicians willing and able to work in impoverished neighborhoods (Hawkins & Proser, 2004). Physicians who practice in low-income minority neighborhoods are less likely to be board certified and less able to provide high quality care and referrals to specialty care (Williams &, Jackson, 2005). Additionally, pharmacies located in segregated areas are less likely to have adequate medication supplies, and hospitals in these neighborhoods are more likely to close (Williams & Jackson, 2005).

For these reasons racial and ethnic groups, which tend to be concentrated in cities and are disproportionately poor and uninsured, are more likely to rely on the safety net system. This system consists of a wide variety of providers delivering care to low-income and other vulnerable populations, including the uninsured and those covered by Medicaid. Major safety net providers include public hospitals, community health centers, teaching and community hospitals, private physicians, and other providers who deliver a substantial amount of care to these populations (Agency for Healthcare Research and Quality, 2003). However, despite federally funded programs like Medicaid and community health centers, many low-income, racial, and ethnic urban residents continue to confront overwhelming obstacles in obtaining adequate health care.

Community Health Centers

For over four decades, community health centers have created the largest national network of safety net primary health care services offering comprehensive community-oriented health care that is accessible and affordable to millions of low-income and medically underserved Americans (Hawkins & Proser, 2004; NACHC, 2005). Community health center patients are disproportionately low-income (92%), depend on Medicaid (35%), are uninsured (40%), are racial and ethnic minorities (64%), and tend to live in inner city communities (50%) (NACHC, 2008). Community health centers serve approximately 17 million patients around the country, offering a range of physical and mental health services, as well as transportation, translation, and culturally sensitive services (NACHC, 2008). Currently, over 1,000 community health centers deliver care in every state and territory, and with the increase of unemployed and uninsured or publicly insured adults in recent months, the need for safety net providers has increased (Proser, Shin, & Hawkins, 2005).

Many studies have recognized community health centers as models for screening, diagnosis, and managing chronic conditions, as well as eliminating health disparities and improving health outcomes for higher-risk populations by establishing themselves as a usual source of care and effectively meeting the needs of low-income and diverse patients who often face multiple and complex barriers (Hawkins & Proser, 2004; Hicks, O'Malley, & Lieu, 2006; NACHC, 2005; Politzer et al., 2001; Shi, Starfield, Politzer, & Regan, 2002; Shi & Stevens, 2007). Further, there is significant evidence demonstrating that the presence of a health center in a community is associated with decreased emergency room visits (Choudhry et al., 2007; Hawkins & Schwartz, 2003). A more recent study found that between 1998 and 2002, health centers experienced "statistically and clinically significant" improvements in diabetes preventive care practices, including hemoglobin A1c and cholesterol levels (Chin et al., 2007).

Yet, despite the overwhelming evidence that community health centers have been successful in providing care to those most in need and in controlling costs, cuts in Medicaid eligibility and benefits jeopardize the ability of health centers to continue to provide their current level of care. This financial strain on health centers is compounded by the ever-growing numbers of uninsured, low-income, and chronically ill patients, usually among the most difficult and costly to treat because they delay needed care (NACHC, 2005). While health centers are able to collect payments from Medicaid, Medicare, and other public insurance programs, they continue to face substantial unpaid charges (NACHC, 2005). As of 2004, community health centers provided almost $1.6 billion in uncompensated care. Therefore, adequate payments from third-party insurers (e.g., Medicaid) are essential in the financial stability of health centers.

Further, despite the passage of Title VI of the Civil Rights Act of 1964 and the subsequent implementation of the Medicare program in 1966, racial and ethnic segregation within the health care system persists (Smith, 2005). As a result of a segregated health care system, many racial and ethnic minorities in metropolitan areas rely on receiving medical care from medical schools, teaching hospitals, and public clinics, where they are less likely than White patients who see private doctors in their offices for outpatient care to establish long-term, consistent, and trusting relationships with providers.

Medicaid

Enacted in 1965 under Title XIX of the Social Security Act and considered the linchpin in our health care system, Medicaid is the nation's publicly financed health coverage program for low-income individuals and families who often lack access to employer-based health insurance, cannot afford private insurance, or are excluded from private insurance based on their health status (Kaiser Commission on Medicaid and the Uninsured, 2009). As of 2005, over 58 million people, approximately 20% of the total U.S. population, were covered by Medicaid (Kaiser Commission on Medicaid and the Uninsured, 2008). A recent report by the Kaiser Commission on Medicaid and the Uninsured estimated that a 1% increase in the national unemployment rate would increase Medicaid and the State Children's Health Insurance Program (SCHIP) enrollment of non-elderly adults and children by 1 million and would result in the number of uninsured adults to rise by 1.1 million (Dorn et al., 2008). The authors also concluded that a 1% increase in unemployment would lead to a 3–4% reduction in Medicaid and SCHIP spending. The Medicaid program is an essential source of financing for safety net providers that serve the uninsured and a significant portion of the low-income population (Kaiser Commission on Medicaid and the Uninsured, 2009). Further, Medicaid is the largest source of third-party payments to community health centers and public hospitals.

Medicaid's dependence on public assistance makes it particularly vulnerable to reductions in financial support. Medicaid is often the first to experience cutbacks, especially as states face limited fiscal capacity, strain during economic turndowns to meet increased demands for Medicaid coverage with declining state revenues, and the pressure to balance their budgets (Dorn et al., 2008). During an economic downturn, many people lose employer-sponsored insurance, which increases the number of uninsured as well as the number of people who qualify for Medicaid (Dorn et al., 2008). Moreover, while unemployment raises caseloads and costs for Medicaid, state revenues decline. Because of state balanced budget requirements, the loss of revenue and increase in expenditures resulting from economic downturn often leads to significant cutbacks in needs-based assistance like Medicaid (Dorn et al., 2008). However, it is during a time when state residents have the greatest need for help that cutbacks in assistance are most likely to occur (Dorn et al., 2008). Implementing cost-containment strategies to Medicaid (e.g., eligibility and benefit reductions or restrictions and provider payment freeze or cut) will inevitably impact the fundamental safety net system that provides much needed services to poorer and sicker populations.

Access to Green Spaces

The built environment, including green spaces, highways, and housing, has a significant influence on physical and mental health. The divestment in resources and services of these communities leads to the deterioration of the physical environment in poor neighborhoods, resulting in disproportionate numbers of factories and landfills in segregated areas (Klitzman, Matte, & Kass, 2006). Because of such decisions, low-income and racially and ethnically segregated communities are disproportionately exposed to toxic physical environments, including airborne pollutants, heavy traffic, and contaminants or other hazardous material from surrounding industrial areas, and are less likely to be able to access places for physical activity (Klitzman, Matte, & Kass, 2006; Schulz et al., 2002).

Additionally, the lack of employment opportunities in impoverished neighborhoods forces inner city residents to travel longer distances, prohibiting any free time to exercise (Lopez & Hynes, 2006). Studies have found that racial and ethnic communities are less likely to access parks and other physical activity settings as compared to White communities, often resulting from decaying sidewalks, parks, and playgrounds (Lee, Mikkelsen, Srikantharajah, & Cohen, 2008; Lopez & Hynes, 2006). Inequities in access to playgrounds are also due to safety issues, such that residents limit their time in public spaces in order to reduce their risk of experiencing crime (Lee et al., 2008).

Access to Healthy Foods

It has been well established that diet plays a critical role in the incidence and prevalence of diabetes. National dietary guidelines recommend diets low in fat and sodium, as well as high in fiber, fruits, and vegetables. However, modern political, cultural, and economic changes have significantly influenced disparities in diabetes in racial and ethnic communities. Referred to as the social production of diabetes, these broader changes have been increasingly recognized as critical factors that add to the burden of diabetes impacting racial and ethnic groups (Liburd & Vinicor, 2003). For example, recent economic forces and social policies have forced adults to work long hours or multiple jobs, resulting in limited time to prepare healthy meals and increasing spending and consumption of fast food. This broader economic pressure has led to a social shift that has eroded traditional family norms of cooking and eating at home, now favoring and even promoting a quick and easy approach to eating outside the home.

Examining how these changes have influenced people's ability to obtain healthy foods in their local neighborhoods and meet the recommended dietary guidelines has gained attention in recent years. Mounting evidence shows that the promotion of unhealthy eating habits in many low-income urban communities of color is influenced by the proliferation of fast food restaurants, a deficiency of supermarkets providing fresh produce, and the higher cost and poorer quality of healthy foods (i.e., low-fat dairy products, fruits, and vegetables) (Andreyeva Blumenthal, Schwartz, Long, & Brownell, 2008; Glanz, Sallis, Saelens, & Frank, 2005; Glanz & Yaroch, 2004; Moore & Diez Roux, 2006). For example, urban residents pay 3–37% more for groceries in their local community compared to suburban residents who buy the same products in large supermarkets (Morland et al., 2002).

Many commercial businesses avoid segregated urban neighborhoods, leading to limited services that are poorer in quality and often higher in price than those available in more integrated urban areas (Williams & Collins, 2001). The exodus of services like banks, restaurants, and large supermarkets from low-income, predominantly minority neighborhoods has forced residents to shop in small grocery or convenience stores, which are often limited in providing fresh produce, are of poor quality, and have high prices (Morland et al., 2002; Schulz et al., 2002). The lack of adequate transportation available in low-income, segregated urban communities has exacerbated malnutrition among the poor by hindering access to healthy foods in surrounding grocery stores (Morland et al., 2002).

Recent studies have also confirmed that inequities in accessing healthy foods are associated with the wealth and racial makeup of neighborhoods (Baker, Schootman, Barnidge, & Kelly, 2006; Moore & Diez Roux, 2006). Segregated urban neighborhoods are often labeled "food deserts," that is, neighborhoods that have an excess amount of fast food restaurants and few, if any, large supermarkets (Baker et al., 2006; Lewis et al, 2005; Moore & Diez Roux, 2006; Powell, Slater, Mirtcheva, Bao, & Chaloupka, 2006; Zenk et al., 2005). Morland and colleagues found over three times as many supermarkets in the wealthier neighborhoods as in the lowest-wealth areas (Morland et al., 2002).

Morland et al.'s (2002) study's findings further showed the impact of residential racial segregation in access to healthy foods. Specifically, they found that supermarkets were four times more common in predominantly White neighborhoods than in predominantly African American neighborhoods. Moreover, wealthier and predominantly White neighborhoods contained fewer small grocery stores, convenience stores without gas stations, and specialty food stores (e.g., organic and kosher food stores) as compared to African American and poor neighborhoods. Other studies have found that most impoverished African American neighborhoods were farther from the nearest supermarket than were the most impoverished White neighborhoods (Zenk et al., 2005).

The number of fast food restaurants in African American neighborhoods, on the other hand, far exceeds that of those in predominantly White neighborhoods (Baker et al., 2006; Morland et al., 2002; Powell, Chaloupka, & Bao, 2007). One study examining racial residential segregation as a fundamental cause of fast food density in racially segregated urban centers suggested that the primary reason for the proliferation of fast food restaurants in African American neighborhoods is that African Americans are specifically targeted by fast food companies and segregation provides easy access to this population (Kwate, 2007). Targeting practices by fast food companies result in increased marketing of poorer quality foods to low-income and minority communities. The author concluded that residential segregation "creates environments ripe for fast food" through the lack of zoning regulations to prohibit disproportionate numbers of fast food restaurants, as well as limited political empowerment of community members (Kwate, 2007).

Health Consequences of Poor Neighborhood Conditions

Residential segregation has played a significant role in shaping neighborhood conditions that damage health, such as modifying built and food environments, as well as the delivery of health care services. These poor neighborhood conditions have been associated with multiple health conditions and behaviors, such as higher rates of all-cause mortality, cardiovascular disease, diabetes, infant mortality, low birth weight, and poor mental health (Schulz et al., 2002). Other studies have found that residential segregation is associated with infant and adult mortality, tuberculosis, cardiovascular disease, homicides, limited availability and access to healthy foods, and exposure to environmental pollutants (Acevedo-Garcia & Lochner, 2003). Below is a summary of the negative health outcomes resulting from the lack of access to health care, green spaces, and healthy foods, all indicated in disparities in diabetes experienced by racial and ethnic populations.

Delayed or Nonreceipt of Care

Racial and ethnic differences in health status are associated with how racial and ethnic groups interact with the health care system in terms of access to care. While individual factors (e.g., ability to pay, health beliefs, cultural practices, and language barriers) contribute to one's ability to obtain care, there is also evidence that environmental determinants, such as the availability and accessibility of health care in the community, play a large role in delay or nonreceipt of care. Between 2003 and 2007, the proportion of Americans delaying or lacking needed medical care increased significantly (Cunningham & Felland, 2008). For example, almost all racial and ethnic minorities were less likely to visit a doctor in the past 12 months than their White counterparts (NCHS, 2007). Previous research has also found that compared to insured adults, uninsured adults are more likely to delay seeking care and less likely to receive preventive services and be referred by primary care physicians for other health services (Diamant et al., 2004; NCHS, 2007). Delay or lack of medical care may cause more serious illness or complications, a worse prognosis, and longer hospital stays (Diamant et al., 2004). This is particularly true for people with uncontrolled diabetes.

The most recent National Healthcare Disparities Report found that disparities in health care access have not improved since 2003 (Agency for Healthcare Research and Quality, 2007). Specifically, African Americans and Hispanics/Latinos were significantly more likely to have worse access to care than Whites. Further, racial and ethnic disparities exist with regard to the burden of disease, quality of care, and treatment. African Americans and Mexican Americans were less likely to have their hemoglobin A1c or blood pressure under control than their White counterparts. Whereas the gap between Whites and Hispanics/Latinos in receiving the three recommended services (i.e., HBA1c testing, eye examination, and foot examination) remained the same, the gap in the rate of lower extremity amputations among persons with diabetes in these same groups increased (Agency for Healthcare Research and Quality, 2008).

Community health centers are considered to be the litmus test that signals the health of the nation's safety net system (NACHC, 2005). Cutbacks to Medicaid can have an immediate and significant impact on safety net providers and the health of their patients by dramatically increasing the number of uninsured patients treated at health centers and reducing much needed revenue from Medicaid to care for the uninsured. The depletion of these revenue sources poses a great threat to the ability of health centers to provide needed health care to the most vulnerable populations and greatly erodes the safety net system, thereby exacerbating health disparities.

Despite overwhelming evidence that community health centers adequately meet the health care needs of its patients and eliminate health disparities, many are threatened with closure. Closing these centers would increase disease and mortality rates and encourage overutilization and inappropriate use of emergency rooms and hospital care. Using limited hospital resources in this manner could further undermine the community safety net as rising emergency room utilization would impact the financial stability of local hospitals, ultimately exacerbating health care disparities among communities served (Hawkins & Proser, 2004).

Chronic Stress

Neighborhood social and economic conditions not only impact physical health but also mental health, particularly as it relates to emotional stress. Recent research has shown that individuals residing in economically disadvantaged neighborhoods have higher levels of chronic stress and poorer mental health (Schulz et al., 2006, 2008; Williams & Jackson, 2005). Residing in segregated neighborhoods disproportionately exposes an individual to stressful environments, yet they lack the ability to access resources to cope with these stressors (Mays et al., 2007). Emotional responses to environmental events like psychological and physical stress have been shown as one pathway for social conditions to "get inside" the body by causing neuroendocrine and physiological changes related to disease processes (Kubzanksy & Kawachi, 2000). Coping with these chronic stressors can result in prematurely wearing down the body and increase risk of disease, otherwise labeled as a weathering effect.

This hypothesis suggests that poor communities and communities of color experience "early health deterioration as a consequence of the cumulative impact of repeated experience with social or economic adversity and political marginalization" (Geronimus, Hicken, Keene, & Bound, 2006). For example, residing in resource-poor neighborhoods that lack adequate employment and educational opportunities, as well as limit access to health care services, healthy foods, and green spaces, can contribute to chronic and acute daily stress. Also, persistent coping with chronic stress resulting from institutional racism can negatively impact health by causing premature physiological deterioration.

A more recent explanation posited by researchers to explain the effects of stress on the body is allostatic load (Mays et al., 2007). The allostatic load hypothesis refers to the association between the psychosocial environment and physical disease. Allostatic load is stress-induced damage, which is considered relevant in cardiovascular disease, cancer, infection, and cognitive decline, and has been associated with accelerated aging (Brunner & Marmot, 2000). Chronic exposure to stress is associated with altered physiological functioning, which may lead to increased risks of disease and other health conditions (Geronimus et al., 2006; Williams & Jackson, 2005). Stress and other negative emotions like anxiety and depression have been shown to evoke physiological processes that are associated with cardiovascular and liver diseases, obesity, hypertension, and diabetes (Geronimus et al., 2006).

Health Outcomes and Behaviors

Negative neighborhood conditions (e.g., proliferation of waste-related facilities, poor infrastructure maintenance, and high crime) caused by residential segregation and neighborhood divestment is positively associated with diabetes and its related risk factors (Lopez & Hynes, 2006). For example, African Americans residing in more segregated metropolitan areas are more likely to be overweight or obese (Chang, 2006). The depletion of resources and opportunities in segregated urban neighborhoods can lead to the inability to walk to work, due to lack of infrastructure maintenance and fear of being a victim of crime, or the lack of adequate time to exercise due to longer commutes to long-distance job sites (Lopez & Hynes, 2006).

The characteristics of the built environment (e.g., accessibility to facilities, opportunities for activity, and aesthetic and safety qualities of the area) can influence an individual's choice to exercise (Auchincloss, Diez Roux, Brown, Erdmann, & Bertoni, 2008). Recent evidence shows that living near walkable green spaces, the presence of sidewalks, and access to facilities increase the likelihood of physical activity, including active transportation (e.g., bicycling and walking) (Frank, Saelens, Powell, & Chapman, 2007; Galea, Freudenberg, & Vlahov, 2005). Creating walkable neighborhoods where significant numbers of people of color live will likely reduce insulin resistance and risk factors for the development of type 2 diabetes (Auchincloss et al., 2008; Frank et al., 2007).

Food choice is influenced by neighborhood environmental factors, such as distance to supermarkets, availability of healthy foods in nearby food stores, proliferation of fast food restaurants, and food prices (Beydoun, Powell, & Wang, 2008; Cassady, Jetter, & Culp, 2007; Flourney & Treuhaft, 2005; Jetter & Cassady, 2006; Powell et al., 2007; Stewart, Blisard, Bhuyan, & Nayga, 2004). All of these neighborhood factors have also been shown to be associated with poor nutrition, obesity, and diabetes in children and adults (Beydoun et al., 2008; Inagami, Cohen, Finch, & Asch, 2006; Morland et al., 2002; Williams & Collins, 2001). Recent studies have also shown that perceived time scarcity (e.g., limited time for food preparation and consumption due to employment, income, and parental demands) can also have a significant influence on diabetes-related disparities (Jabs & Devine, 2006).

CONCLUSION

Despite the overwhelming evidence demonstrating the significant effects that residential racial segregation has on neighborhood conditions and health outcomes, many large cities and their surrounding suburban areas are not expected to meet the Healthy People 2010 goals of eliminating racial and ethnic health disparities, which may be due in part to the failure of addressing this issue (U.S. Department of Health and Human Services, 2006). As our nation's urban neighborhoods continue to face deleterious effects from residential segregation, divestment of municipal services, and exacerbating health inequities, researchers are calling for the need to reconceptualize disparities in a broader scope that goes beyond individual factors like diet and physical activity and considers the multiple social determinants of health, in turn emphasizing the attention on developing strategies that change social and economic policies, social and physical environments, and the potential impact they have on health outcomes. Utilizing a socioecological approach to such interventions will enable public health practitioners to intervene at various levels and settings.

Researchers suggest that in order to effectively eliminate the negative effects of segregation, major investments must be infused into disadvantaged communities to improve their social, physical, and economic infrastructures (Williams & Jackson, 2005). However, the process of revitalizing and integrating urban neighborhoods that promote healthy eating must not perpetuate the displacement of its original residents through gentrification. Gentrification, the process by which higher-income households move into low-income neighborhoods, can greatly benefit a community by establishing new stores and resources in previously rundown neighborhoods (Levy, Comey, & Padilla, 2006). However, despite the benefits the revitalization of such neighborhoods may also impose significant financial and social consequences for those already residing in those areas (e.g., inability to pay higher rents, mortgages, or property taxes and social isolation or conflicts) (Kennedy & Leonard, 2001).

Promoting mixed-income or inclusionary zoning polices that offer a variety of housing prices or a percentage of housing units for low- and moderate-income residents can minimize residential displacement. Mitigating the negative consequences of gentrification in previously neglected neighborhoods through such strategies will not only minimize residential displacement but also allow low-income residents the opportunity to access health care services, healthy foods, and green spaces; gain employment, and thus health insurance coverage; and obtain a quality education—all essential contributors to good health.

Further, effective programs and policies addressing residential segregation must provide opportunities for active participation from community residents in land planning and neighborhood revitalization processes in order to ensure equitable outcomes. Public health researchers and practitioners are increasingly recognizing the need for approaches that build equitable partnerships between decision makers, health advocates and other practitioners, and community members to develop strategies that actually address local needs as well as broader community and social change. One such approach may be community-based participatory research, which is founded on several key principles, including establishing a collaborative approach that equitably involves all partners in the decision making process, recognizing the unique strengths that each partner brings, promoting co-learning and capacity building among all partners, achieving a balance between knowledge and action, and emphasizing local relevance of public health problems and ecological perspectives that recognize and attend to the multiple determinants of health and disease (Israel et al., 1998).

It is critical that efforts to eliminate health disparities focus on addressing conditions and forces, such as institutional racism and residential segregation, that perpetuate such disparities. The study of place, in this respect, can redirect our efforts to examine neighborhood contexts in order to better understand structural barriers and avoid the perpetuation of "victim blaming" by solely focusing on individual behavior interventions. Efforts to address these social and economic determinants of health does not preclude the need to also address short-term outcomes, such as providing information and resources related to diet, physical activity, and health care services. However, examining the political, social, and economic processes that create and perpetuate racial differences in access to social and economic resources is crucial. Thus, understanding and addressing discriminatory institutional policies and practices and their impact on health will play a profound role in improving population health and reducing disparities in the prevalence of diabetes in communities of color.

REFERENCES

Acevedo-Garcia, D., & Lochner, K. A. (2003). Residential segregation and health. In I. Kawachi and L. F. Berkman (Eds.), *Neighborhoods and health* (pp. 265–287). New York: Oxford University Press.

Agency for Healthcare Research and Quality. (2003). *Safety net monitoring initiative: Fact sheet.* Rockville, MD: Agency for Healthcare Research and Quality, U.S. Department of Health and Human Services. AHRQ Publ. No. 03-P011.

Agency for Healthcare Research and Quality. (2007). *National healthcare disparities report 2008.* Rockville, MD: Agency for Healthcare Research and Quality, U.S. Department of Health and Human Services. AHRQ Publ. No. 08-0041.

Anderson, L. M., St. Charles, J., Fullilove, M. T., Scrimshaw, S. C., Fielding, J. E., Normand, J., & the Task Force on Community Preventive Services. (2003). Providing affordable family housing and reducing residential segregation by income: A systematic review. *American Journal of Preventive Medicine, 24(3S)*, 47–67.

Andreyeva, T., Blumenthal, D. M., Schwartz, M. B., Long, M. W., & Brownell, K. D. (2008). Availability and prices of foods across stores and neighborhoods: The case of New Haven, Connecticut. *Health Affairs, 27(5)*, 1381–1388.

Auchincloss, A. H., Diez Roux, A. V., Brown, D. G., Erdmann, C. A., & Bertoni, A. G. (2008). Neighborhood resources for physical activity and healthy foods and their association with insulin resistance. *Epidemiology, 19(1)*, 146–157.

Baker, E. A., Metzler, M. M., & Galea, S. (2005). Addressing social determinants of health inequities: Learning from doing. *American Journal of Public Health, 95(4)*, 553–555.

Baker, E. A., Schootman, M., Barnidge, E., & Kelly, C. (2006). The role of race and poverty in access to foods that enable individuals to adhere to dietary guidelines. *Preventing Chronic Disease, 3,* 1–11.

Beydoun, M. A., Powell, L. M., & Wang, Y. (2008). The association of fast food, fruit and vegetable prices with dietary intakes among US adults: Is there modification by family income? *Social Science & Medicine, 66,* 2218–2229.

Bocian, D. G., Ernst, K. S., & Li, W. (2006). *Unfair lending: The effect of race and ethnicity on the price of subprime mortgages.* A report from the Center for Responsible Lending.

Brunner, E., & Marmot, M. (2000). Social organization, stress, and health. In M. Marmot & R. Wilkinson (Eds.), *Social determinants of health* (pp. 17–43). London: Oxford University Press.

Campen, J., Nafici, S., Rust, A., Smith, G., Stein, K., & van Kerkhove, B. (2007). *Paying more for the American dream: A multi-state analysis of higher cost home purchase lending.* A joint report by the California Reinvestment Coalition, Community Reinvestment Association of North Carolina, Empire Justice Center, Massachusetts Affordable Housing Alliance, Neighborhood Economic Development Advocacy Project, & Woodstock Institute.

Cassady, D., Jetter, K. M., & Culp, J. (2007). Is price a barrier to eating more fruits and vegetables for low-income families? *Journal of the American Dietetic Association, 107,* 1909–1915.

Chang, V. W. (2006). Racial residential segregation and weight status among US adults. *Social Science & Medicine, 63,* 1289–1303.

Charles, C. Z. (2003). The dynamics of racial residential segregation. *Annual Reviews for Sociology, 29,* 167–207.

Chin, M. H., Drum, M. L., Guillen, M., Rimington, A., Levie, J. R., Kirchhoff, A. C., Quinn, M. T., & Schaefer, C. T. (2007). Improving and sustaining diabetes care in community health centers with the health disparities collaboratives. *Medical Care, 45(12),* 1135–1143.

Choudhry, L., Douglass, M., Lewis, J., Olson, C. H., Osterman, R., & Shah, P. (2007). *The impact of community health centers and community-affiliated health plans on emergency department use.* National Association of Community Health Centers & Association for Community Affiliated Plans Report. Retrieved from http://www.nachc.com/research-reports.cfm

Cunningham, P. L., & Felland, L. E. (2008). *Falling behind: Americans' access to medical care deteriorates, 2003–2007.* Center for Studying Health System Change. Tracking Report No. 19. Retrieved from http://www.hschange.com/CONTENT/993/?topic=topic06

Diamant, A. L., Hays, R. D., Morales, L. S., Ford, W., Calmes, D., Asch, S., Duan, N., Fielder, E., Kim, S., Fielding, J., Sumner, G., Shapiro, M. F., Hayes-Bautista, D., & Gelberg, L. (2004). Delays and unmet need for health care among adult primary care patients in a restructured urban public health system. *American Journal of Public Health, 94(5),* 783–789.

Dorn, S., Garrett, B., Holahan, J., & Williams, A. (2008). *Medicaid, SCHIP and economic downturn: Policy challenges and policy responses.* Kaiser Commission on Medicaid and the Uninsured Report. Retrieved from http://www.kff.org/medicaid/7770.cfm

Flournoy, R., & Treuhaft, S. (2005). *Healthy food, healthy communities: Improving access and opportunities through food retailing.* PolicyLink & The California Endowment Report.

Frank, L. D., Saelens, B. E., Powell, K. E., & Chapman, J. E. (2007). Stepping towards causation: Do built environments or neighborhood and travel preferences explain physical activity, driving, and obesity? *Social Science & Medicine, 65(9)*, 1898–1914.

Freudenberg, N. (2000). Health promotion in the city: A review of current status and future prospects in the United States. *Annual Review of Public Health, 21,* 473–503.

Freudenberg, N., Galea, S., & Vlahov, D. (2005). Beyond urban penalty and urban sprawl: Back to living conditions as the focus of urban health. *Journal of Community Health, 21(3),* 949–957.

Freudenberg, N., Galea, S., & Vlahov, D. (2006). Changing living conditions, changing health: U.S. cities since World War II. In N. Freudenberg, S. Galea, & D. Vlahov (Eds.), *Cities and the health of the public* (pp 19–45). Nashville, TN: Vanderbilt University Press.

Freudenberg, N., & Ruglis, J. (2007). Reframing school dropout as a public health issue. *Preventing Chronic Disease, 4(4).*

Fullilove, M. T. (2003). Neighborhoods and infectious diseases. I. Kawachi & L. F. Berkman (Eds.), *Neighborhoods and health* (pp. 211–222). New York: Oxford University Press.

Galea, S., Freudenberg, N., & Vlahov, D. (2005). Cities and population health. *Social Science & Medicine, 60,* 1017–1033.

Gee, G. C. (2002). A multilevel analysis of the relationship between institutional and individual racial discrimination and health status. *American Journal of Public Health, 92,* 615–623.

Geronimus, A. T., Hicken, M., Keene, D., & Bound, J. (2006). "Weathering" and age patterns of allostatic load scores among Blacks and Whites in the United States. *American Journal of Public Health, 96(2),* 1–7.

Glanz, K., Sallis, J. F., Saelens, B. E., & Frank, L. D. (2005). Healthy nutrition environments: Concepts and measures. *American Journal of Health Promotion, 19(5),* 330–333.

Glanz, K., & Yaroch, A. L. (2004). Strategies for increasing fruit and vegetable intake in grocery stores and communities: Policy, pricing and environmental change. *Preventive Medicine, 39,* S75–S80.

Hawkins, D., & Proser, M. (2004). *A nation's health at risk: A national and state report on America's 36 million people without a regular healthcare provider.* National Association of Community Health Centers. Special Topics Issue Brief No. 5. Retrieved from http://www.nachc.com/research-reports.cfm

Hawkins, D., & Schwartz, R. (2003). Health centers and the states: Partnership potential to address the fiscal crisis. *Journal of Ambulatory Care Management, 26(4),* 285–295.

Hicks, L. S., O'Malley, J., & Lieu, T. A. (2006). The quality of chronic disease care in US community health centers. *Health Affairs, 25(6),* 1713–1723.

Hofrichter, R. (2003). The politics of health inequities: Contested terrain. In R. Hofrichter (Ed.), *Health and social justice: Politics, ideology, and inequity in the distribution of disease* (pp. 1–56). San Francisco: Jossey-Bass.

House, J. S., & Williams, D. R. (2003). Understanding and reducing socioeconomic and racial/ethnic disparities in health. In R. Hofrichter (Ed.), *Health and social justice: Politics, ideology, and inequity in the distribution of disease* (pp. 89–131). San Francisco: Jossey-Bass.

Iceland, J., Weinberg, D. H., & Steinwetz, E. (2002). *U.S. Census Bureau Series CENSR-3: Racial and ethnic residential segregation in the United States: 1980–2000.* Washington, DC: U.S. Government Printing Office.

Inagami, S., Cohen, D. A., Finch, B. K., & Asch, S. M. (2006). You are where you shop: Grocery store locations, weight, and neighborhoods. *American Journal of Preventive Medicine, 31(1),* 10–17.

Institute of Medicine. (2002). Understanding population health and its determinants. In *The future of the public's health in the 21st century* (ch. 2, pp. 46–95). Washington, DC: National Academies Press.

Israel, B. A., Schulz, A. J., Parker, E., & Becker, A. B. (1998). Review of community-based research: Assessing partnership approaches to improve public health. *Annual Review of Public Health, 19,* 173–202.

Jabs, J., & Devine, C. M. (2006). Time scarcity and food choices: An overview. *Appetite, 47(2),* 196–204.

Jetter, K. M., & Cassady, D. L. (2006). The availability and cost of healthier food alternatives. *Amerian Journal of Preventive Medicine, 30(1),* 38–44.

Jones, C. P. (2000). Levels of racism: A theoretical framework and a gardener's tale. *American Journal of Public Health, 90(8),* 1212–1215.

Kain, J. F. (1992). The spatial mismatch hypothesis: Three decades later. *Housing Policy Debate, 3(2),* 371–460.

Kaiser Commission on Medicaid and the Uninsured. (2008). *Medicaid enrollment as a percent of total population, 2005.* Retrieved from http://www.statehealthfacts.org/comparemaptable.jsp?ind=199&cat=4

Kaiser Commission on Medicaid and the Uninsured. (2009). *Medicaid: A primer.* Publ. No. 7334-03. Retrieved from http://www.kff.org/medicaid/7334.cfm

Kennedy, M., & Leonard, P. (2001). *Dealing with neighborhood change: A primer on gentrification and policy choices.* Discussion paper.

Klitzman, S., Matte, T. D., & Kass, D. E. (2006). The urban physical environment and its effects on health. In N. Freudenberg, S. Galea, & D. Vlahov (Eds.), *Cities and the health of the public* (pp. 61–84). Nashville, TN: Vanderbilt University Press.

Kubzansky, L. D., & Kawachi, I. (2000). Affective states and health. In L. F. Berkman & I. Kawachi (Eds.), *Social epidemiology* (pp. 213–241). New York: Oxford University Press.

Kwate, N. O. A. (2007). Fried chicken and fresh apples: Racial segregation as a fundamental cause of fast food density in Black neighborhoods. *Health & Place, 14(1),* 32–44.

Lee, V., Mikkelsen, L., Srikantharajah, J., & Cohen, L. (2008). *Promising strategies for creating healthy eating and active living environments.* Healthy Eating Active Living Convergence Partnership Report. Retrieved from http://www.convergencepartnership.org/site/c.fhLOK6PELmF/b.3917533/

Lethbridge-Cejku, M., & Vickerie, J. (2005). Summary health statistics for U.S. adults: National Health Interview Survey, 2003. National Center for Health Statistics. *Vital and Health Statistics, 10(225).*

Levy, D. K., Comey, J., & Padilla, S. (2006). *In the face of gentrification: Case studies of local efforts to mitigate displacement.* The Urban Institute Report.

Lewis, L. B., Sloane, D. C., Nascimento, L. M., Diamant, A. L., Guinyard, J. J., Yancey, A. K., et al. (2005). African Americans' access to healthy food options in South Los Angeles. *American Journal of Public Health, 95(4),* 668–673.

Liburd, L.C., & Vinicor, F. (2003). Rethinking diabetes prevention and control in racial and ethnic communities. *Journal of Public Health Management and Practice, 9(Suppl),* S74–S79.

Logan, J. R., Stults, B. J., & Farley, R. (2004). Segregation of minorities in the metropolis: Two decades of change. *Demography, 41(1),* 1–22.

Lopez, R. P., & Hynes, H. P. (2006). Obesity, physical activity, and the urban environment: Public health research needs. *Environmental Health, 5(25),* 1–10.

Lubell, J., Crain, R., & Cohen, R. (2007). Framing the issues: The positive impact of affordable housing on health. Washington, DC: Center for Housing Policy. Retrieved from www.nhc.org/pdf/chp_int_litrvw_hsghlth0707.pdf

Maantay, J. (2001). Zoning, equity, and public health. *American Journal of Public Health, 91(7),* 1033–1041.

Macintyre, S., & Ellaway, A. (2003). Neighborhoods and health: An overview. In I. Kawachi and L. F. Berkman (Eds.), *Neighborhoods and health* (pp. 20–44). New York: Oxford University Press.

Mays, V. M., Cochran, S. D., & Barnes, N. W. (2007). Race, race-based discrimination, and health outcomes among African Americans. *Annual Reviews of Psychology, 58,* 201–225.

Moore, L. V., & Diez Roux, A. V. (2006). Associations of neighborhood characteristics with the location and type of food stores. *American Journal of Public Health, 96(2),* 325–331.

Morland, K., Wing, S., Diez Roux, A., & Poole, C. (2002). Neighborhood characteristics associated with the location of food stores and food service places. *American Journal of Preventive Medicine, 22(1),* 23–29.

National Association of Community Health Centers. (2005). *The safety net on the edge.* Retrieved from http://www.nachc.com/research-reports.cfm

National Association of Community Health Centers. (2008). *America's health centers.* Fact Sheet No. 0108. Retrieved from http://www.nachc.com/research-factsheets.cfm

National Association of Community Health Centers & The Robert Graham Center. (2007). *Access denied: A look at America's medically disenfranchised.* Retrieved from http://www.nachc.com/research-reports.cfm

National Center for Health Statistics. (2007). *Health, United States, 2007 with chartbook on trends in the health of Americans.* Hyattsville, MD: Centers for Disease Control and Prevention. DHHS Publ. No. 2007-1232. Retrieved from http://www.cdc.gov/nchs/hus.htm

Perdue, W. C., Stone, L. A., & Gostin, L. O. (2003). The built environment and its relationship to the public's health: The legal framework. *American Journal of Public Health, 94(9),* 1390–1394.

PolicyLink. (2008). *Healthy food retailing: History.* Retrieved from http://www.policylink.org/EDTK/HealthyFoodRetailing/Why.html#8

Politzer, R., Yoon, J., Shi, L., Hughes, R., Regan, J., & Gaston, M. (2001). Inequality in America: The contribution of health centers in reducing and eliminating disparities in access to care. *Medical Care Research and Review, 58(2),* 234–248.

Pompay, J., Williams, G., Thomas, C., & Gatrell, A. (2003). Theorizing inequalities in health: The place in lay knowledge. In R. Hofrichter (Ed.), *Health and social justice: Politics, ideology, and inequity in the distribution of disease* (pp. 385–409). San Francisco: Jossey-Bass.

Powell, L. M., Chaloupka, F. J., & Bao, Y. (2007). The availability of fast-food and full-service restaurants in the United States. *American Journal of Preventive Medicine, 33(4S),* S240–S245.

Powell, L. M., Slater, S., Mirtcheva, D., Bao, Y., & Chaloupka, F. J. (2006). Food store availability and neighborhood characteristics in the United States. *Preventive Medicine, 44,* 189–195.

Proser, M., Shin, P., & Hawkins, D. (2005). *A nation's health at risk III: Growing uninsured, budget cutbacks challenge President's initiative to put a health center in every poor county.* National Association of Community Health Centers. Special Topics Issue Brief No. 9. Retrieved from http://www.nachc.com/research-reports.cfm

Schootman, M., Andresen, E. M., Wolinsky, F. D., Malmstrom, T. D., Miller, J. P., Yan, Y., & Miller, D. K. (2007). The effect of adverse housing and neighborhood conditions on the development of diabetes mellitus among middle-aged African Americans. *American Journal of Epidemiology, 166,* 379–387.

Schulz, A. J., Israel, B. A., Zenk, S. N., Parker, E. A., Lichtenstein, R., Shellman-Weir, S., & Klem, A. B. L. (2006). Psychosocial stress and social support as mediators of relationships between income, length of residence and depressive symptoms among African American women on Detroit's eastside. *Social Science & Medicine, 62,* 510–522.

Schulz, A. J., Williams, D. R., Israel, B. A., & Lempert, L. B. (2002). Racial and spatial relations as fundamental determinants of health in Detroit. *The Milbank Quarterly, 80(4),* 677–707.

Schulz, A. J., Zenk, S. N., Israel, B. A., Mentz, G., Stokes, C., & Galea, S. (2008). Do neighborhood economic characteristics, racial composition, and residential stability predict perceptions of stress associated with the physical and social environment? Findings from a multilevel analysis in Detroit. *Journal of Urban Health, 85(5),* 642–661.

Schulz, A. J., Zenk, S., Odoms-Young, A., Hollis-Neely, T., Nwankwo, R., Lockett, M., Ridella, W., & Kannan, S. (2005). Healthy eating and exercising to reduce diabetes: Exploring the potential of social determinants of health frameworks within the context of community-based participatory diabetes prevention. *American Journal of Public Health, 95(4),* 645–651.

Shi, L., Starfield, B., Politzer, R., & Regan, J. (2002). Primary care, self-rated health, and reductions in social disparities in health. *Health Services Research, 37(3),* 529–550.

Shi, L., & Stevens, G. D. (2007). The role of community health centers in delivering primary care to the underserved. *Journal of Ambulatory Care Management, 30(2),* 159–170.

Smith, D. B. (2005). *Eliminating disparities in treatment and the struggle to end segregation.* The Commonwealth Fund Report, No. 775.

Stewart, H., Blisard, N., Bhuyan, S., & Nayga, R. M. (2004). *The demand for food away from home: Full service or fast food?* U.S. Department of Agriculture. Agriculture Economic Report No. 829.

U.S. Department of Health and Human Services. (2006). *Healthy people 2010 midcourse review.* Washington, DC: U.S. Government Printing Office.

Vlahov, D., Gibble, E., Freudenberg, N., & Galea, S. (2004). Cities and health: History, approaches, and key questions. *Academic Medicine, 79(12),* 1133–1138.

Wallace, D., & Wallace, R. (1998). Scales of geography, time, and population: The study of violence as a public health problem. *American Journal of Public Health, 88(12),* 1853–1858.

Wallace, R. (1988). Synergism of plagues: "Planned shrinkage," contagious housing destruction, and AIDS in the Bronx. *Environmental Research, 47,* 1–33.

White, K., & Borrell, L. N. (2006). Racial/ethnic neighborhood concentration and self-reported health in New York City. *Ethnicity & Disease, 16,* 900–908.

Wilkes, R., & Iceland, J. (2004). Hypersegregation in the twenty-first century. *Demography, 41(1),* 23–36.

Williams, D. R. (1999). Race, socioeconomic status, and health: The added effects of racism and discrimination. *Annals of the New York Academy of Sciences, 896,* 173–188.

Williams, D. R., & Collins, C. (2001). Racial residential segregation: A fundamental cause of racial disparities in health. *Public Health Reports, 116,* 404–416.

Williams, D. R., & Jackson, P. B. (2005). Social sources of racial disparities in health. *Health Affairs, 24(2),* 325–334.

Woodward, S. E. (2008). *A study of closing costs for FHA mortgages.* Washington, DC: U.S. Department of Housing and Urban Development.

World Health Organization. (2007). *A conceptual framework for action on the social determinants of health: A discussion paper for the Commission on Social Determinants of Health.* Retrieved from http://www.who.int/social_determinants/resources/latest_publications/en/

Zenk, S. N., Schulz, A. J., Israel, B. A., James, S. A., Bao, S., & Wilson, M. L. (2005). Neighborhood composition, neighborhood poverty, and the spatial accessibility of supermarkets in metropolitan Detroit. *American Journal of Public Health, 95(4),* 660–667.

7

Community Change: Its Importance in Evaluating Diabetes Programs in Communities of Color[1]

MARK D. RIVERA AND PATTIE J. TUCKER

INTRODUCTION

The Institute of Medicine (IOM) has defined public health as what we as a society do collectively to assure conditions in which people can be healthy (IOM, 1988). In practice, however, community members are not sought out and adequately engaged in shaping, implementing, and sustaining policies and programs. While addressing these gaps, it has become increasingly common for community members, community-based organizations, and local health departments to work collaboratively to address community health issues. (IOM, 2003; Schwab & Syme, 1997).

This chapter explores community change as defined on subsequent pages and within the context of diabetes health disparities and the social determinants of health in communities of color. Our discussion of community change as a relevant focus in the evaluation of efforts to eliminate health disparities is organized through a melding of the National REACH 2010 Program Logic Model (Tucker, Liao, Giles, & Liburd, 2006) with a socioecological Model (SEM) (Dahlberg & Krug, 2002). The need to maximize community involvement and build inter-organizational

---

[1] The findings and conclusions in this chapter are those of the authors and do not necessarily represent the official position of the Centers for Disease Control and Prevention.

relationships is also discussed, along with the benefits of, and the need to evaluate, multilevel program and policy interventions.

We argue that the quality and focus of the initial community assessment sets up the rigor and value of the subsequent evaluation of community change. We propose a number of potential policy change targets, and suggest community level resources that can be measured to document social and policy changes that support the elimination of diabetes disparities. Community changes that reflect an emphasis on shared capacity and outcomes are highlighted. Capacity and outcomes are not simple; they result from complex clusters of organizational resources and efforts across levels of a community. To ground this discussion, we, along with other authors in this text, consider the concepts of social determinants of health and health equity.

SOCIAL DETERMINANTS OF DIABETES AND HEALTH EQUITY

Broad agreement exists on the impact of social determinants on health (Brennan Ramirez, Baker, & Metzler, 2008; Jong-wook, 2005; Kelly & Bonnefoy, 2007; Marmot, 2005; Smedley, Stith, & Nelson, 2003; World Health Organization, 2008). Social determinants of health include contextual factors, such as features of neighborhoods and broader communities (e.g., income distribution, segregation, access to resources linked to health, and exposure to hazards), as well as individual factors (e.g., family structure, education, occupation, and social support) (Brennan Ramirez et al., 2008). Framing the diabetes disparities discussion in terms of social determinants of health fosters a broader discussion of potential public health solutions (Schulz et al., 2005) and issues of health equity and social justice in communities of color (IOM, 2003; World Health Organization, 2008).

Health equity is an inherent right of all people to the resources and opportunities that help to ensure good health. In response to mounting evidence of a strong relationship between health equity and social determinants of health (Blas et al., 2008; Inagami, Cohen, & Finch, 2007; Prah Ruger, 2004; Working Group on Health Disparities 2005), the Commission on Social Determinants of Health was formed by the World Health Organization (WHO). Building on earlier work of the IOM (2003) and others, this commission has moved beyond immediate causes of diseases to examine "causes of the causes" and the structures and socially determined conditions where people grow, live, work, and age (WHO, 2008).

The commission concluded that social determinants affect access to healthy food and safe environments. Further, they concluded that social determinants lead to health disparities across social groupings with respect to race, ethnicity, socioeconomic position, geographic location, disability status, gender, and sexual orientation. The commission's findings support the idea that these health disparities are avoidable and therefore an issue of health equity and social justice (WHO, 2008).

A better understanding of the influences of social determinants on population health and health equity can inform the development and assessment of interventions and other forms of targeted action (WHO, 2008). Sustaining targeted action will then require investments from a range of stakeholders (Krieger, 2001). To better understand the types of investments necessary to address social determinants of health, we explore what constitutes community change and the structures and capacities needed within communities to bring them about.

Defining Community

Before we can pursue community change as a viable outcome for population health and achieving health equity, it is useful to establish what we mean by community and how communities factor into the health of their members. Liburd more extensively describes meanings of community and relationships between community and health in chapter 5. For this chapter, we define a community as people and organizations that are governed by a local administration in the same geographic area. The people share social interactions, a sense of belonging, and political and social responsibilities. They also share culture and language, norms, interests, experiences, values, means of problem solving, and health risks and conditions (Brennan Ramirez et al., 2008; Hassinger & Pinkerton, 1986; Hawe, 1994; IOM, 2003). Healthy communities collaborate across sectors and value contributions of ethnically, socially, and economically diverse community members. Communities consider and address a broad array of determinants of health and enable individuals to make informed, positive choices in the context of health-protective and supportive environments, policies, and systems (IOM, 2003).

Supportive relationships within a community allow greater participation in community life through social networks. Civic engagement is enabled and health status is better (Metzler, 2007). These relationships are shaped by the history, culture, and demographics of people living in the community. Community organizations rely on social networks to influence policies, launch or institutionalize programs, and leverage resources to sustain them. Community relationships are also shaped by factors often associated with places in communities, as discussed at length by Navarro in chapter 6. These factors include walkability, access to public transportation, parks, a full-service grocery store, and physical characteristics of businesses. We will revisit in this chapter the importance of place in efforts to achieve community change that reduces diabetes disparities.

Community Change

In recent years, there has been a shift from a focus on changes in public health awareness, behavioral change, and clinical measures to a greater emphasis on the development of community capacity, effective resource mobilization, and increased sustainability of community changes (Bruner, Bell, Brindis, Chang, & Scarbrough, 1993; Flora, Emery, Fey, & Bregendahl, 2008; Kretzmann & McKnight, 1993). In the process, there has been a growing interest in programs and practices that build community capacity to create policies and other system-level changes, as well as changes in the capacities of governmental bodies, agencies, businesses, and other sectors of the community that support population health (KU Work Group on Health Promotion and Community Development, 2007, (ch. 38). These changes are often described within levels of a SEM (Dahlberg & Krug, 2002), ranging from changes at the level of health-related behaviors of individuals to changes at the organizational, community, and societal system levels. The primary focus of this chapter will be achieving and assessing change at the larger socio-ecological level.

Social ecology is the study of people in an environment and how those people influence one another (Hawley, 1950). The SEM has been used widely in pubic health and modified for different contexts (Dahlberg & Krug, 2002; IOM, 2003). Each version can be seen as a heuristic that helps to guide our thinking regarding how best to affect the public's health. With regard to social determinants of health, a SEM can help us think about the multiple determinants of population health, whereas a focus on any one level would underestimate the effects of other contexts (Klein, Tosi, & Cannella, 1999; Stokols, 1996).

THE REACH 2010 NATIONAL PROGRAM MODEL

The Racial and Ethnic Approaches to Community Health (REACH) 2010 logic model illustrates how local coalitions can take action to bring about reductions in health disparities in racial and ethnic groups. The sections of this chapter consider the stages of the REACH 2010 model with a primary focus on the first three stages: Planning, implementation, and evaluation (see Figure 7.1).

The planning phase includes four components and begins with "understanding context, causes, and solutions for health disparity." This understanding of context is continually emerging and helps the coalition to more effectively address health disparities. Further, the "planning and capacity building" component highlights those activities that prepare the coalition for action and result in a "community action plan" that, in turn, informs further coalition development. The coalition uses this plan, within the context of "existing activities" and "external influences" (e.g., demographic changes) to inform "targeted REACH action," the first component of the implementation and evaluation phase. Targeted actions lead to "community and systems change" and, in the process, "change agents change." That is, in addition to affecting programs, policies, and practices within the community and broader systems, executing against the action plan causes changes that are internal to the coalition and its partners (e.g., increases in inter-organizational capacities and depth of relationships) that may increase effectiveness in addressing health disparities. "Widespread change in risk/protective behaviors" are hoped to be the result of community, systems, and change agent changes and, in turn, are linked to the ultimate goal of "reduced health disparity" and "other outcomes." Finally, there is an arrow connecting these last two components to "coalition," emphasizing a feedback loop where coalitions use ongoing assessment of their progress to modify plans and target their capacity building efforts (Tucker et al., 2006).

In this chapter, the primary focus is placed on three components of the REACH 2010 logic model. Planning and capacity building places emphasis on the readiness of a coalition and its members to take action toward transforming community conditions and systems. Targeted REACH action addresses intervention activities believed to bring about desired effects. Community and systems change is directed toward changing risk conditions by altering the environment within which individuals and groups behave. (Tucker et al., 2006). Taken together, these

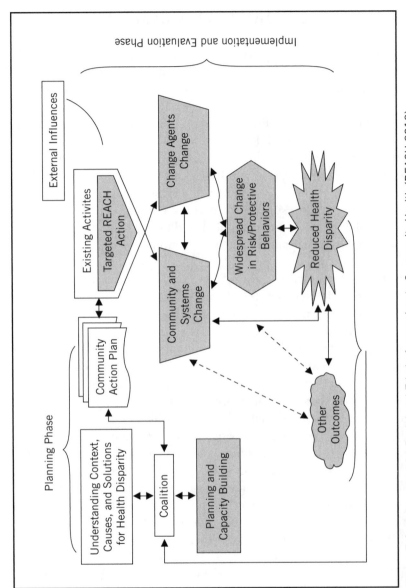

Figure 7.1 Logic model for Racial and Ethnic Approaches to Community Health (REACH 2010).

three areas for community change increase community capacity to eliminate health disparities.

Community Assessment

Strategic Planning

Identifying the needs and assets of community members is an important step in determining the key issues to guide strategic planning and mobilization to address diabetes disparities (Watson-Thompson, Fawcett, & Schultz, 2008). Therefore, it is important to include a diverse group of community representatives to ensure the needs across the community are considered. It is essential that change agents within communities develop comprehensive strategic plans to implement, sustain, and evaluate these efforts. The IOM Committee on Using Performance Monitoring to Improve Community Health (1997) discusses the development of a community health improvement plan (CHIP). As part of the process of developing a CHIP, communities assess health needs and priorities, formulate a health improvement strategy, and collaboratively identify and use indicators to monitor and make adjustments to the CHIP and its implementation. Assessment is often carried out at the organizational level and can facilitate the development of a strategic plan, identification of priority programs, and mobilization of community resources.

Needs

Needs assessments help communities target their programmatic efforts. Communities also find it helpful to periodically re-assess the needs of their target populations, since needs change over time (Myers, 1999; Petersen & Alexander, 2001). Supplementing this periodic review with other community indicators related to the economic, social, and physical community context is necessary to further assist communities in setting public health priorities.

The IOM Committee on Using Performance Monitoring to Improve Community Health (1997) recommended creating a community health profile composed of indicators of basic demographic and socioeconomic characteristics, health status, and health risk factors proposed by the coalition or other community level organization. This profile offers a broad overview of a community's characteristics, health status, and resources. For an added valuable dimension to these assessments, the community health status indicators (CHSI) (U.S. Department of Health and Human Services, 2008) web-based tool has mapping capabilities that allow users to visually compare peer counties. The report generated by the CHSI tool can serve as a starting point for a community assessment of needs, quantification of disadvantaged populations, and measurement of preventable diseases, disabilities, and deaths.

Many have argued that needs assessments fall short in some respects. They consider what is missing (i.e., a deficit orientation) (Tatian, 2000) and may be conducted in a way that does not honor the understanding that mobilizing existing community assets can be an effective tool (Metzler, 2007).

Assets

Asset-based approaches draw from the literature on risk-protective factors, termed "assets" (University of Arizona, 2008). Kretzmann and McKnight (1993) advocate for an asset-based approach to assist communities in finding ways to empower themselves and to sustain change. Further, Kretzmann and McKnight have underscored the considerable assets that communities often possess and argue that it is helpful when assessing a community's needs to simultaneously locate assets to help address them. Assets within a community may include physical resources, skill sets (including problem solving) among community members, and structures and relationships at all levels of the community. By placing the focus on resources within a community's individuals and organizations, it becomes possible not only to utilize these strengths but also to build on them (Tatian, 2000).

Identifying unacknowledged assets and needs can be empowering to communities. Making known both strengths and gaps helps communities to identify and implement home-grown solutions. Communities can draw from the scientific literature, as well as the knowledge and experience of community members, when identifying program priorities to address social determinants of health (Monsey, Owen, Zierman, Lamberb, & Lyman, 1995).

Community Participation

Community-based participatory data collection strategies provide an even greater degree of specificity with regard to the community's context and a better understanding of the often indirect influences of social determinants on a community's health. Building this understanding through community dialogue (e.g., through town hall meetings, focus groups, and other discussions) can inform the selection and targeting of activities in ways that better meet community needs.

For example, Darrow et al. (2004) used community discussions to identify the types of intervention approaches most desired. These were found to include horizontal outreach to residents, vertical outreach to stakeholders and gatekeepers, strategic communications, capacity building, and infrastructure development. Ultimately, the process for identifying intervention approaches, that is, having significant community engagement, led to them being well received. These discussions can also be structured to identify gaps in community resources and factors that may contribute to disease burden and, if addressed, may improve the community's health (Aronson, Wallis, O' Campo, Whitehead, & Schafer, 2007).

Participating community members also gain valuable skills in the assessment process, and their involvement helps ensure the sustainability of this new knowledge within the community (Watson-Thompson et al., 2008) and feelings of empowerment (Butterfoss, 2004; Butterfoss, Goodman, & Wandersman, 1996) and can enhance a community's ability to effectively mobilize its resources (Watson-Thompson et al., 2008). As can be seen, the strategic planning process establishes what constitutes success in regard to community change. This, in turn, informs the selection of targeted actions.

Targeted Action

As part of the planning phase, targeted actions within the context of a SEM are often selected to address community needs and with assets in mind (e.g., Bergstrom et al., 1995; Chappell, Funk, Carson, MacKenzie, & Stanwick, 2006; Dailly & Barr, 2008; English, Fairbanks, Finster, Rafelito, Luna, & Kennedy, 2006; Kegler, Twiss, & Look, 2000; KU Work Group on Health Promotion and Community Development, 2007, ch. 8; Tucker et al., 2006; Watson-Thompson et al., 2008). Brenan Ramirez, Baker, and Metzler (2008) offer a workbook that can help communities identify targeted actions. Using a case study approach, they provide examples that illustrate community programs and approaches to increase health equity by addressing social determinants of health.

Before turning to the organizational, community, and societal levels of the SEM, four areas for targeted action are briefly reviewed: process development, intervention development and implementation, policy development and implementation, and citizen and resource development. These are adapted from the collaboration framework for addressing community capacity (Bergstrom et al., 1995).

Multilevel Intervention Development and Implementation

Targeted actions may take the form of multilevel community interventions. Ideally they reflect the community needs and assets identified during the assessment and planning phase. Lafferty & Mahoney (2003) found that multilevel interventions include goals that focus on individual, /family, neighborhood, and systems change. Programmatically, their focus tends to be social support, education and /training, and economic development (Aspen Institute, 1997; Lafferty & Mahoney, 2003; Rosenberg, Kerr, King, Moore, Patrick, & Sallis, 2008; Schensul & Trickett, 2009). Interventions may target a specific health area, (e.g., type 2 diabetes) within a priority population (e.g., African American adults). Efforts are then made to ensure intervention content and delivery match the preferences of the target audience and are culturally competent. Clearly defining the program and its intended population, and documenting its implementation, helps the community identify changes attributable to the program and apply lessons learned to other populations.

The benefits of comprehensive, multilevel interventions are well-established (Glasgow, Vogt, & Boles, 1999; IOM, 2003; Lafferty & Mahoney, 2003; Lasker, Weiss, & Miller, 2001; Pentz, 2000). Consistent with the spectrum of prevention (Hanni, Mendoza, Snider, & Winkleby, 2007), they utilize activities at multiple levels, including strengthening individual knowledge and skills, promoting community education, educating providers, fostering coalitions and networks, changing organizational practices, and influencing policy and legislation. Multilevel interventions partly reflect the need to address multiple factors that influence a community's health. They also reflect a need to work (and leverage resources) across community sectors to bring about change. These interventions can build community capacity through improving approaches to governance, funding, staffing, technical assistance, and evaluation. Multilevel interventions may more effectively use social networks that cut across multiple community levels and thereby increase their effectiveness in addressing barriers by involving those with influence over circumstances and events that fall outside a community's control at any one level. These interventions also honor the goal of involving and reaching all members across a community.

The use of activities and interventions in combination with one another, and at multiple levels, is one of the reasons that multilevel interventions are likely to produce more lasting community change than single activities or interventions. (Cohen & Swift, 1999; Hanni et al., 2007). Whereas effectively implementing and evaluating multilevel and multi-component interventions poses challenges (Lafferty & Mahoney, 2003), there is wide support for their use to affect community change.

Policy Development and Implementation

Some interventions may entail new or expanded services (the plan itself may imply a policy change) with or without a stated intention that the programmatic policy will contribute to changes in health-related behaviors or outcomes (Pentz, 2000). Other interventions are directed at a policy process. Policies are action plans that are used to guide decision making to reach a desired goal. The steps making up the policy process may include issue definition, setting objectives and priorities, defining options, options appraisal, policy implementation and evaluation, and assessment of community capacity to develop and influence policies and actions related to implementing and evaluating policy changes (Breinbauer & Maddaleno, 2005; Hill et al., 2007). A targeted action directed at policy change may include one or more steps in the policy process. Overall, attributes identified by Breinbauer and Maddaleno (2005) for an effective policy process, are the need for flexibility, transparency, and openness to broad public participation.

There are different types of policies. For example, regulatory policies include formal laws, regulations, and ordinances. They can also guide rather than prescribe actions. Some or all of these types of policies may have implications for eliminating diabetes disparities. Programmatic (or implementation) policies may be geared toward institutionalizing programs (e.g., allowing employees time off from work to exercise and allotting resources to make stairwells safer and more appealing to encourage their use). Overall, regulatory policies may show the most immediate effect, whereas programmatic ones have the most potential for long-term impact (Pentz, 2000).

The relationship between social determinants of health and health outcomes can be quite complex, indirect, and embedded in a range of contextual factors. In addition, the time often required to affect policy changes, as well as the often significant lag to reap benefits, may be seen as prohibitive. Documenting the impact of policy change on the public's health also remains a challenge (Chaloupka & Johnston, 2007; Hill, Sallis, Peters, 2004; Mackenbach; 2003), especially with regard to the impact of policy changes on social determinants and health equity (Kelly & Bonnefoy, 2007). However, there is general agreement that both policy and programmatic targeted actions strengthen the ability of multilevel interventions to produce sustained effects and, in turn, sustain community prevention efforts (Pentz, 2000). Community-based diabetes programs are encouraged to develop, implement, enforce, and evaluate policy changes directed at reducing diabetes disparities.

Capacity Development

Building community capacity to sustain targeted action toward community change is critical. In addition to training and technical assistance, effective interventions require increased community participation. Participatory approaches recognize the rights of community members to make decisions about issues that affect their collective health.

These approaches help partnerships build on local strengths and resources (Cargo & Mercer, 2008). Throughout the process, from determining community needs and assets through implementation and evaluation of targeted action, a community-based participatory approach is strongly encouraged. These approaches foster social justice through the inclusion of individual community members, community organizers, public health workers, policy makers, and others (Cargo & Mercer, 2008).

THE COMMUNITY-BASED SOCIOECOLOGICAL MODEL

The socioecological model used here will be referred to as the community-based socioecological model (CBSEM). The CBSEM is a conceptual, multilevel model that depicts health related behaviors as not only how an individual's knowledge, beliefs, and behaviors influence their health status but also how efforts at multiple community levels can influence long-term healthy options for an entire population (Ammerman & Mansourch, 2005; Dahlberg & Krug, 2002; IOM, 2003). The CBSEM is closely aligned conceptually with the IOM determinants of health model provided in chapter 3. The CBSEM's five levels are: (a) individual, (b) family and social networks, (c) organizational, (d) community and inter-organizational, and (e) systems.

Efforts to reduce and eliminate diabetes disparities begins at the individual level. In addition, the family and social networks level includes an individual's closest network of people (i.e., family, friends, peers, providers, etc.) who promote healthy behaviors and encourage the individual to make healthy choices. An individual's social network may vary in size, stage of the life cycle, frequency of contact, relationship quality, and geographical proximity. These networks may also influence an individual's norms and values (Ammerman & Mansourch, 2005; Dahlberg & Krug, 2002; IOM, 2003).

Although the lifestyle factors and social networks of individuals with diabetes are clearly important to address health disparities, we now focus on change within and brought about by community organizations and through their inter-organizational relationships within and outside the community. In turn, we frame the discussion of community change at the level of an individual organization, an inter-organizational or community level, and a systems level. As with the model introduced by Liburd in chapter 3, we see the lines between CBSEM levels as dotted, indicating that their relationship is dynamic, with individual organizational capacities and having direct implications for what is accomplished inter-organizationally and at the systems level.

Organizational Level of the CBSEM

At the organizational level there are local entities and organizations that influence community conditions. They include government (e.g., state and local health departments, federal agencies, schools, and law enforcement), non-profits (e.g., faith-based institutions, voluntary organizations, and associations), and businesses and industries (e.g., barbershops, beauty salons, grocers, and chambers of commerce) (Ackermann, Finch, Brizendine, Zhou, & Marrero, 2008; McKeever, Koroloff, & Faddis, 2006). Various organizations provide the public with diabetes information and materials to increase awareness on the prevention, treatment, and control of diabetes. Some national, regional, and statewide organizations and associations exist to provide evidence-based guidelines and resources to health professionals and practitioners.

Structure

Formal organizations existing in the U.S. are typically categorized as (a) government, including federal, state, and local government (i.e., county, sub-county, etc.); (b) non-profit organizations with a tax-exempt status (i.e., private foundations, professional association, faith-based organizations, etc.); or (c) business and industry, or for-profit organizations (i.e., restaurants, convenience stores, barbershops, etc.). Members of U.S. communities are served by one or more of these organizations where the resources offered may vary from one community to the next. For example, one community may have access to a supermarket where a variety of fresh fruits and vegetables are sold, whereas another community's access to fruits and vegetables is limited to a local convenience store. Planners of community-based diabetes interventions should examine the engagement of these institutions in supporting a broad range of efforts that reduce the burden of diabetes in communities of color.

Government

Several federal agencies and national organizations serve as clearinghouses for people seeking diabetes information (National Institute of Diabetes and Digestive and Kidney Diseases, 2007). They also provide evidenced-based clinical practice guidelines and information regarding federal regulations to community health professionals (U.S. Department of Veteran's Affairs, 2007). Federal organizations may also provide funds to state-based diabetes prevention and control programs to develop and maintain local programs (Centers for Disease Control and Prevention, 2008) and resources to support diabetes research (Juvenile Diabetes Research Foundation International, 2009; National Institute of Diabetes and Digestive and Kidney Diseases, 2009; National Kidney Foundation, 2009).

Local entities like schools must now serve the diabetes management needs of their students (Kaufman, 2002), but this does not always happen. Instead there are children with diabetes enrolled in schools and daycare centers with personnel who are not equipped to make good diabetes management possible for their students (Kaufman, 2002). It is therefore essential for families to understand their children's legal rights in schools. In turn, schools are charged with meeting federal laws that provide protection to school children with diabetes (Kaufman, 2002).

Non-Profit Organizations

The reach of non-profit organizations to promote diabetes awareness can extend well into the community. A number of national non-profit diabetes organizations produce and disseminate educational materials and publications to respond to frequent inquiries, including those from health professionals, regarding the prevention and treatment of diabetes (e.g., The American Diabetes Association, Diabetes Exercise and Sports Association, National Diabetes Education Program, National Kidney and Urologic Diseases Information Clearinghouse Program, National Kidney Disease Education, and Weight-Control Information Network). They also play a significant role supporting, funding, and advocating for diabetes research and programs (Centers for Disease Control and Prevention, 2008).

Faith-based institutions are also involved in local health promotion strategies that support diabetes prevention and control. One example is Project Diabetes Interventions Reaching and Educating Communities Together (Project DIRECT), which is described in more detail in chapter 8. This multi-year participatory research project, sponsored by the Centers for Disease Control and Prevention, examined how social and environmental changes to support diabetes prevention and control were achieved by a North Carolina historically Black university and Black churches in southeast Raleigh (Reid, Hatch, & Parrish, 2003). Other types of non-profit organizations have also demonstrated their capacity to implement diabetes prevention programs. For example, the Young Men's Christian Association (YMCA) participated in a study to evaluate the delivery of a group-based diabetes prevention program lifestyle intervention in a YMCA facility located in a semi-urban community. The YMCA was found to be a promising conduit for disseminating diabetes interventions to adults at risk of diabetes (Ackermann et al., 2008). Another type of non-profit organization is the Association of Community Organizations for Reform Now (ACORN), a grassroots community organization of low- and moderate-income people addressing community issues, including affordable housing, quality education, and access to health care services. An example of their work takes place in California where ACORN elected to "organize statewide for affordable, quality coverage for all Californians," regardless of age and immigration status (ACORN, 2007). It was reported in April 2007 that the efforts of ACORN members led to the San Francisco Board of Supervisors landmark legislation requiring medium and large businesses to provide health coverage for their workers. (ACORN, 2007).

Business and Industries

People often spend the majority of their working hours at worksites. Worksite health promotion programs are making significant contributions to improved diabetes control (Glasgow et al., 1999). For example, Burton and Connerty (1998, 2002) found that worksite-based patient education programs for employees resulted in significant improvements in diabetes control. Such programs are expected to lead to lower health care costs and improved quality of life (Burton & Connerty, 1998, 2002).

One result is that businesses of all sizes and from various industries are implementing health promotion interventions. The African American Health Coalition, a REACH 2010 project in Portland, OR, implemented several interventions to reduce disparities among African Americans. The Lookin' Tight Livin' Right intervention is implemented in local beauty salons and barbershops. Based on established relationships with their clients, trained hair stylists used motivational interviewing techniques to educate clients about cardiovascular disease, a co-morbidity of diabetes (McKeever et al., 2006).

Organizational Policy

Policy determines the rules by which opportunities are framed, that is, what is allowed, encouraged, discouraged, and prohibited (Bell & Standish, 2005). Flexibility in government, non-profit, for-profit, and other decentralized community-level organizational structures can support differing community change needs (Hamilton & Tesh, 2002). Increases in organizational flexibility at the community level may represent a significant change. Communities also benefit when organizations are familiar with key community issues and understand how its functions can serve community needs (Tatian, 2000). A community organization's targeted actions that contribute to local strengths and resources will in turn experience social engagement and growing levels of community trust (Cargo & Mercer, 2008).

Policies affect a range of community characteristics. For example, they influence the types of businesses in a geographic area, their proximity to residential neighborhoods, and residential neighborhood density. The policy development process, which includes defining the issue, establishing objectives and priorities, determining options, assessing the options, and implementing and evaluating the policy, shapes these and other neighborhood characteristics (Breinbauer & Maddaleno, 2005). The policy process can be influenced by the efforts of local businesses and advocacy groups, as well as government agencies and other entities within and outside the community.

Organizational policies vary and are typically aligned with the goals and objectives of the organization. The reasons an organization might develop policies include: to institutionalize programs and services; create environments that are more supportive of behavioral changes; adopt health-enhancing standards and guidelines for delivery of programs, practices, and services; conform to laws and regulations; connect to an intervention component of another organization; and respond to community concerns. Policies that affect community environments present organizations with opportunities to eliminate health disparities (Bell & Standish, 2005).

Improved enforcement of regulatory policies, including formal laws, regulations, and ordinances, may constitute a significant policy change. For example, Section 504, a civil rights law, prohibits any school receiving federal funds from discriminating against people on the basis of disability (e.g., having diabetes). This law has resulted in qualified schools developing diabetes management strategies for students (Kaufman, 2002). All of these organizational policy changes and community efforts represent promising new avenues for affecting the determinants of health and improving health status. With concerted long-term attention and support, they can reduce the severity and incidence of diabetes health disparities, thus charting a new and much-needed pathway for change.

Organizational Capacity

The capacity of an organization is based on its resources, possession or awareness of information or facts, and processes. For example, capacity includes the organization's leadership, programs, linkages with other groups or organizations, staff, and financial resources (International Development Research Centre, 2008). A local health center offers diabetes self-management education by a certified diabetes educator in the language primarily spoken in the majority of homes in the community. This enhances the health center's capacity to deliver a culturally tailored intervention. In turn, changes to staff training and development opportunities enhance the organization's capacity to deliver such interventions. Collecting data regarding these interventions' delivery can constitute an important organizational change; distilling lessons learned can shape organizational strategies, enhance their level of readiness, and ultimately improve their public health impact (Potapchuck, 2007).

An organization's capacity can be greatly enhanced through partnerships with a diverse group of stakeholders, including political allies (the community's power brokers and policy makers) like local governing boards and elected leaders, nonpolitical individuals of influence (Potapchuck, 2007) or change agents (Tucker et al., 2006), and community advocates). Another key ingredient to organizational capacity is community-level participation in local decision making, involvement is important regardless of the level of the organization. The community's involvement can result in leadership opportunities, a shared sense of belonging, and increased trust in local government and other community organizations. These in turn are all reflections of increased organizational capacity (Potapchuck, 2007). Organizations also benefit from increased personal commitment from leaders, employees, clients, and constituents (Potapchuck, 2007).

Social networks between community organizations can increase individual organization effectiveness in meeting community needs (Brieger, 2008). Through inter-organizational linkages, organizations learn of other community programs providing services to the same community— services that might enhance one another. These intersections between organizational efforts can provide partnership opportunities (Community Research Partners, 2008; IOM, 2003; Metzler, 2007). In communities with comprehensive initiatives that address the needs of large populations, partnering with organizations at many levels (e.g., neighborhood, city, county, and region) may help address barriers to what they can accomplish (Tatian, 2000). These partnership opportunities constitute important community change as new inter-organizational relationships.

Community Level of the CBSEM

The community level of the CBSEM includes the formation and maintenance of community and inter-organizational relationships. These are often created to address community health issues and are seen as falling toward the collaborative end of Himmelman's continuum. Himmelman

(1996) places collaboration at the most demanding end of a continuum of working together. Among collaborating organizations, each serves a particular function that defines their contribution and through which they provide leadership. Agreement around organizational functions requires mutual interest in collaborating. It also requires a similar understanding of collaborative purpose and desired outcomes, the presence of specific skills, and consideration of contextual factors affecting collaborative success.

These community-level relationships (CLRs) consist of individuals and organizations, often facilitated by a central coordinating organization. As with the previous level of the CBSEM, these relationships depend on individuals and organizations having an interest in working together toward a common goal, such as the elimination of diabetes disparities in communities of color (Butterfoss, 2007; Kegler, Norton, & Aronson, 2008; KU Work Group on Health Promotion and Community Development, 2007, ch. 5). The formation of these strong yet flexible relationships can constitute an important community change, encouraging participatory decision making and supporting better integration of community efforts and resources (Kegler, Steckler, McLeroy, & Malek, 1998; Potapchuck, 2007).

Bergstrom et al. (1995) recommend the use of collaborative processes to achieve rapid changes in beliefs, behaviors, and policies. They see collaboration as particularly effective in the areas of public safety, education, economic well-being, family support, health, and environment. These areas of collaboration appear consistent with multilevel interventions addressing social determinants of health. For this reason, collaboration in itself may constitute an important community change.

Community Level Relationships

A CLR may take many forms, including that of a nonprofit organization, advisory board, consumer rights and advocacy group, coalition, or partnership. For the present discussion, a CLR can be one or more of these community structures, each containing representatives from multiple organizations and working toward a common goal. Formation of CLRs may include a large number of organizations over time, with the CLR periodically convening to make decisions around inter-organizational efforts.

In addition to its involvement of residents (Potapchuck, 2007), a CLR brings together members from diverse community sectors (Potapchuck, 2007), including businesses, racial and ethnic groups, faith-based organizations, and various public agencies (IOM, 2003; Johnston, Marmet, Coen, Fawcett, & Harris, 1996; Potapchuck, 2007). The CLR may involve health regulators, providers, advocates, and experts (Hamilton & Tesh, 2002). In turn, they may include the local health department, public health officials, health care and mental health services providers, social service and community development agencies, educators, faith-based leaders, a chamber of commerce representative, and others (IOM, 2003; Kegler et al., 2000; Potapchuck, 2007).

A CLR may include a large inter-organizational network and require a significant level of community involvement in the planning process and for targeted action (Watson-Thompson et al., 2008). Perkins, Florin, Rich, Wandersman, and Chavis (1990) offer examples of individual-level factors (e.g., years of residence, race, ethnicity, income, and home ownership) and characteristics of the built environment (e.g., neighborhood parks, architecture, transportation routes, street lights, and grocery stores) that influence levels of participation. In communities of color, where demographic and environmental factors may be associated with lower levels of participation (IOM, 2003; World Health Organization, 2008), the structure provided by a CLR helps encourage participation in decision making. This and other CLR attributes have been associated with greater civic engagement, member participation and satisfaction, action plan quality, resource mobilization, implementation effectiveness, and neighborhood outcomes (Kegler et al., 1998; Potapchuck, 2007).

Increased participation in the inter-organizational CLR constitutes an important community-level change by better enabling the CLR to have an accurate understanding of diverse community needs and assets. This provides assurance that any subsequent targeted actions will address the most pressing of community needs. Also as a result, the plan for targeted action may more fully consider and incorporate community assets (IOM, 2003) where use of asset mapping can serve as evidence of a CLR's concerted effort to accomplish this goal. Increased participation in program design and delivery provides community members with detailed program knowledge, thereby providing needed capacity to deliver and sustain public health efforts.

Member organizations can experience greater levels of interest in collaborating and have a clearer sense of the key health issues and their individual functions (Tatian, 2000). One result may be a collective vision and goals (IOM, 1997; Potapchuck, 2007; Tatian, 2000). They may also experience the process as having a higher level of social engagement and have greater feelings of inter-organizational trust.

The CLR represents a diverse set of the community's organizations and encourages targeted actions that are community-directed and build on local strengths and resources (Cargo & Mercer, 2008). It may also foster feelings of inclusiveness, indicated by greater levels of participation by organizations and community residents in assessments of program planning, delivery, and outcomes (Potapchuck, 2007; Watson-Thompson et al., 2008). Ultimately, community change efforts benefit from increased community leader commitment (Potapchuck, 2007).

Structures and Relationships

Sustained inter-organizational collaboration toward a common goal strengthens feelings of empowerment, which are associated with perceptions of inclusive and equitable decision making (Hamilton & Tesh, 2002), feelings of social engagement, social cohesion, and efficacy (Foster-Fishman, Berkowitz, Lounsbury, Jacobson, & Allen, 2001; Shediac-Rizkallah & Bone, 1998; Watson-Thompson et al., 2008). Higher levels of functioning among these community-level groups is also associated with degree of civic engagement, member participation and satisfaction, quality of action plans, effectiveness of resource mobilization and intervention implementation, and neighborhood health outcomes (Kegler et al., 1998; Potapchuck, 2007).

Sustaining CLRs is, in large part, about the sharing of inter-organizational capacities. Organizations may choose to collaboratively coordinate their efforts and combine resources to deliver or improve services. These partnerships help maximize capacity to address community health needs and enable the CLR to capitalize on the reach of their combined social networks across sectors to other political, commercial, clinical/patient, and community partners (Weech-Maldonado, Benson, & Gamm, 2003). CLRs are often better positioned than individual organizations to change the root causes of health inequalities (Cargo & Mercer, 2008). Public-private partnerships, such as empowerment zones and enterprise communities, can also infuse significant government resources and ensure collaboration at the local level to improve health in communities. These entities may also already be oriented toward community health issues (Beck, Wingard, Zúñiga, Heifetz & Gilbreath, 2008; Public Health Foundation, 2000; U.S. Department of Housing and Urban Development, 2005; U.S. Department of Housing and Urban Development, 2009).

Once a CLR is established around a specific goal, considerable efforts are dedicated to strengthening and sustaining the CLR. In the present context, the CLR represents an agreement between a number of organizations to address priority health issues together. Relationships may falter if organizational members do not continue to feel that the CLR membership represents the diversity of organizations across community sectors; member organization roles and responsibilities become unclear (Watson-Thompson et al., 2008); there is an inappropriate level of inter-organizational involvement (Nelson, Chapko, Reiber, & Boyko, 2005); or the originally identified goals are no longer seen as addressing the highest community health priorities (Potapchuck, 2007).

The CLR may conduct periodic assessments of its processes, program activities, and early outcomes and review these findings in concert with community-level indicators (Community Research Partners, 2008; Metzler et al., 2008). The findings can inform inter-organizational decisions regarding how best to use its limited resources. Assessment of activities and outcomes as they are unfolding can help explain and address low community involvement, build capacity to sustain culturally competent interventions, and foster their consistent delivery across the community (when this is a goal).

Ultimately, the evidence of whether a community's organizational structures and governance are effective is whether it is able to bring about environmental and policy changes (Meister & De Zapien, 2005). Meanwhile, member organizations can document any efficiencies resulting from their integrated program efforts (Potapchuck, 2007) and examples of how inter-organizational relationships have affected their sense of ownership and empowerment. They might also document the inter-relationships between these individual organizational stories to begin to paint a picture of how community change occurs. For example, community redevelopment efforts, in partnership with local agencies and businesses, may bolster employment levels that, in turn, improve personal income. This may support access to health insurance and tax revenues that can be used to improve neighborhood parks, city transit, and so forth (IOM, 2003; National Association of City and County Health Officials, 2000).

Policy

As a result of their participation, CLR member organizations may exhibit increases in their abilities and interests in policy development. There may also be evidence, in formal documents such as a strategic or community health improvement plan, of a transition from a predominantly programmatic focus to one that is intentional regarding policy change (Hill et al., 2007). A growing policy focus may also be evidenced by advocacy activities associated with policy shifts (Hill et al., 2007).

A CLR can influence policy change within individual member organizations, for example, to develop, expand, or institutionalize programs and services that promote health in the workplace (Kegler, Norton, & Aronson, 2008; Kegler et al., 2000; Sorensen, Emmons, Hunt, & Johnston, 1998). It can encourage member organizations to support internal policies related to one or more multilevel intervention components identified by the CLR as high priority. For example, larger organizations may be asked to disclose the approximate calorie content of food served in their cafeteria or to offer time off to employees for physical activity. The CLR may also advocate for adoption of program standards and guidelines to help ensure quality program implementation of programs across member organizations (Pentz, 1994). Influence through the regulatory process by advocating for formal laws, regulations, and ordinances is another policy impact of the CLR. For example, the CLR may advocate for closer monitoring and stronger enforcement of school lunch and vending machine content (Pentz, 2000).

A variety of factors have been found to influence whether a community policy is ultimately enacted. Pentz (2000) found that coalition achieving policy goals had identified and developed local resources to sustain the policies, assessed program effects, and included policy changes among their stated objectives. Some included policies explicitly stating the intention to contribute to changes in the social determinants of diabetes. CLRs also influence the regulatory process by advocating for ordinances, regulations, and formal laws that have, in turn, been coupled with improved enforcement (Kegler et al., 2000, 2008).

Policy support is more effective when CLRs use mass media to keep issues (e.g., community racial and ethnic disparities) in the local media (Pentz, 2000; Potapchuck, 2007). Effectiveness of mass media is also evidenced by improvements over time in the ability to convey messages to priority populations with greater accuracy, efficiency, and effectiveness. (Shediac-Rizkallah & Bone, 1998).

More generally, effective inter-organizational policy processes tend to emphasize flexibility, since organizational policies can differ significantly. Transparency is important and can be achieved through broad and public participation. There is also a growing emphasis to close the policy process loop through the evaluation of CLR policy efforts and incorporating what is learned into subsequent planning and targeted action. Finally, studies show the identification of an influential program champion to be associated with policy success, program sustainability, feelings of empowerment, higher levels of interpersonal communication, and even the level of specificity of a coalition's objectives (Butterfoss, Goodman, & Wandersman, 1996; Pentz, 2000; Saxe et al., 1997).

Possibly reflecting a previous programmatic emphasis, many community members and organizations will not fully understand the policy process in a community decision making context. The development of this understanding may constitute a realistic community change milestone as a prerequisite for other targeted actions toward policy change. The CLR organizational structure can help to build this civic capacity with inter-organizational partnerships serving as a learning network in which partners receive mutual support through structured opportunities to share experiences. They can use the shared information to assess their capacities and intervention strategies and, in turn, can help disseminate best practices instilled through workshops, curricula, web-based clearinghouses, and tool kits designed for community leaders and local elected officials (Potapchuck, 2007). Community member participation in the advocacy process also serves to build capacity for ongoing change efforts (Meister & De Zapien, 2005), as do the CLR policies and practices that define and encourage community member involvement in decision making.

While some CLRs have developed primarily with a programmatic focus, for others the policy focus may change significantly over time. In either case, CLR membership may include a large number of public health experts and organizations but few with expertise in public management or education. These may be areas in which the CLR hopes to have a larger policy impact. In addition to CLR membership expertise, strategic plans and structures may also need to be supplemented to address the growing or changing policy focus.

CLRs may seek out community organizations with policy expertise and may partner with community redevelopment efforts, public-private partnerships (e.g., empowerment zones and enterprise communities), or other efforts that can contribute policy experience toward addressing root causes of health inequalities. The CLR may also supplement its own organizational structure with a special action group charged with championing key policy and advocacy activities. These and other workgroups can be helpful to identify and prioritize policy issues and secure new resources to support policy changes (Cohen, Meister, deZapien, Zuckerman, & Zuckerman, 2004; Meister & De Zapien, 2005).

Community Capacity

CLRs leverage capacity for community-level change through joint programs and other relationships between their multiple organizations. In addition to expanding financial resources to sustain diabetes efforts (Graber et al., 2008; Huang et al., 2007; Shediac-Rizkallah & Bone, 1998), they may share social (e.g., expertise) and human (e.g., staff time) capital across organizations and intervention activities (Kegler et al., 2000). In addition to these in-kind contributions, much of the capacity needed to sustain interventions may be generated by the interventions themselves—for example, by strengthening individual knowledge and skills through community and provider education.

Communities of Practice

The CLR may also serve as a community of practice through which member organizations receive mutual support and opportunities to share experiences. Through this learning community, CLRs may share resources and provide training to build understanding of diabetes, social determinants of health, policy processes, and race relations.

They may also seek to enhance skills in leadership, cultural competency, community building, engagement strategies, and framing community problems and goals in racial-equity terms (Potapchuck, 2007).

Building this capacity may occur through workshops and tool kits targeting community leaders, institutional allies, elected officials, and partners; a web-based clearinghouse for reports, tools, tip sheets, and other resources for organizations; satellite broadcasts or webcasts, community-level data; and strategies for improving the community health system (Cahn et al., 2007; Potapchuck, 2007). As with program and policy interventions, there are a number of frameworks that CLRs can draw from to inform capacity-building efforts. For example, Potapchuck's framework (2007) summarizes current thinking regarding key community actions to bring about health equity.

As a result of training, the CLR might expect increases in policy advocacy among its member organizations. For example, there may be an increase in the frequency and visibility with which organizational leaders take a formal position within the community's decision making processes (Potapchuck, 2007). Efforts to document its learning opportunities, inter-organizational actions, and changes can help the CLR to "connect the dots" between the capacity and leadership it provides and the policy impact.

In addition to reflection on the CLR inter-organizational capacity, structures, and activities, the CLR must also document its delivery of the multilevel intervention and establish the level of progress toward stated health-related goals. Complex interventions that incorporate policy, environmental, and individual components should be evaluated with measurements suited to their settings, goals, and purpose (Glasgow et al., 1999) and, ultimately, program impact is likely to be among the critical questions asked. Toward these ends, Glasgow et al. (1999) offer the RE-AIM framework. They propose that in order to determine population-based impact, programs and policies are often effectively assessed across levels of the SEM with a focus on their reach, efficacy, adoption, implementation, and maintenance. In addition to this impact focus, documenting program intensity, duration, and penetration into the community can also be important (IOM, 2003). This provides evidence regarding the degree to which the targeted action plan is fully implemented to address community needs.

Documenting these aspects of the program also helps to communicate more clearly what it entails. For those instances in which a previously developed program was adopted, indicators may already exist (that can be adopted) to assess its impact and help gauge the degree to which program fidelity was maintained. However, the value of program fidelity must also consider that initiatives evolve over time so they can respond to the changing community needs (Lafferty & Mahoney, 2003). Assessing the allocation of resources over time to each of the major components of a complex programmatic effort can also help ensure the highest priority community changes are realized by providing a means to prioritize resources.

Even with a comprehensive, multilevel evaluation plan, a frequent challenge is the need for local area data that accounts for neighborhood-level variation. This challenge has resulted in an over-reliance on secondary data analysis and the use of administrative areas and aggregate census data to characterize neighborhoods (Diez Roux, 2007). However, these data may not accurately portray associations between neighborhood characteristics and health effects. For example, many less formal community networks and other processes are likely to operate at the block level and not be accurately represented or understood at other levels of analysis (Perkins et al., 1990). Block boundaries are easily identifiable. They tend to be more culturally similar than larger geographic areas and allow for better estimates of the level of participation across groups within a community.

It has also been pointed out that when assessing the impact of neighborhood programs on community health, impact measures should be broadened. For example, a study by Diez Roux (2007) underscores the preponderance of evidence linking neighborhood characteristics to community mental health. Even so, policy makers infrequently incorporate mental health as a measure for evaluating neighborhood improvement programs.

In addition to supporting staff and organizational development, the CLR encourages evaluation and reflection to reveal progress toward key goals, strategies that have been most and least effective, key areas of difference in community readiness, and so forth (Potapchuck, 2007). As a result, the CLR may continue to promote specific issues or strategies and minimize its involvement with and use of others (Potapchuck, 2007; Tatian, 2000). Assessment and reflection by the CLR is critical as a supportive feedback loop between targeted action, community change, and ongoing inter-organizational strategic planning.

Systems Level of the CBSEM

Community-level diabetes prevention and control efforts may depend on the simultaneous engagement of multiple networks of health professionals positioned in a range of community organizations and across multiple sectors and systems. They exist at the local, state, and national levels and interact and influence one another (Lafferty & Mahoney, 2003; Porche, 2004). The CBSEM systems level is all-encompassing, involving individuals, communities, organizations, and local, state, and federal governments working together to produce change. Local policies, statewide legislation, and federal laws each have a role in comprehensive approaches for supporting the elimination of diabetes health disparities and addressing health equity. Other overlapping systems exist as well (e.g., health, economic, educational, and social policy) and each is essential to achieving and sustaining health equity.

Multilevel interventions reflect the need to work (and leverage resources) across community organizations and sectors. These interventions honor the goal of involving and reaching all members of a community and considering system-level factors that contribute to or hinder community change efforts. In their comprehensiveness, they can help communities transform their institutions by changing policies and practices to eliminate racial and ethnic disparities (Potapchuck, 2007).

Structures and Relationships

Communities, as both change agents and those affected by social determinants of health inequity, empower themselves by partnering across disciplines and levels of political and social organization (Metzler, 2007). To alter constraints placed by the external environment on what they can accomplish, and because community-level organizations may not associate directly with broader public health systems (Hassinger & Pinkerton, 1986), communities partner with outside stakeholders. These external partners may include city- or county-wide, state-level, regional, and national organizations (Brennan Ramirez et al., 2008; Hassinger & Pinkerton, 1986; Metzler, 2007; Potapchuck, 2007; Tatian, 2000). The Kansas Leadership to Encourage Activity and Nutrition Coalition is one example of how a local effort can grow over several years. It was eventually able to foster the development of a statewide coalition of more than 60 organizations. It includes participation from state and local public health departments, extension offices, nonprofit community and professional organizations, and businesses like supermarkets to prevent chronic disease through dietary change and exercise (Johnston et al., 1996).

The scope of assessing community- and system-level efforts can be staggering. The IOM Committee on Using Performance Monitoring to Improve Community Health (1997) discusses the role of performance monitoring in the community change process (Community Research Partners, 2008; Potapchuck, 2007). As mentioned earlier, this IOM committee proposes the CHIP as one tool for community partners to develop and implement a well-integrated community health approach. The CHIP was developed on the premise that social and economic conditions are strong determinants of health outcomes and require involvement of less traditional public health partners (Community Research Partners, 2008; IOM, 1997) and a cross-sector response (Tatian, 2000). When communities implement a CHIP, it helps monitor responsibilities that are shared across sectors in a manner that considers a variety of health determinants (IOM, 1997) and in turn promotes collaboration and accountability. There are also comprehensive community indicator data sources available to communities at no cost (e.g., Metzler et al.,

2008). These sources can help establish a sense of urgency for action and inform program planning, implementation, and evaluation.

Policy

CLRs also advocate for system-level policy changes because of their potential impact on the community. A community-level organization may help establish and participate in a state-level health disparities collaborative and in turn support the enactment of system-level policies (Texas Association of Community Health Centers, 2008). They also may work to influence policies geared to institutionalize programs by advocating structural or financial resources to support the administration of a program.

Through CLRs, organizations can have a larger policy influence on community leaders than they can alone. They are better positioned to influence funding decisions and build awareness at the community and system levels in ways that influence land use plans and policies regarding density of fast food restaurants and the location of full-service grocery stores. Together they may advocate more effectively for increasing the mixed use of neighborhoods—not only because these neighborhoods can provide greater opportunities for healthful behaviors but also because they may increase civic participation and social capital, key ingredients for sustaining community change.

Capacity

Some barriers outside the community reduce the possibility of community change and organizational effectiveness. Only at the system level can these barriers be effectively addressed. In addition, inter-organizational partnerships that extend beyond the community can lead to much more expansive networks that offer access to needed resources to sustain community change. For this reason, multi-sectoral, inter-organizational partnerships can be central to securing diverse financial resources (Hassinger & Pinkerton, 1986). This can include corporate sponsors and foundations that bring valuable perspectives to community development systems, long-standing community relationships with civic leaders, and familiarity in broad programmatic areas (Potapchuck, 2007).

As with the community level of the CBSEM, there may be a need to build systems-level capacity within the CLR by seeking involvement from organizations with system-level expertise, providing leadership training of institutional allies and partners, and offering opportunities to share systems-level lessons learned. Community assessment activities previously described, including the use of a CHIP (IOM, 1997), adoption of comprehensive, multilevel evaluation approach such as the RE-AIM Framework (Glasgow et al., 1999), and use of existing community indicator systems (Community Research Partners, 2008; Metzler et al., 2008), play equally important roles with regard to system-level change. Further, just as a CHIP represents an agreement regarding a formal inter-organizational partnership, community development corporations promote a shared agenda across sectors like health, workforce development, education, and criminal justice,—reaching beyond the community to engage public and private partners at the city, county, and regional levels. These relationships may allow organizations to share their combined expertise in ways that limit the need for each to develop and maintain all areas of expertise internally.

Inter-organizational structures also foster greater inclusiveness and encourage nontraditional partnerships. This can lead to innovative and resource-efficient solutions to public health problems. For example, Cahn at al. (2007) describe the benefits of communities partnering with health sciences libraries to gain access to historical information and strategies for improving and protecting the public's health. Inter-organizational partnerships can also increase access to cross-sectoral expertise, policy influence, and resources that in turn promote increases in the scale, stability, and sustainability of community changes (Potapchuck, 2007).

CONCLUSION

Evaluations of community change efforts need to place greater emphasis on assessment of a community's ability to develop and leverage its capacity through inter-organizational relationships. These relationships with new and nontraditional partners within and outside the community should help these entities develop a clearer sense of themselves as part of the public health system and their role(s) within it. Measures must reflect the shared capacity and outcomes that result from complex clusters of organizational resources and efforts across levels of a community. Evaluations should also reflect the time needed to address social determinants of health and focus primarily on contribution rather than attribution due to the typically indirect path between programmatic and policy interventions addressing health outcomes through social determinants of health. They will also need to consider those milestones that help to ensure that the longer-term social determinants of health outcomes are realized. Tables 7.1–7.3 highlight content presented in this chapter as one starting point for identifying such milestones.

Table 7.1

STRUCTURAL CHANGE

ORGANIZATIONAL LEVEL	COMMUNITY LEVEL	SYSTEMS LEVEL
• Organization serves as an intermediary for dissemination of program materials (Ackerman et al., 2008). • Implementing and enforcing federal regulations. This may involve educating staff regarding standards and guidelines (Kaufman, 2002). • Serving as a context for diabetes public health research	• Negotiated community-level organization goals and roles (Foster-Fishman et al., 2001; Shediac-Rizkallah & Bone, 1998) • New and deeper relationships with nontraditional partners, influential leaders for innovative and resource-efficient solutions (Lafferty & Mahoney, 2003; Scott & Proeschold-bell, 2008) • Structures reflect emerging community needs and priorities (Meister & De Zapien, 2005).	• New and deeper relationships with nontraditional partners, influential leaders, institutional allies outside the sectors (Hassinger & Pinkerton, 1986; Lafferty & Mahoney, 2003; Scott & Pro-escholdbell, 2008; Tatian, 2000)

Table 7.2

POLICY CHANGE

ORGANIZATIONAL POLICY CHANGE	COMMUNITY POLICY CHANGE	SYSTEMS POLICY CHANGE
• Intra-organizational changes in physical and social programs, policies, or practices (e.g., increase resources for health programs, building-level decisions for healthy food options, and employee allowed time off for physical activity leave to exercise) (Nelson, et al., 2005; Potapchuck, 2007; Watson-Thompson et al., 2008) • Greater policy focus in organization structures and plans (Brieger, 2008; Hill, et al., 2007)	• Adopting or modifying community-level policies, programs, and practices (e.g., adopting a resource across wellness programs and inter-organizational agreements) (Scott & Proescholdbell, 2008; Watson-Thompson et al., 2008) • Increased inter-organizational policy focus in structures and plans and inter-organizational agreements (Brieger, 2008; Hill et al., 2007; IOM, 2003) • Changing community norms for health behavior (Kegler et al., 2000). • Enacting and enforcing policies (Kaufman, 2002)	• Adoption of new or modified policies by entities whose boundaries include the entire community and often extend beyond it (e.g., city budget for neighborhood improvements that facilitate exercise, access to healthy food and healthcare, job creation, and better quality housing and education) • Improved policy enforcement (Scott & Proescholdbell, 2008; Watson-Thompson et al., 2008)

Table 7.3

CHANGES IN RESOURCES AND CAPACITY

ORGANIZATIONAL LEVEL	COMMUNITY LEVEL	SYSTEMS LEVEL
• Expansion and better integration of organizational financial capital (University of Arizona, 2008; Watson-Thompson et al., 2008) • Expansion and better integration of intra-organizational social and human capital (University of Arizona, 2008; Watson-Thompson et al., 2008) • Knowledge and skill-building opportunities (Madison, Hung, & Jean-Louis, 2004; Potapchuck, 2007; Watson-Thompson et al., 2008)	• Expansion and integration of financial resources shared across organizations (Shediac-Rizkallah & Bone, 1998; Watson-Thompson et al., 2008) • Expansion and better integration of inter-organizational (in-kind) support (Kegler et al., 2000; Potapchuck, 2007; University of Arizona, 2008) • Development and use of learning communities (Cahn et al., 2007; Tatian, 2000; Tucker et al., 2006) • Program fidelity, evaluation, and reflection (Butterfoss & Francisco, 2004; Lafferty & Mahoney, 2003; Potapchuck, 2007)	• Expansion of partnerships beyond community to multisectoral nontraditional public health agencies/organizations, groups, and individuals to access cross-sectoral expertise, for accountable reassessment of resources usage, and to sustain community change (Hassinger & Pinkerton, 1986; Potapchuck, 2007) • Knowledge and skill-building in cultural competency (IOM, 2003; Potapchuck, 2007) • Enactment of system level polices that support diabetes prevention and control (Texas Association of Community Health Centers, 2008)

Addressing diabetes health disparities in communities of color will require focussed attention on the development, implementation, and evaluation of multilevel interventions that directly address social determinants of health. This focus needs to be paired with approaches that maximize community (i.e., individuals and organizations) involvement in all phases of these efforts as a means to build the community capacity needed and sustain efforts long enough to produce and maintain desired changes in these "causes of the causes" (World Health Organization, 2008).

Addressing social determinants of health is essential to eliminating diabetes health disparities among African Americans. This will require greater community involvement, stronger community inter-organizational relationships, and the design, integration, and evaluation of multilevel program and policy interventions that specifically address social determinants of health. These elements of shared capacity will promote lasting community change.

REFERENCES

Ackermann, R. T., Finch, E. A., Brizendine, E., Zhou, H., & Marrero, D. G. (2008). Translating the diabetes prevention program into the community: The DEPLOY pilot study. *American Journal of Preventive Medicine, 35,* 357–363.

Ammerman, A., & Mansourch, T. (2005). Treatment adherence at the community level: Moving toward mutuality and participatory action. In H. B. Bosworth, E. Z. Oddone, & M. Weinberger (Eds.), *Patient treatment adherence: Concepts, interventions, and measurement* (pp. 393–420). New York: Routledge.

Aronson, R. E., Wallis, A. B., O'Campo, P. J., & Schafer, P. (2007). Neighborhood mapping and evaluation: A methodology for participatory community health initiatives, *Maternal and Child Health Journal, 11,* 373–383.

Aronson, R. E., Wallis, A. B., O'Campo, P. J., Whitehead, T. L., & Schafer, P. (2007). Ethnographically informed community evaluation: A framework and approach for evaluating community-based initiatives. *Maternal and Child Health Journal, 11,* 97–109.

Aspen Institute (1997). Voices from the field: learning from the early work of comprehensive community initiatives. *Roundtable on Comprehensive Community Initiatives for Children and Families.* Washington, DC : Aspen Institute.

Association of Community Organizations for Reform Now. (2007). *San Francisco passes universal health care ordinance.* Retrieved October 10, 2008, from http://www.acorn .org/index.php?id=11008&L=0%3Fid%3D8144&tx_ttnews(tt_news)=19055&tx_ ttnews(backPid)=10821&cHash=0354b1710a

Beck, E., Wingard, D.L., Zúñiga, M.L., Heifetz, R., & Gilbreath, S. (2008). Addressing the health needs of the underserved: A national faculty development program. *Academy of Medicine, 83,* 1094-1102.

Bell, J., & Standish, M. (2005). Communities and health policy: A pathway for change. *Health Affair, 24,* 339–342.

Bergstrom, A., Clark, R., Hogue, T., Iyechad, T., Miller, J., Mullen, S. et al. (1995). *Collaboration framework: Addressing community capacity.* The National Network of Collaboration. Retrieved August 17, 2008, from http://www.cyfernet.org/nnco/framework.html

Blas, E., Gilson, L., Kelly, M. P., Labonté, R., Lapitan, J., Muntaner, C. et al. (2008). Addressing social determinants of health inequities: What can the state and civil society do? *Lancet, 372,* 1684–1689.

Breinbauer, C., & Maddaleno, M. (2005). *Youth: Choices and change. Promoting healthy behaviors in adolescents.* Washington, DC: Pan American Health Organization.

Brennan Ramirez, L. K., Baker, E. A., & Metzler, M. (2008). *Promoting health equity: A resource to help communities address social determinants of health.* Atlanta: U.S. Department of Health and Human Services, Centers for Disease Control and Prevention. Atlanta, GA.

Brieger, W. (2008). *Community change models.* Retrieved August 5, 2008, from http://ocw.jhsph.edu/courses/SocialBehavioralFoundations/PDFs/Lecture12.pdf

Brownson, R.C., P. Riley, and T.A. Bruce. 1998. Demonstration projects in community-based prevention." *Journal of Public Health Management and Practice 4,* 66–77.

Bruner, C., Bell, K., Brindis, C., Chang, H., & Scarbrough, W. (1993). *Chartering a course: Assessing a community's strengths and needs.* New York: National Center for Service Integration, Columbia University

Burton, W. N., & Connerty, C. M. (1998). Evaluation of a worksite-based patient education intervention targeted at employees with diabetes mellitus. *Journal of Occupational and Environmental Medicine, 40,* 702–706.

Burton, W. N., & Connerty, C. M. (2002). Worksite-based diabetes disease management program. *Disease Management, 5,* 1–8.

Butterfoss, F. D. (2004). The coalition technical assistance and training framework: Helping community coalitions help themselves. *Health Promotion Practice, 5,* 118–126.

Butterfoss, F. D. (2007). *Coalitions and partnerships in community health.* San Francisco, CA: Jossey-Bass.

Butterfoss, F., & Francisco, V. T. (2004). Evaluating community partnerships and coalitions with practitioners in mind. *Health Promotion Practice, 5,* 108–114.

Butterfoss, F. D., Goodman, R. M., & Wandersman, A. (1996). Community coalitions for prevention and health promotion: Factors predicting satisfaction, participation, and planning. *Health Education Quarterly, 23,* 65–79.

Cahn, M. A., Auston, I., Selden, C. R., Cogdill, K., Baker, S., Cavanaugh, D., et al. (2007). The Partners in Information Access for the Public Health Workforce: A collaboration to improve and protect the public's health, 1995–2006. *Journal of the Medical Library Association, 95,* 301–309.

Cargo, M., & Mercer, S. L. (2008). The value and challenges of participatory research: Strengthening its practice. *Annual Review of Public Health, 29,* 325–350.

Carver, V., Reinert, B., & Range, L.M. (2007). Sustaining tobacco control coalitions amid declining resources. *Health Promotion Practice, 8,* 292–1988

Centers for Disease Control and Prevention. (2008). *Directory of diabetes organizations.* Division of Diabetes Translation. Retrieved January 2, 2009, http://www.cdc.gov/diabetes/

Chaloupka, F.J., & Johnston, L. D. (2007). Bridging the gap: research informing practice and policy for healthy youth behavior. *American Journal of Preventive Medicine. 33,* S147–S161.

Chappell, N., Funk, L., Carson, A., MacKenzie, P., Stanwick, R. (2006). Multilevel community health promotion: How can we make it work? *Community Development Journal, 41,* 352–366.

Cohen, L. & Swift, S. (1999). The Spectrum of Prevention: developing a comprehensive approach to injury prevention. *Injury Prevention, 5,* 203–207.

Cohen, S. J., Meister, J. S., deZapien, J. G., Zuckerman, M., & Zuckerman, E. (2004). Special action groups for policy change and infrastructure support to foster healthier communities on the Arizona-Mexico border. *Public Health Reports, 119,* 40–47.

Community Research Partners. (2008). *Community indicators project.* Retrieved September 2, 2008, from http://centralohioindicators.org/site/indicators/indicators.html

Dahlberg, L. L., & Krug, E. G. (2002). Violence: A global public health problem. In E. G. Krug, L. L. Dahlberg, J. A. Mercy, A. B. Zwi, & R. Lozano (Eds.), *World report on violence and health* (pp. 1–21). Geneva: World Health Organization.

Dailly, J. & Barr, A. (2008). Understanding a Community Led Approach to Health Improvement. Retrieved June 11, 2009, from http://www.scdc.org.uk/uploads/under standing_community_led_approach_to_health_jane_dailly_and_alan_barr.pdf

Darrow, W. W., Montanea, J. E., Fernández, P. B., Zucker, U. F., Stephens, D. P., & Gladwin, H. R. (2004). Eliminating disparities in HIV disease: Community mobilization to prevent HIV transmission among Black and Hispanic young adults in Broward County, Florida. *Ethnicity & Disease, 14,* S108–S116.

DiClemente, R. J., Crosby, R. A., & Kegler, M. C. (Eds.). (2002). *Emerging theories in health promotion practice and research: Strategies for improving public health* (ch. 7, pp. 157–193). San Francisco: Jossey-Bass.

Diez Roux, A. V. (2007). Neighborhoods and health: Where are we and where do we go from here? *Revue d'Epidemiologie et de Sante Publique, 55,* 13–21.

English, K.C., Fairbanks, J., Finster, C.E., Rafelito, A., Luna, J., Kennedy, M. A. (2006). Socioecological approach to improving mammography rates in a tribal community. *Health Education Behavior. 20,* 1–14.

Flora, C., Emery, M., Fey, S., & Bregendahl, C. (2008). *Community capitals: A tool for evaluating strategic interventions and projects.* Retrieved September 1, 2008, from http://www.ag.iastate.edu/centers/rdev/projects/commcap/

Foster-Fishman, P. G., Berkowitz, S. L., Lounsbury, D. W., Jacobson, S., & Allen, N. A. (2001). Building collaborative capacity in community coalitions: A review and integrative framework. *American Journal of Community Psychology, 29,* 241–261.

Glasgow, R. E., Fisher, E. B., Anderson, B. J., LaGreca, A., Marrero, D., Johnson, S. B., Rubin, R. R., & Cox, D. J. (1999). Behavioral science in diabetes: Contributions and opportunities. *Diabetes Care, 22,* 832–843.

Glasgow, R. E., Vogt, T. M., & Boles, S. M. (1999). Evaluating the public health impact of health promotion interventions: The RE-AIM framework. *American Journal of Public Health, 89,* 1323–1327.

Graber, J. E., Huang, E. S., Drum, M., Chin, M., Walters, A., & Heuer, L. (2008). Predicting changes in staff morale and burnout at community health centers participating in the health disparities collaboratives. *Health Services Research, 43,* 1403–1423.

Hamilton, N., & Tesh, A. S. (2002). The North Carolina Eden Coalition: Facilitating environmental transformation. *Journal of Gerontological Nursing, 28,* 35–40.

Hanni, K. D., Mendoza, E., Snider, J., & Winkleby, M. A. (2007). A methodology for evaluating organizational change in community-based chronic disease interventions. *Preventing Chronic Disease, 4(4),* A105. Retrieved September 4, 2008, from http://www.pubmedcentral.nih.gov/articlerender.fcgi?artid=2099270

Hassinger, E. W., & Pinkerton, J. R. (1986). *The human community.* New York: Macmillan Publishing Company.

Hawe, P. (1994). Capturing the meaning of 'community' in community intervention evaluation: Some contributions from community psychology. *Health Promotion International, 9,* 199–210.

Hawley, A. (1950). *Human ecology.* New York: The Ronald Press Company.

Heath, E.M., & Coleman, K.J. (2003). Adoption and Institutionalization of the Child and Adolescent Trial for Cardiovascular Health (CATCH) in El Paso, Texas Health Promotion Practice, 4; 157–164.

Hill, A., Guernsey de Zapien, J., Staten, L., Moore-Monroy, M., Elenes, J., & McClelland, D. (2007). From program to policy: Expanding the role of community coalitions. *Preventing Chronic Disease, 4.* Retrieved from http://www.pubmedcentral.nih.gov/articlerender.fcgi?artid=2099268

Hill, J. O., Sallis, J. F, Peters, J. C. (2004). Economic analysis of eating and physical activity: A next step for research and policy change. *American Journal of Preventive Medicine. 27,* 111–116.

Himmelman, A. (1996). *On the theory and practice of transformational collaboration: Collaboration as a bridge from social service to social justice.* In C. Huxham (Ed.), *Creating collaborative advantage.* London: Sage Publishers.

Huang, E. S., Zhang, Q., Brown, S., Drum, M. L., Meltzer, D. O., & Chin, M. H. (2007). The cost-effectiveness of improving diabetes care in U.S. federally-qualified community health centers. *Health Services Research, 42,* 2174–2193.

Inagami, S., Cohen, D. A., & Finch, B. K. (2007). Non-residential neighborhood exposures suppress neighborhood effects on self-rated health. *Social Science & Medicine, 65,* 1779–1791.

Institute of Medicine. (1988). *The future of public health.* Washington, DC: National Academy of Sciences.

Institute of Medicine. (1997). *Improving health in the community: A role for performance monitoring.* Committee on Using Performance Monitoring to Improve Community Health. Washington, DC: National Academy Press.

Institute of Medicine. (2003). *The future of the public's health in the 21st century.* Committee on Assuring the Health of the Public in the 21st Century. Washington, DC: National Academy Press.

The International Development Research Centre. (2008). *The basics of capacity, organizational capacity development, and evaluation: Evaluating Capacity Development.* Retrieved December 20, 2008, from http://www.idrc.ca/en/ev-43616-201-1-DO_TOPIC.html

Johnston, J. A., Marmet, P. F., Coen, F. S., Fawcett, S. B., & Harris, K. J. (1996). Kansas LEAN: An effective coalition for nutrition education and dietary change. *Journal of Nutrition Education, 28,* 115–118.

Jong-wook, L. (2005). Public health is a social issue. *Lancet, 365,* 1005–1006.

Juvenile Diabetes Research Foundation International. (2009). Retrieved January 2, 2009, from http://www.jdrf.org/index.cfm?page_id=100686

Kaufman, F. R. (2002). Diabetes at school: What a child's health care team needs to know about federal disability law. *Clinical Diabetes, 20,* 91–92.

Kegler, M., Norton, B. L., & Aronson, A. R. (2008). Achieving organizational change: Findings from case studies of 20 California healthy cities and communities coalitions. *Health Promotion International, 23,* 109–118.

Kegler, M. C., Steckler, A., McLeroy, K., & Malek, S. H. (1998). Factors that contribute to effective community health promotion coalitions: A study of 10 Project ASSIST coalitions in North Carolina. *Health Education & Behavior, 25,* 338–353.

Kegler, M. C., Twiss, J. M., & Look, V. (2000). Assessing community change at multiple levels: The genesis of an evaluation framework for the California Healthy Cities Project. *Health Education & Behavior, 27,* 760–779.

Kelly, M. P., & Bonnefoy, J. (2007). *The social determinants of health: Developing an evidence base for political action.* World Health Organization, Commission on the Social Determinants of Health. Retrieved from http://www.who.int/social_determinants/resources/mekn_report_10oct07.pdf

Klein, K. J., Tosi, H., & Cannella, A. A. (1999). Multilevel theory building: Benefits, barriers, and new developments. *Academy of Management Review, 24,* 243–248.

Kretzmann, J., & McKnight, J. (1993). *Building communities from the inside out: A path toward finding and mobilizing a community's assets.* Chicago: ACTA Publications.

Krieger, N. (2001). Theories for social epidemiology in the 21st century: An ecosocial perspective. *International Journal of Epidemiology, 30,* 668–677.

KU Work Group on Health Promotion and Community Development. (2007). Identifying community assets and resources. In *The community tool box* (ch. 8). Lawrence, KS: University of Kansas. Retrieved October 26, 2008, from http://ctb.ku.edu/en/tablecontents/sub_section_main_1043.htm

KU Work Group on Health Promotion and Community Development. (2007). Coalition building: Starting a coalition. In *The community tool box* (ch. 5). Lawrence, KS: University of Kansas. Retrieved October 26, 2008, from http://ctb.ku.edu/tools/en/sub_section_tools_1364.htm

KU Work Group on Health Promotion and Community Development. (2007). Gathering information: Monitoring your progress. *The community tool box* (ch. 38). Lawrence, KS: University of Kansas. Retrieved October 26, 2008, from http://ctb.ku.edu/tools/en/sub_section_tools_1364.htm

Lafferty, C. K., & Mahoney, C. A. (2003). A framework for evaluating comprehensive community initiatives. *Health Promotion Practice, 4,* 31–44.

Lasker, R. D., Weiss, E. S, & Miller, R. (2001). Partnership synergy: A practical framework for studying and strengthening the collaborative advantage. *The Milbank Quarterly, 79(2),* 179–205.

Mackenbach, J. P. (2003). Tackling inequalities in health: the need for building a systematic evidence base *Journal of Epidemiology and Community Health, 57,* 162.

Madison, A., Hung, R., & Jean-Louis, E. (2004). The Boston Haitian HIV Prevention Coalition formative evaluation: A participatory approach to community self-assessment. *Ethnicity & Disease, 14(Suppl 1),* 20–26.

Marmot, M. (2005). Social determinants of health inequalities. *Lancet, 365,* 1099–1104.

McKeever, C., Koroloff, N., & Faddis, C. (2006). The African American Wellness Village in Portland, Oregon. *Preventing Chronic Disease, 3,* A104. Retrieved from http://www.pubmedcentral.nih.gov/articlerender.fcgi?artid=1637792

Meister J., & De Zapien, J. (2005). Bringing health policy issues front and center in the community: Expanding the role of community health coalitions. *Preventing Chronic Disease, 2.* Retrieved September 20, 2008, from http://www.pubmedcentral.nih.gov/articlerender.fcgi?artid=1323319

Metzler, M. (2007). Social determinants of health: What, how, why, and now. *Preventing Chronic Disease, 4.* Retrieved September 20, 2008, from http://www.cdc.gov/pcd/issues/2007/oct/07_0136.htm.

Metzler, M., Kanarek, N., Keisher, H., Straw, R., Bialek, R., Stanley, J., Auston, I., & Klein, R. (2008). Community health status indicators project: The development of a national approach to community health. *Preventing Chronic Disease, 5,* A94. Retrieved from http://www.pubmedcentral.nih.gov/articlerender.fcgi?artid=2483544

Monsey, B., Owen, G., Zierman, C., Lamberb, L., & Lyman, J. (1995). *Community report card. What works in preventing rural violence: Strategies, risk factors and assessment tools.* St. Paul, MN: Amherst H. Wilder Foundation.

Myers, A. M. (1999). *Program evaluation for exercise leaders.* Champaign, IL: Human Kinetics.

National Association of City and County Health Officials. (2000). *Community revitalization and public health: Issues, roles and relationships for local public health agencies.* Washington, DC: National Association of City and County Health Officials.

National Institute of Diabetes and Digestive and Kidney Diseases. (2007). *Directory of diabetes organizations.* National Diabetes Information Clearinghouse. Retrieved October 24, 2008, from http://diabetes.niddk.nih.gov/resources/organizations.htm

National Institute of Diabetes and Digestive and Kidney Diseases. (2009). *National Diabetes Information Clearinghouse.* Retrieved January 2, 2009, from http://diabetes.niddk.nih.gov/

National Kidney Foundation. (2009). *Research Grants.* Retrieved January 2, 2009, from http://www.kidney.org/professionals/research/

Nelson, K. M., Chapko, M.K., Reiber, G., & Boyko, E. J. (2005). The association between health insurance coverage and diabetes care: Data from the 2000 Behavioral Risk Factor Surveillance System. *Health Services Research, 40,* 361–372.

Pentz, M. A. (1994). Adaptive evaluation strategies for estimating effects of community-based drug abuse prevention programs. *Journal of Community Psychology, CSAP Special Issue,* 26–51.

Pentz, M. A. (2000). Institutionalizing community-based prevention through policy change. *Journal of Community Psychology, 28,* 257–270.

Perkins, D. D., Florin, P., Rich, R. C., Wandersman, A., & Chavis, D. M. (1990). Participation and the social and physical environment of residential blocks: Crime and community context. *American Journal of Community Psychology, 18,* 83–115.

Petersen, D. J., & Alexander, G. R. (2001). *Needs assessment in public health: A practical guide for students and professionals.* New York: Kluwer Academic/Plenum Publishers.

Public Health Foundation (2000). *EZ/EC Health Planning Capacity Survey: Final Report.* Washington, DC: Public Health Foundation.

Porche, D. J. (2004). *Public and community health nursing practice.* Thousand Oaks, CA: Sage Publications Inc.

Potapchuck, M. (2007). *Community changes processes and progress in addressing racial inequities.* M. P. Associates & Aspen Roundtable. Retrieved October 2, 2008, from http://www.aspeninstitute.org/site/c.huLWJeMRKpH/b.612045/k.4BA8/Round table_on_Community_Change.htm

Prah Ruger, J. (2004). Ethics of the social determinants of health. *Lancet, 364,* 1092–1097.

Reid, L., Hatch, J., & Parrish, T. (2003). The role of a historically Black university and the Black church in community-based health initiatives: The Project DIRECT experience. *Journal of Public Health Management, 9,* S70–S73.

Renaud, L., Chevalier, S., & O'Loughlin, J. (1997). Institutionalization of community programs: review of theoretical models and proposal of a model. *Canadian Journal of Public Health. 1997 88(2),* 109–113.

Rosenberg, D., Kerr, J., King, A., Moore, D., Patrick, K., Sallis, J., (2008). Feasibility and outcomes of a multilevel place-based walking intervention for seniors: a pilot study. *Health and Place, 15,* 173–179.

Saxe, L., Reber, E., Hallfors, D., Kadushin, C., Jones, D., Rindskopf, D. et al. (1997). Think globally, act locally: Assessing the impact of community-based substance abuse prevention. *Evaluation and Program Planning, 20,* 357–366.

Schensul, J. J., & Trickett E. (2009). Multilevel Community-Based Culturally Situated Interventions and Community Impact: An Ecological Perspective. *American Journal of Community Psychology, 43,* 232–240.

Schulz, A. J., Zenk, S., Odoms-Young, A., Hollis-Neely, T., Nwankwo, R., Lockett, M. et al. (2005). Healthy eating and exercising to reduce diabetes: Exploring the potential of social determinants of health frameworks within the context of community-based participatory diabetes prevention *American Journal of Public Health, 95,* 645–651.

Schwab, M., & Syme, S. L. (1997). On paradigms, community participation, and the future of public health. *American Journal of Public Health, 87,* 2049–2051.

Scott, S. A., & Proescholdbell, S. (2008). Informing best practice with community practice: The community change chronicle method for program documentation and evaluation. *Health Promotion Practice, 10,* 102–110, 1–9.

Shediac-Rizkallah, M., & Bone, L. (1998). Planning for the sustainability of community-based health programs: Conceptual frameworks and future directions for research, practice and policy, *Health Education Research, 13,* 87–108.

Smedley, B. D., Stith, A. Y., & Nelson, A. R. (Eds.). (2003). *Unequal treatment: Confronting racial and ethnic disparities in healthcare.* Washington, DC: National Academies Press.

Sorensen, G., Emmons., K., Hunt., M. K., & Johnston, D. (1998). Implications of the results of community intervention trials. *Annual Review of Public Health, 19,* 379–416.

Stokols, D. (1996). Translating social ecological theory into guidelines for community health promotion. *American Journal of Health Promotion, 10,* 282–298.

Tatian, P. (2000). *Indispensable information: Data collection and information management for healthier communities.* National Neighborhood Indicators Partnership Report. Washington, DC: The Urban Institute. Retrieved October 7, 2008, from http://www.urban.org/nnip/publications.html

Texas Association of Community Health Centers. (2008). *Health disparities collaboratives.* Retrieved July 15, 2008, from http://www.tachc.org/HDC/Overview.asp

Tucker, P., Liao, Y., Giles, W. H., & Liburd, L. (2006). The REACH 2010 logic model: An illustration of expected performance. *Preventing Chronic Disease, 3.* Retrieved November 2, 2008, from http://www.cdc.gov/pcd/issues/2006/jan/05_0131.htm

University of Arizona. (2008). *Evaluating the national outcomes: Introduction and model for community programming and evaluation.* Retrieved June 15, 2008, from http://ag .arizona.edu/fcs/cyfernet/nowg/comm_index.html

U.S. Department of Health and Human Services. (2008). *Data sources, definitions, and notes: Community health status indicators 2008 report.* Retrieved from http://www .communityhealth.hhs.gov

U.S. Department of Housing and Urban Development (2005). *Capturing Successes in Renewal Communities and Empowerment Zones: Spotlight of Results.* Retrieved June 12, 2009 from http://www.nls.gov/offices/cpd/economicdevelopment/library/ spotlight508.pdf

U.S. Department of Housing and Urban Development. *HUD's Initiative for Renewal Communities and Urban Empowerment Zones.* Retrieved June 12, 2009 from http://www.hud.gov/offices/cpd/economicdevelopment/programs/rc/index.cfm

U.S. Department of Veteran's Affairs. (2007). *V.A. Diabetes Program.* Retrieved December 5, 2008, from http://www1.va.gov/diabetes/#veterans

Weech-Maldonado, R., Benson K.J., & Gamm, L.D. (2003). Evaluating the effectiveness of community health partnerships: A stakeholder accountability approach. *Journal of Health and Human Services Administration, 26,* 58–92.

Watson-Thompson, J., Fawcett, S. B., & Schultz, J. A. (2008). A framework for community mobilization to promote healthy youth development. *American Journal of Preventive Medicine, 34,* S72–S81.

Working Group on Health Disparities. (2005). *Health disparities and the body politic: A series of international symposia.* Harvard University, School of Public Health Disparities.

World Health Organization. Commission on Social Determinants of Health (2008). *Closing the gap in a generation: Health equity through action on the social determinants of health.* Geneva: World Health Organization, Commission on Social Determinants of Health.

Innovative Case Studies from the Field

The framework for eliminating diabetes disparities set forth in this text is visionary, ambitious, cross-cutting, and comprehensive. It challenges us to develop community-based public health approaches that address the broader social, political, economic, and cultural determinants of diabetes and individual behavior change. While practitioners and researchers have long been aware of the influence of history and the social determinants of health on the shaping of risks for diabetes, effective policy and environmental, economic, and community change strategies are still emerging.

The following chapters feature diabetes programs currently underway that have been conducted in urban and rural communities of color across the United States, including the Pacific Basin. Representing over 20 years of collective experience, these programs are funded wholly or in part by three Centers for Disease Control and Prevention initiatives, namely, the REACH U.S. program, the Prevention Research Centers Program, the Division of Diabetes Translation's state-based Diabetes Prevention and Control Program, and the National Diabetes Education Program. Leadership for these programs comes from state and local health departments, universities, community-based organizations and institutions, and community members. They demonstrate the necessity and benefits of galvanizing and sustaining a broad-based community effort focused on reversing the growing tide of diabetes in communities of color.

The leaders of the case studies were invited by the editor to demonstrate the range of community-based approaches currently underway in racial and ethnic communities. The case studies are a sample of a much bigger universe of community-based diabetes programs. The authors were asked to describe the origins and components of their programs; how the community was engaged in the program design, implementation, and evaluation; challenges the program confronted; its impact to date in reducing diabetes disparities; how the program will be sustained; and so forth. Each case study begins with an editor's note that includes questions to challenge the reader to consider community-based approaches in a broader framework that privileges attention to the social determinants of diabetes.

The case studies reflect the voice and experience of the communities. There are few opportunities in the peer-reviewed literature to chronicle a community diabetes program in such rich and reflective detail. We are hopeful that these case studies will spark new ideas, strengthen methods of intervention research and evaluation, and inspire new opportunities to eliminate diabetes disparities in communities of color in the U.S. and internationally.

8

Project DIRECT (Diabetes Interventions Reaching and Educating Communities Together)

JOYCE C. PAGE, JOHN W. HATCH, LAVERNE
REID, AND LUCILLE H. WEBB

Collaboration is especially important when each party has a stake in the design
of studies and the orientation and interpretation of research findings . . . The
importance of this collaboration also arises from the fact that if those who form
hypotheses are from different cultures from those being studied, ambiguity
resulting from a limited understanding of local culture can cause a biased
interpretation of observed behavior.

—Dr. John Hatch, DrPH, MSW (Hatch, 1993, p. 31)

Editor's Note: One of the most important keys to a successful community-based approach to diabetes prevention and control in racial and
ethnic populations is the active engagement, leadership, and ownership
of program and evaluation efforts by affected community members. As
we think about the diversity of community norms, structures, and political economies across the U.S., it can be a bit daunting to conceptualize
and implement a community mobilization plan. Imagine that you have
been hired to implement a community-based diabetes program. You are
a newcomer to a mid-size city in the southeastern region of the U.S. and
have the responsibility for convening a diabetes coalition charged with
eliminating diabetes disparities in a cluster of zip codes where available
epidemiological data documents a disproportionate burden of diabetes,
its risk factors, and associated complications. You discover that approximately 25,000 African Americans live in these neighboring zip codes and

are considered mixed-income and stable, (i.e., there is very little in- or out-migration from this area). While there are social class distinctions and separations (e.g., the more affluent members of the community live together in a neighborhood close to one of the historically Black colleges located in the area), there is strong social cohesion and a sense of caring about everyone's quality of life. The multi-class nature of this community gives some members access to governmental power structures and the state's elite institutions of higher education. Community members with this access leverage their influence to achieve social change that benefits their neighbors. You have the challenge of identifying the community stakeholders who should be members of the coalition and guide the development, implementation, and evaluation of the program. This scenario characterizes our first case study and the community that launched Project Diabetes Intervention Reaching and Educating Communities Together (DIRECT).

Project DIRECT represents the first bold attempt by the Centers for Disease Control and Prevention to develop a community-based diabetes demonstration project intended to reduce the burden of diabetes in an African American community. In this case study, you will learn the history of the development of this program from the community's perspective and the processes they engaged in to mobilize southeast Raleigh to address type 2 diabetes. The actual names of community members involved in selected aspects of the project are given to both honor and celebrate the role they played, as well as to authenticate the influence of the many voices of the community that shaped this groundbreaking public health effort.

As you read this case study, consider these questions:

- The primary theoretical orientation for much of this community-based diabetes program was based on a premise of patterns of association having an influence on health beliefs and behaviors. In other words, if we are able to tap into those indigenous networks that shape health beliefs and perpetuate health behaviors through social practices (e.g., foods served during church events across several generations) and shift those norms toward health promotion and disease prevention, then we can reduce the burden of diabetes. In addition to focusing on changing community cultural norms, what are some other policy or community change strategies that Project DIRECT could implement to eliminate diabetes disparities?

■ Project DIRECT has been in place in this community for over a decade. The demographics of southeast Raleigh are beginning to shift toward greater racial and ethnic diversity. How might the established leaders of the project sustain their focus on reducing the burden of diabetes among African Americans while also broadening their work to benefit newcomers to the community? On the other hand, should Project DIRECT ignore their new neighbors and maintain a focus on African American health? What are the pros and cons of either approach?

■ Should community diabetes coalitions do succession planning to sustain the vision and work of the original coalition members? Is it ever advisable to disband an established and effective coalition after a decade-long commitment? If yes, under what circumstances? If no, why not?

BACKGROUND

Project Diabetes Interventions Reaching and Educating Communities Together (DIRECT) began in 1995 as the largest comprehensive community-based diabetes demonstration project in the United States in an African American community. It focused on improving self-care, access to care, and quality of care for residents in the Southeast Raleigh (SER) community. The Centers for Disease Control and Prevention (CDC) funded the project and hoped to determine if planning and implementing a project with the community as a partner could significantly affect the burden of diabetes. Southeast Raleigh, with a population of approximately 25,000, is predominantly African American and is defined by seven census tracts in Raleigh.

Project DIRECT has been a partner with the CDC, the North Carolina Department of Health and Human Services (NC DHHS), Wake County Human Services (WCHS), and many organizations and individuals in SER. Through contractual agreements, additional partnerships were formed with local universities. The project was governed by a 13-member executive committee, representing WCHS, NC DHHS, and residents of Southeast Raleigh. While the research phase of Project DIRECT ended in 2003, the project continues interventions in community outreach, health promotion, and diabetes care. In 2007 Project DIRECT became part of Strengthening the Black Family (STBF), a nonprofit organization in Southeast Raleigh. STBF has a mission to improve the quality of life for families, with a special emphasis on Black families.

Southeast Raleigh Community

It's the most intriguing community, diverse in any aspect that you can imagine. . . . It tends to be seamless, and for that reason things can happen here that might not easily happen elsewhere.

—Dr. Dudley Flood, Chair, Project DIRECT Community
Coalition (Project DIRECT, 2002)

Southeast Raleigh, near downtown, has been known as the center of African American presence since post-Civil War. Church congregations (of particular importance to African Americans) and two historically African American universities are located in Southeast Raleigh. Developed as a culturally and economically diverse community from its founding, many civic and social organizations are based here. Patterns of leadership and the web of diverse interaction in Southeast Raleigh have not been common in urban African American communities. Small African American-owned businesses and professional service providers have continued to live in and service the area. Prior to desegregation of public services and private businesses, many communities similar to Southeast Raleigh dotted the landscape of cities in the South and some northern places with substantial African American populations. Those that retained their community and business culture, as well as a residential mix of lower-, middle-, and upper-class families, appeared better able to build effective and sustainable actions needed to reduce the risk of disease and other dangers that compromise the quality of life, and indeed the length of life itself. There has been a long history and tradition of civic action and involvement to draw from in Southeast Raleigh.

Burden of Diabetes in Wake County and Southeast Raleigh

A 1993 pilot study involving household interviews and medical examinations was conducted among persons 20–74 years of age in Wake County. Diagnosed diabetes was two times more common in African Americans than in other races (5.2% vs. 2%) and undiagnosed diabetes was five times higher among African Americans (5.5% vs. 1.1%). African Americans were more likely to smoke, use an emergency room for medical care, and have uncontrolled hypertension. African Americans had a high prevalence of obesity and physical inactivity (Herman et al., 1998).

In 1996–1997 a pre-intervention survey was conducted among persons 18–75 years of age in Southeast Raleigh. The prevalence of diabetes was 10.5%. A 2003–2004 post-intervention survey found the prevalence rate for diabetes increased to 16.7% (American Diabetes Association, 2007). Blacks had greater risk factors for diabetes and were more likely to be obese (51%). Obesity was most prevalent among Black women (60%). Blacks were also more likely to be inactive (52%), which was most prevalent among Black women (60%). Compared to non-Blacks, Blacks with diagnosed diabetes were less likely to report having a private health-care provider, less likely to report having health insurance, and more likely to report using an emergency room for medical care. Retinopathy, nephropathy, and amputations tended to be more common among Blacks with diagnosed diabetes than non-Blacks with diagnosed diabetes (Herman, et al., 1998).

The 1996–1997 pre-intervention survey found that African Americans, in both the intervention and control communities, with diabetes and without health insurance were more than twice as likely to have inadequate preventive care and poorer HbA1c and LDL values as those with health insurance. African Americans without a particular health care provider for diabetes care were twice as likely to receive inadequate preventive care. Glycemic and lipid control in African Americans with diabetes were poor: 60% had HbA1c levels >8% and LEL cholesterol levels were >130 mg/dL. Of African Americans without insurance, 50% had HbA1c levels >9.5% and 60% had an LDL level >130 mg/dL (Gregg et al., 2001).

In addition, a study of perceptions of managing and coping with diabetes among African American men as part of Project DIRECT found that participants characterized having diabetes as inescapable and a form of social inequality, a "private hell" (Liburd, Namageyo-Funa, Jack, & Gregg, 2004).

Diabetes Disparities in Southeast Raleigh

In Wake County, African Americans have been socioeconomically less advantaged than Caucasians. The 1990 census data shows that the average White family earned $26,885 annually, whereas the average Black family earned $15,347. Poverty data for 1989 show 19% of Blacks lived in poverty as opposed to 5.3% of Whites (Wake County Department of Health, 1996).

To describe the burden of diabetes in the community, data was collected from the 1993 Project DIRECT Pilot Study, the 1996–1997 Project DIRECT Pre-Intervention Baseline Survey, the 1995 Community Leaders Survey, Wake County Department of Health's 1996 Community Diagnosis: A Statistical Analysis of Wake County, NC, and the community focus groups and key informant interviews conducted in 1996–1997. Data was collected on gender, age, income, education, disease duration, medications, hypertension, health insurance coverage, whether respondents had a doctor, whether they needed medical care or medications and could not get them, preventive care services received, obesity, prevalence of diagnosed and undiagnosed diabetes, prevalence of impaired glucose tolerance, dietary and physical activity habits, diabetes complications, diabetes care practices, participation in diabetes education, and receipt of counseling for diabetes management.

ORIGINS AND HISTORY OF PROJECT DIRECT

The 1985 Secretary of Health and Human Services' Task Force on Black and Minority Health identified diabetes as a major cause of disability and death for minorities. Two years later, the National Diabetes Advisory Board called for an evaluation of community-based interventions to reduce risks for diabetes. The CDC called for proposals to implement multiyear community demonstration projects. Following a pilot study in Wake County, SER was selected as the intervention site and a community in Greensboro, NC, was selected as the control group. The CDC contracted with the Research Triangle Institute to conduct a pre-intervention survey.

A community advisory board was created with the local health department to mobilize the community. In 1994 the CDC awarded a cooperative agreement to the North Carolina Department of Environmental, Health and Natural Resources (NC DEHNR) to demonstrate and document the effectiveness of the project model. The NC DEHNR contracted with the WCHS to implement the project's interventions. The NC DEHNR and WCHS both had existing large networks of county contacts who were crucial in identifying other community partners to support and sustain the project. An executive committee, comprised of seven community, two state, and two county representatives, was formed to develop policies and guidelines, review and endorse action plans, promote the project, and provide consultation on interventions.

STAFFING

After the project began, Mrs. Lucille H. Webb, chair of the executive committee and a resident of the SER with years of voluntary leadership in planning and developing community initiatives, requested the involvement of North Carolina Central University's (NCCU) Department of Health Education. NCCU, an historically Black institution, had faculty members raised in African American communities in North Carolina with expertise and understanding of the cultural dynamics of the community. From the Health Education Department, a senior community organization specialist joined as the co-principal investigator. Specialists in organization theory and small group dynamics joined as consultants for community outreach. A specialist in fitness promotion from the NCCU Department of Physical Education joined as a physical activity consultant. In addition, several NCCU students served as interns.

FUNDING

In 1994 an initial award was made through a CDC cooperative agreement with the NC DEHNR to plan the project with community involvement. Throughout the study, funding was provided by the CDC for community engagement in the project's design, implementation, and evaluation phases. Over the years of the project, funding averaged about $900,000 per year.

COMMUNITY AND INSTITUTIONAL PARTICIPANTS

We need to be there [at the table] because it's really the community where the work is being done. I see the community as the laboratory for the researchers. So I think it's very important that we have a say in what the research is going to be and how it's going to be conducted.

—*Mrs. Lucille H. Webb (Project DIRECT, 2002)*

Multiple partners, collaborators, and supporters created a community concern about diabetes from all levels of government (federal, state, and local), SER, private and state-supported universities, fraternities and sororities, local businesses, faith-based organizations, medical care facilities, professional medical groups, recreation facilities, and public housing. The roles of key partners and collaborators are described below:

- **African-American churches.** Hosted interventions and promoted diabetes awareness through pastor messages and presentations.
- **CDC Division of Diabetes Translation.** Conceptualized, funded, guided, and evaluated the project.
- **Community advisory board.** A pre-intervention advisory board that promoted the project and facilitated its acceptance and ownership by the community.
- **Community coalition.** Volunteers who served on committees and work groups to plan interventions, recruit participants, stimulate media and public relations, and hold highly visible community events.
- **Executive committee.** The 13-member project governing body responsible for policies and guidelines, linkages with the community, review and advice on implementation and evaluation of interventions, and dissemination of study findings.
- **Health care providers.** Comprised of doctors and other providers, medical facilities, medical associations (e.g., The Old North State Medical Society, the nation's oldest association of Black physicians) who were participants in the Continuous Quality Improvement Program and referred patients to project interventions.
- **Media.** Provided public service announcements, television and radio broadcasts, and articles promoting project activities.
- **NCCU.** Provided a co-principal investigator and consultants, for community engagement and physical activity, and student interns.
- **NC DHHS.** Formerly under NC DEHNR, the state health department administered the CDC cooperative agreement, collaborated to design protocols, staffed committees, documented activities, facilitated communication, and assured Institutional Review Board approval.

- **Southeast Raleigh community.**   Targeted community whose representatives provided understanding of community structure and function and whose volunteers served on boards, committees, and work groups.
- **WCHS.**   Local health department that conducted interventions, housed project, staffed committees, gathered data, hosted coalition committees and work groups, and engaged the community.

STRATEGIES FOR COMMUNITY ENGAGEMENT

We went not only to the churches, we went to the barber shops . . . to the beauticians, we went to the fraternities . . .we touched base with every organization within the Black community in Southeast Raleigh that we could find.
> **—Rev. Paul Anderson, first Chair, Project DIRECT**
> **Executive Committee (Project DIRECT, 2002)**

Multiple-level interventions and strategies were used for community engagement. The conceptual model used to plan interventions with community involvement was adapted from the CDC's Planned Approach to Community Health program. It involved three basic guidelines: (a) involve the target population in planning, (b) plan interventions that coordinate multiple approaches, and (c) develop interventions for the total community and sites in the community. Other approaches and strategies used for community engagement are discussed below.

Conducting Key Informant Interviews and Focus Groups

Interviews and focus groups were conducted throughout SER with persons from doctors' offices, businesses, churches, fraternal groups, public housing, and service organizations. The snowball sampling technique was used to identify community members perceived as influential. The interviewer asked, "Who in this community do you think needs to be involved in Project DIRECT?" (Parks, 1995). An extensive list of organizations and groups (see Table 8.1) was developed and included a network of social interactions and influential community members who propelled the project's recognition and acceptance.

Table 8.1

SOME ORGANIZATIONS SUPPORTING PROJECT DIRECT

ORGANIZATIONS CONTRIBUTING TO PROJECT DIRECT	CONTRIBUTIONS
American Diabetes Association (African American Program)	Educational materials
Barbershops	Volunteers, host focus groups
Beauty Salons	Volunteers, host focus groups
Churches (African American)	Diabetes awareness, interventions, project promotion
City of Raleigh, Parks and Recreation	Walking path, host Ready Set Walk (RSW) programs, diabetes awareness
Crosby Clinic	Host focus groups
General Baptist State Convention of North Carolina	Host diabetes awareness sessions
Hargett St. Homeless Shelter	Host focus groups
Le Count's Catering Service	Healthy menu selections
Media (newspaper, radio, and television)	Public service announcements, articles, broadcasts
North Carolina Central University	Principal investigators, consultants, interns, IRB approval
North Carolina Cooperative Extension	Nutrition demonstrations
North Carolina Department of Health and Human Services	Project administration, documentation, liaison between partners, IRB approval
North Carolina State University	Volunteers from African-American Science and Health Society, consultants, data analysis, IRB approval
Open Door Clinic	Host focus groups, diabetes awareness programs
Pan-Hellenic Council of eight Greek letter organizations	Volunteers (community ambassadors)
Professional Black Nurses' Society (Chi Eta Phi)	Ambassadors, screening volunteers
Raleigh City Council	Project acceptance and promotion
Raleigh Housing Authority	Site for screenings, outreach interventions

(continued)

Table 8.1 (continued)

ORGANIZATIONS CONTRIBUTING TO PROJECT DIRECT	CONTRIBUTIONS
Rex Senior Center	Host diabetes self-management classes, RSW program
Shaw University	Host diabetes awareness programs, student volunteers
Southlight (Substance Abuse Services)	Host focus groups
St. Augustine College	Host RSW program
Strengthening the Black Family	Diabetes awareness sessions through member organizations, houses project after research phase ends
Triangle RETRADE (association of diabetes educators)	Diabetes care class instructors
University of North Carolina at Chapel Hill	Consultants, student interns
Wake County Housing Authority	Diabetes awareness sessions, referrals
Wake County Human Services	Interventions, project office, IRB approval
Wake Forest University	Co-principal investigator, IRB approval
Wake Health Services	Patient referrals, outreach interventions
Wakeview Clinic (Substance Abuse Services)	Host focus groups
Women's Center	Host focus groups, intervention referrals
YMCA and YWCA	Referrals, host diabetes awareness programs

Hiring a Culturally Sensitive Community Organizer

The hiring of an African American community organizer who grew up in the area and whose family was well-known and respected in the general and medical communities opened many doors into the community. Serving on the community advisory board, she developed a plan to promote the project, educate the public about project goals, and ensure community involvement. She explained her approach to engaging the community by her perception of them as VIPs.

Involving the Black Church

Health promotion interventions focused largely on reaching the most significant institution in the Black community, the church. Focus group interviews conducted by NCCU in 1997 found that 97% of respondents had church affiliations and most believed churches should be involved. The largest association of Black churches in North Carolina has been the General Baptist State Convention (GBSC) of North Carolina. The Health and Human Services (HHS) Program of the GBSC had a history of working with university researchers and state program managers to address chronic illnesses and maternal and child health through the use of lay health educators.

Project DIRECT's church outreach interventions were based on the work of the HHS that found learning took place at two levels: (a) church lay leaders increased their understanding of specific diseases and (b) health professionals learned about community perceptions of healthcare (Holmes, 2004). Two important outreach tools were the Congregational Health Assessment Tool (CHAT) and Church Health Action Plan (CHAP). These tools were created by NCCU as a result of Dr. John Hatch's observation that changes in patterns of daily life are more likely to occur when at-risk populations have basic technical understanding of risks and are convinced that recommended changes are efficacious, available, and appropriate. The CHAT questionnaire was used to engage ministers and other church leaders in a dialogue to identify health and related problems of church members. Information was gathered on church demographics, health-related lifestyle issues, funerals, food events, theological understanding of health, and existing health programs and resources. The CHAP was provided to churches after completion of the CHAT to identify health resources and provide guidance to plan and implement a health promotion program, thus transferring responsibility from the agency or health professional to the faith community (Hatch, Reid, Parrish, & Hoyo, 2000).

Involving Influential Community Members

Project DIRECT involved a number of influential community members (many served on boards, committees, and work groups) who helped convince the community that diabetes prevention and treatment should be a priority. A few are described below:

- Mrs. Dorothy Sanders is an outreach work group chair, SER resident, outstanding church worker, volunteer, and advocate with over 30 programs locally and statewide.
- Rev. H. B. Pickett is an executive committee member, SER resident, president of the local chapter of the National Association for the Advancement of Colored People, pastor, retired school counselor, and community advocate.
- Mrs. Lucille H. Webb is an executive committee chair (for 10 years), retired educator and administrator, Kellogg Foundation's Community-Based Public Health Initiative consultant and advisor to the School of Public Health, University of North Carolina at Chapel Hill, and STBF president.

THEORETICAL FRAMEWORK

Approaching public health problems at multiple levels and stressing the interaction and integration of factors within and across levels is known as an ecological perspective. The following ecological approaches were used for Project DIRECT's interventions:

- **Stages of Change Model.**   Ready Set Walk (RSW) is a comprehensive walking program designed to teach adults how to walk safely and encourage walking for exercise on a regular basis. The program's design was based on the Stages of Change Model that considers an individual's readiness to change toward health-promoting behaviors. The Lay Exercise Leader (LEL) program was designed to institutionalize RSW by teaching those who have completed the program the skills and knowledge needed to begin and maintain other community walking groups. Approximately 1,000 persons participated in RSW.
- **Social Learning Theory.**   This theory posits that people and their environments are influenced by and influential within their unique social environments. It was used to create interventions in which staff provided technical advice and encouragement and helped launch and maintain healthy behaviors. Interventions included the CHAT, the CHAP, RSW, LEL, diabetes self-management (DSM),

and church nutrition training (CNT) (Reid, Hatch, & Parrish, 2003). CNT taught church kitchen committees and other persons responsible for congregation meals to prepare favorite dishes like collards, crunchy chicken, and fruit punch with less sugar and fat.

■ **Organizational Change Theory.** This theory is based on the belief that organization structures and processes influence health behaviors and motivation. It was used to help organizations establish policies and environments that support health behavior change. Greater emphasis was given to changing indigenous institutions' structures versus changing corporate structures external to grassroots community control. Churches were approached and interventions (CHAT, CHAP, RSW, LEL, and CNT) were held to promote policy changes. The diffusion of innovation theory (the belief that new ideas, behaviors, products, and social practices spread from one group to another) was used to identify community messengers to spread ideas and act as motivational role models. This led to the creation of community ambassadors who spread diabetes awareness messages in churches, businesses, recreation centers, and other community settings of opportunity. This theory was used to engage a physician and television personality, radio show hosts, pastors, and local political leaders as advocates to inform and stimulate community involvement. Staff and supporters often wore shirts with the project logo while visiting in the community or attending special events. They often heard onlookers shout, "Go Project DIRECT!," an indication of the community's proud identification with the project.

PROGRAM COMPONENTS

It's positive, it's like an intimate little family. You get to meet people . . . You share so much . . . you think you're all alone with the disease, but when you are among other people, you are not alone.
   —Desiree Petersen, Project DIRECT participant (Project DIRECT, 2002)

Project DIRECT interventions were funded through the CDC cooperative agreement and provided without charge for residents of the Southeast Raleigh community and the general public. Interventions were conducted mostly in the targeted Southeast Raleigh community, although occasionally interventions were held in the surrounding communities.

Outreach and health promotion interventions were held at churches, public housing complexes, doctors' offices, parks and recreation centers, and local businesses. Diabetes care interventions were held at the Project DIRECT office, doctors' offices, the local hospital, the Area Health Education Center (AHEC), and the local community health center of Wake Health Services, which serviced approximately half of the people in SER.

Although most financial support came from the CDC, diabetes testing supplies and education materials were often provided by businesses (e.g., pharmaceutical and diabetes supply companies). Donations were received from service organizations with mostly African American memberships and included:

- Order of the Eastern Star, an adoptive rite of Masonry with male and female members
- Delta Sigma Theta Sorority, a Greek letter organization of college-educated women
- The Links, a service organization of women

Project Interventions and Levels of Preventive Care

Outreach Interventions (Primary and Secondary Prevention)

Increased awareness of diabetes and its risk factors, number of high-risk persons screened for diabetes, number of persons with diabetes who received regular care. Local support included:

- Radio announcements, newspaper articles, and television reports
- Diabetes awareness and participant recruitment sessions
- A diabetes education resource center at the Project DIRECT office
- Town hall meetings to share and receive feedback on project activities
- The 2002 National Forum on Project DIRECT held in Southeast Raleigh
- The 2006 Community Forum on Project DIRECT to disseminate final project results
- Annual community coalition meetings to inform and receive feedback

- Community ambassador awareness presentations
- The 1995 Chavis Park Kick-off Festival to launch the project (attended by hundreds)
- Physician referrals to project interventions (over 700 received)
- A project information booth at Wake Health Services (manned by staff)
- The 1996–1999 community diabetes screenings (>3,000 persons screened at 183 events)

The CHAT and the CHAP were developed by health education faculty at NCCU as strategies for increasing knowledge of risk factors for diabetes and providing information needed to tailor a diabetes prevention and control program for each participating congregation.

Health Promotion (Primary and Secondary Prevention)

Decreased the prevalence and risk factors for diabetes by improving dietary practices, reducing obesity and increasing physical activity. Interventions were designed to be sustained by community volunteers and organizations; aspects of these interventions included:

- Food articles in newspapers crafted with knowledge of education and interest levels
- CNT that helped congregations prepare healthier meals and healthier versions of favorite dishes of the congregation
- Community food demonstrations held during educational and social events
- The RSW community walking program and the LEL program that equipped members of congregations with the skills needed to lead exercise programs within churches
- DSM classes to increase understanding of diabetes
- The CHAT needs assessment and CHAP corresponding action plan to foster healthier diets and increase physical activity among church members

Diabetes Care Interventions (Tertiary Prevention)

Activities focused on improving self-care practices among persons living in Southeast Raleigh with diagnosed diabetes and improving the access to and level of diabetes care received by these individuals from their providers. Interventions included:

- DSM classes, which trained over 700 people to increase their understanding of how to manage the disease
- The Quality Care Improvement Program, designed to improve providers' diabetes care skills through workshops and distribution of American Diabetes Association (ADA) clinical guidelines

COMMUNITY RESPONSE TO PROJECT DIRECT

You have people who don't [see] themselves as belonging. 'They really don't want me because I'm not articulate, don't use the grammar well.' [Project DIRECT] has cut across that better than anything I worked with for a while.
                                    —*Project DIRECT Executive Committee member (Goodman,*
                                    Liburd, & Green-Phillips, 2001, p. 24)

The community involvement and their desire to be involved from the very beginning is one of the strongest things for Project DIRECT.
                                    —*CDC representative (Goodman et al., 1998, p. 24)*

There was community-wide acceptance and excitement about this project. This was evidenced by attendance at the kick-off event, the high level of participation at community coalition meetings, the number of community volunteers, community representation on committees and work groups, and members of organizations becoming community ambassadors. The project was welcomed by political leaders, community organizations, businesses, churches, and local care providers.

Numerous internal influences propelled the project to successful completion, including:

- Community involvement and support in every aspect of the project
- Support from the CDC to continue the project despite unanticipated delays
- Commitment of community leaders and residents to volunteer their services over an 8-year period, working numerous hours alongside staff and consultants

- Dedicated staff who believed the program was the best job they have ever had
- Local health care professionals who welcomed the operation of a community-based program serving high-risk and socioeconomically disadvantaged persons

There appeared to be very few external influences that propelled the program, since the list of internal collaborators and partners was so extensive.

CHALLENGES TO PROGRAM IMPLEMENTATION

The greatest challenges were issues of autonomy and control as a result of the complexity of the project design and numerous partners. Lack of communication, coordination, and cooperation in the early stages resulted in role confusion and goal conflict. Placement of the project director at the state health department and staff implementing the project at the local health department created additional bureaucratic challenges.

The CDC hired two consultants to analyze the conflicts experienced in the project's formative years. Dr. Robert Goodman used the rapid evaluation, consultation, and systems technique (Goodman et al., 1998) and Dr. William Ronco used the design and construction partnership method, which is used by the Army Corps of Engineers. These exercises resulted in ongoing communication between partners and increased understanding of partners' role (Ronco, 1997).

Challenges were also addressed by hiring culturally sensitive staff and consultants raised in African American communities in North Carolina. In addition, community involvement was a neutralizer for many potential conflicts. The community's presence was a constant reminder of the program's purpose and motivated staff to work around complexities.

No resistance to implementing the program was observed. From grant award through implementation and evaluation, the greatest challenge was the ability of the multiple partners to operate within a complex model in which leadership roles and responsibilities were not clearly delineated. The co-principal investigator and consultants for community outreach strongly objected to the patterns of oversight on human subjects (required for institutional board approval) from the CDC and viewed these as misdirected. These actions sometimes clashed with scheduled events and resulted in program cancellations that reduced confidence by the community that Project DIRECT would follow through.

PROGRAM EVALUATION

Evaluation results of Project DIRECT show improvements have been achieved in all project components: outreach, health promotion, and diabetes care (CDC, 2006). The project influenced a significant change in behavior related to diabetes prevention and care and reduced the expected rate of increase in the prevalence of type 2 diabetes. Although the incidence of diabetes rose, the rate of increase was significantly lower in SER than in the control community (10.5% to 16.7% vs. 9.3% to 18.6%). The prevalence of sedentary behavior in SER fell from 39.4% to 29%, whereas in the control community the rate only fell from 35.5% to 32.7% (ADA, 2007).

Policy and Environmental Changes

Changes were made at local, state, and federal levels. Many churches started health promotion programs (Hoyo et al., 2004) and added low-fat and sugar-free selections to congregation meals. Walking sessions became established programs in churches, community centers, and local businesses.

At the state level (NC DHHS), a SER representative from Project DIRECT was appointed to the North Carolina Diabetes Advisory Council and SER community volunteers have become faculty members for the annually conducted Project DIRECT Academy. The academy is a 2-day workshop that brings together teams of community volunteers and local health department representatives to learn effective methods of community engagement based on the lessons learned from Project DIRECT. The workshop has been taught by Project DIRECT partners since 2004 and has received a 96% approval rating by participants.

On the federal level, community members were included on the Research Triangle Institute Advisory Committee for the evaluation of interventions. In addition, Southeast Raleigh community members have been invited to present at numerous conferences (e.g., national conferences of the CDC, the ADA, and the National Association of Chronic Disease Directors).

New Partnerships

With the project's relocation to STBF, another partnership formed with their board. This was demonstrated when a team of community, county, state, and STBF representatives attended the Management Academy for Public Health at the University of North Carolina at Chapel Hill's School of Public Health and Kenan-Flager School of Business. These partners developed DIRECT Solutions for Diabetes Control, a plan to create the ADA recognition program that began in 2008.

Changed Perceptions

Outreach interventions changed the perception of diabetes. People with diabetes now feel comfortable telling others they have diabetes. They no longer see it as a disease to be ashamed of but rather a disease to control. Project participants often said that friends and family had progressed from having "a touch of sugar" to having diabetes.

Access to Care

Access to care increased as staff identified sources of medical care, which was especially helpful for persons with low incomes, limited education, and no health insurance.

Quality of Care

Diabetes care interventions increased the quality of care through health care providers and the health care delivery system (Din-Dzietham et al., 2004). The Quality Care Improvement Program provided doctors with current diabetes care guidelines and a resource for patient education, the DSM classes.

Lifestyle Behaviors

Health promotion interventions fostered an environment conducive to reducing risk factors for type 2 diabetes. DSM classes encouraged people to pursue healthy lifestyles.

Increased Knowledge

Outreach and diabetes care interventions increased knowledge of diabetes, including risk factors, signs, symptoms, treatment, and management techniques.

LESSONS LEARNED

Having the community involved in this way creates dialogue across these different realms that can strengthen the research.

> —*Dr. Kristina Ahlen, Research Triangle Institute Project Director of Survey Research (RTI International, 2007)*

Those of us who wish to improve a community's health must learn to think like the people of that community. All people have ways of coping with sickness. These habits and beliefs . . . are elements in a broader system of meaning that may not be apparent to persons outside the cultural system.

> —*Dr. John Hatch (2002 National Forum on Project DIRECT)*

Numerous lessons have been learned and include:

- By spending time in the community and communicating routinely with community members, public health workers and researchers gain insight and perspectives required for effecting health promotion and partnerships.
- Project DIRECT experiences influenced the design of a number of CDC programs, including Project REACH (Racial and Ethnic Approaches to Community Health) and Diabetes Today.
- Students and faculty of historically Black colleges and universities can play a major role in health promotion in African American communities because of their understanding of the culture and ability to gain acceptance in the community (Reid et. al., 2003).
- Teamwork developed a unified approach to community engagement. As reported by Naomi Penny, a doctoral candidate at Cornell University in her 2002 research study on community coalitions, "As a whole, this coalition seems to have a really good grasp as to how to reach their community and how to work with the community. This is not common" (Penny, 2002).

- Establishing partnerships requires a long phase of ongoing communication and cooperation. "Often the most serious challenges facing an effective health program is not the content of the program but the ability of the organizations implementing it to work together" (Ronco, 1997, p. 4).
- Everyone learned from working together. Public health practitioners increased their knowledge and understanding of community engagement and community members increased their knowledge of diabetes and skills for health promotion planning.

PROGRAM SUSTAINABILITY

We have just begun to transition Project DIRECT to independent operation, and we hope to continue and expand interventions to improve quality of life.
     —Mrs. Lucille H. Webb, Chair of the Executive Committee (ADA, 2007)

Project DIRECT was conceived as a partnership with a community ready to take on the responsibilities and demands. After nurturing this relationship over 13 years, mutual respect and bonds of trust were established. Sustaining the project is a priority for this partnership and has been placed in motion by:

- creation of the Project DIRECT Academy to disseminate lessons learned,
- transitioning the project to STBF, a community-based organization, and
- recognizing the program as a recognized ADA education program.

SUMMARY

Project DIRECT successfully involved community members in the design, implementation, and evaluation of the project. The greatest challenge was getting researchers and public health practitioners to recognize and respect the expertise of each partner, especially the community, and to maintain ongoing and open communication. The selection of staff and consultants who respected and valued the community's involvement improved the partnership's dynamics and was essential for survival. The community embraced its role as an equal partner throughout the project. Research tends to exclude communities from influence over the research process; however, Project DIRECT proved that involvement of the community gave the project acceptance in the community and enhanced the knowledge and understanding of researchers and public health practitioners. Community partnering is long-term work. We, the Project DIRECT partners, must be prepared to stay the course to assure sustainability of the project and dissemination of findings.

REFERENCES

American Diabetes Association. (June 23, 2007). *Rates of increase in diabetes prevalence reduced in Raleigh, NC over 8 years.* Archived Press Releases, 67th Annual Scientific Sessions. Retrieved from http://professional.diabetes.org/UserFiles/File/Scientific%20Sessions/Media/2007/Project%20DIRECT%20Final.doc

Centers for Disease Control and Prevention (2006). Improvement in lipid and glycated hemoglobin control among black adults with diabetes—Raleigh and Greensboro, North Carolina, 1997–2004. *Morbidity and Mortality Weekly Report, 55(46),* 1248–1251.

Din-Dzietham, R., Porterfield, D. S., Cohen, S. J., Reaves, J., Burrus, B., & Lamb, B. M. (2004). Quality care improvement program in a community-based participatory research project: Example of Project DIRECT. *Journal of the National Medical Association, 96(10),* 1310–1321.

Goodman, R. M., Speers, M. A., McLeroy, K., Fawcett, S., Kegler, M., Parker, E., Smith, S. R., Sterling, T. D., & Wallerstein, N. (1998). Identifying and defining the dimensions of community capacity to provide a basis for measurement. *Health Education & Behavior. 25(3),* 258–278.

Goodman, R. M., Liburd, L. C., & Green-Phillips, A. (2001). The formation of a complex community program for diabetes control: Lessons learned from a case study of Project DIRECT. *Journal of Public Health Management Practice, 7(3),* 19–29.

Gregg, E. W., Geiss, L. S., Saaddine, J., Fagot-Campagna, A., Beckles, G., Parker, C., Visscher, W., Hartwell, T., Liburd, L., Narayan, K. M., & Engelgau, M. M. (2001). Use of diabetes preventive care and complications risk in two African-American communities. *American Journal of Preventive Medicine, 21(3),* 197–202.

Hatch, J., Moss, N., Saran, A., Presley-Cantrell, L., & Mallory, C. (1993). Community research: Partnership in Black communities. *American Journal of Preventive Medicine, 9(6 Suppl),* 27–31.

Hatch, J., Reid, L., Parrish, T., & Hoyo, C. (2000). *Promoting healthy behaviors in African-American faith communities: The Project DIRECT experience.* Retrieved from http://www.ncdiabetes.org/_pdf/CHATCHAP.pdf

Herman, W. H., Thompson, T. J., Visscher, W., Aubert, R. E., Engelgau, M. M., Liburd, L., Watson, D. J., & Hartwell, T. (1998). Diabetes mellitus and its complications in an African-American community: Project DIRECT. *Journal of the National Medical Association, 90(3),* 147–156.

Holmes, A. (2004). Health disparities, the faith agenda, and health promotion/disease prevention: The General Baptist State Convention of North Carolina model. *North Carolina Journal of Medicine, 65(6),* 373–376.

Hoyo, C., Reid, L., Hatch, J., Sellers, D., Ellison, A., Hackney, T., Porterfield, D., Page, J., & Parrish, T. (2004). Program prioritization to control chronic diseases in African-American faith-based communities. *Journal of the National Medical Association, 96(4),* 524–532.

Liburd, L. C., Namageyo-Fuma, A., Jack, L., & Gregg, E. (2004). Views from within and beyond: Illness narratives of African-American men with type 2 diabetes. *Diabetes Spectrum, 17(4),* 219–224.

Parks, C. P. (1995). *Community leaders survey: Results and summary.* Southeast Raleigh Center for Community Health and Development. Raleigh, NC.

Penny, N. (2002). *Raleigh, NC Project DIRECT, conceptualizing community input.* A Cornell University student research report.

Project DIRECT. (2002). *Project DIRECT: A community partnership* (video). Diabetes Prevention and Control, NC Department of Health and Human Services. [Shown April 2, 2002, at the Project DIRECT National Forum].

Reid, L., Hatch, J., & Parrish, T. (2003) The role of a historically Black university and the Black church in community-based health initiatives: The Project DIRECT experience. Commentary. *Journal of Public Health Management Practice 9(Suppl),* S70–S73.

Ronco, W. (July 1997). *Improving partnering effectiveness in CDC diabetes programs: A case study of a partnering pilot program.* Gathering Pace, Inc. A report submitted to the Project DIRECT partners.

RTI International. (2007). *Project DIRECT: Community-based interventions to fight diabetes.* Retrieved July 7, 2008, from http://www.rti.org/page.cfm?objectid=16D78878-8B83-4962-A37D952F6A685505

Wake County Department of Health. (1996). *1996 community diagnosis: A statistical analysis of Wake County, NC.*

9

REACH Charleston and Georgetown Diabetes Coalition: Improving Outcomes for African Americans with Diabetes[1]

CAROLYN JENKINS, GAYENELL MAGWOOD,
BARBARA CARLSON, VIRGINIA THOMAS, AND
FLORENE LINNEN

Editor's Note: History, as kind or unkind as it is, tells many stories about the lives of African Americans. Descendants of those who were forcibly brought into the U.S. and sold as slaves in the southern states have remained in many of these areas, including Charleston and Georgetown counties in South Carolina. These counties are known today as the gateway for African American slavery. We find within these communities a rich history and culture reflecting a legacy of people who have overcome great struggles. However, many find themselves faced with burdens beyond race. Gaining access to the basic necessities of life and equal access to adequate health care has proven difficult for African Americans. Imagine the impact on this country if this reality were true for all communities in America.

[1] We would like to thank the following persons for their work, which contributed to this paper: Charleston and Georgetown Diabetes Coalition partners and community members; Dr. John Colwell, Chair of the Diabetes Initiative of South Carolina; and Ms. Pamela Arnold of the Diabetes Initiative of South Carolina. The project described in this chapter is funded by the REACH Charleston and Georgetown Diabetes Coalition CDC Grant/Cooperative Agreements U50/CCU422184-05 and 1U58DP001015-01 from the Centers for Disease Control and Prevention, the Medical University of South Carolina College of Nursing, and the Diabetes Initiative of South Carolina. The contents of this article are solely the responsibility of the authors and do not necessarily reflect the official views of the funding agencies.

237

In reading this case study, you will find how people internalized racism but still overcame the legacy of slavery by focusing on the empowerment of a community. As a result of this community-based diabetes program, African Americans were able to take charge of their diabetes through partner and community interventions. Many factors contributed to the success of this program. Educating the providers as well as the patients played a major role in setting the stage for trust building within the community. This community-based approach focused on eliminating health care disparities and linking the health care system with the community.

It was not an easy task for those involved. Individuals within the community and providers had to adjust to change, whether they perceived that change as good or bad. In these counties, African American communities adapted to the lack of access to adequate health care, knowledge regarding diabetes care, and transportation to receive health care and other needed resources, to name a few. Community partners and others committed to a healthier Charleston and Georgetown addressed diabetes disparities with the intent of achieving lasting change that would improve the lives of those who lived in these communities. Many residents had become accustomed to outsiders coming into the community with big ideas and plans to positively impact their way of life, resulting in little or no improvement to the burdens the residents face. Communities are often left to pick up the pieces themselves as the outsiders with the big ideas vanish. Trust is a huge factor in the success or failure of programs geared toward helping a community thrive. When public health professionals work with community organizations to eliminate health disparities, the rewards are great. Partners, community organizations, and other leaders embarked on enormous, cross-cutting efforts to achieve a health care system that helped people with diabetes receive the preventive care they needed.

As you read through this case study, consider the following questions:

- South Carolina has historically been ranked in the top 10% of all states for diabetes prevalence. Significant financial and human resources have been invested in reducing the burden of diabetes in the state. Thinking broadly, what additional resources would you identify to help the community move toward better diabetes prevention and control?

- With the success that the Racial and Ethnic Approaches to Community Health (REACH) Charleston and Georgetown Diabetes Coalition, other partners, and community leaders have had in educating the community and providers, what plans for sustainability would you propose?
- African American communities in Charleston and Georgetown counties have been characterized as medically underserved and as health professional shortage areas. What changes can be made to the health care system at the structural, policy, and practice levels to eliminate health care disparities and ensure ongoing access to high-quality diabetes care for these communities?

BACKGROUND

Geographic Area

The REACH Charleston and Georgetown Diabetes Coalition is a community-campus partnership between the Medical University of South Carolina and community agencies and organizations to improve health and health care outcomes among more than 12,000 African Americans with diabetes.

Charleston and Georgetown counties are located in South Carolina on the southeastern coast of the United States and are home to one of the most historic and diverse regions of the South. Culture, history, and environmental beauty are woven into a rich tapestry, which makes the area one of the most distinguished in the nation. Picturesque streets and antebellum mansions are reminders of Charleston and Georgetown's historical status as a premier center of southern culture and wealth. However, the area is also known as the gateway for African American slavery. Many descendants of the early African Americans who entered America as slaves still live along the Carolina coast. About 128,000 people, or 32–34.5% of the population, in the two counties were identified as African American (U.S. Census, 2009) and most still live in largely segregated communities. Most African American communities in both counties are designated as medically underserved and as health professional shortage areas.

Based on data from the National Health Interview Survey, the National Health and Nutrition Examination Survey, the National Hospital

Discharge Survey, and surveys conducted through the Behavioral Risk Factor Surveillance System (BRFSS), the reported prevalence rate for diabetes in South Carolina has historically been in the top 10% of all states. In the 2006 REACH Risk Factor Survey, 21% of African American adults in the two counties reported that they had been told by a health care provider that they had diabetes, as compared to the national prevalence of 13.3% (American Diabetes Association, 2008; Centers for Disease Control, 2005).

Prior to REACH, focus group participants in Charleston's Enterprise (inner city) Community reported diabetes as the second most prevalent health problem that they wanted to improve, with hypertension as the most prevalent. These qualitative data were supported by community health center ($n = 3$) and outpatient sites ($n = 12$) that reported diabetes as the most frequent diagnosis for primary care visits. Greater than 80% of all people with diabetes also had diagnosed hypertension. Two area hospitals, Roper Hospital and Medical University Hospital, had active outreach programs; two research programs, the Sea Islands Genetic African-American Registry Project (Project SuGAR) and the Hypertension and Diabetes Management and Education Program. The Tri-County Black Nurses Association offered screening and education programs in the Charleston area, and the Georgetown Diabetes CORE Group, a grassroots coalition in Georgetown County, recognized diabetes as a major problem in their community. The South Carolina Legislature also recognized problems related to diabetes and had created the Diabetes Initiative of South Carolina in 1994 to improve professional education, outreach, and surveillance related to diabetes and its complications. Other community groups were also organizing educational activities and ways to meet needs related to diabetes.

Community Needs Assessment

Community needs assessment methods are listed in Table 9.1 and described below. The Institutional Review Board for Human Subjects reviewed and approved community assessment methods. One of the first challenges was to objectively document the number of people with diabetes in our communities, as currently diabetes is not a reportable disease (to state health departments) and only estimates exist. Data could be self-reported by people with diabetes, small sample surveys could provide an estimate that could be extrapolated to the population, or health systems could report the number of users with documented diagnosis of diabetes, based on the International Statistical Classification of Diseases and Related Health Problems code 250 for diabetes mellitus (World Health Organization, 2007). To document the number of people with diabetes, partner health provider organizations, the federally-qualified health centers ($n = 3$), and university and hospital outpatient facilities ($n = 2$) examined existing data and reported more than 11,000 African American primary care users with diabetes in 1999 (Jenkins, 2003). If data from private physicians were included, the numbers would increase significantly. We noted that some may have used multiple systems and thus could have been counted more than once.

Table 9.1

COMMUNITY NEEDS ASSESSMENT METHODS

Focus Groups, Interviews, and Surveys
People with diabetes
Health care providers
Community leaders and key informants
Public health experts
Medical Record Audits in Five Health Systems
Persons with diabetes
Epidemiological Data
Use of health care systems (e.g., emergency medical services, ER, and hospital)
Costs of care
Costs of complications
Primary and contributing causes of death
Secondary Data
People with diabetes
Health care providers
Community leaders and key informants
Public health experts

We also examined available (secondary) data from the South Carolina Department of Health and Environmental Control's Diabetes Prevention and Control Program (BRFSS and deaths related to diabetes), South Carolina Budget and Control Board's Office of Research and Statistics (emergency room [ER] visits, hospitalizations, complications, and costs of care), U.S. Census data for the two-county area, a community survey by the Roper Hospital Foundation, Enterprise Community focus

Table 9.2

NUMBER AND RATE* OF DIABETES-RELATED CONDITIONS BY RACE AND GENDER

MEASUREMENT	LOCATION COUNTY	WHITE MALES		WHITE FEMALES		NON-WHITE MALES**		NON-WHITE FEMALES**	
		NUMBER	RATE	NUMBER	RATE	NUMBER	RATE	NUMBER	RATE
Deaths with diabetes as underlying factor	Charleston	12	25	18	24	17	72	37	114
	Georgetown	4	36	3	17	2	67	9	128
Deaths with diabetes as underlying or contributing factor	Charleston	64	132	66	88	57	273	76	235
	Georgetown	16	144	14	106	12	267	25	341
ER visits with diabetes as primary diagnosis	Charleston	70	99	47	62	135	451	191	474
	Georgetown	12	80	11	78	23	366	28	312
ER visits with diabetes as any diagnosis	Charleston	209	308	268	359	370	1,277	727	1,880
	Georgetown	76	600	129	895	127	2,093	297	3,590
Hospitalizations with diabetes as primary diagnosis	Charleston	121	175	132	160	180	647	272	669
	Georgetown	34	266	38	276	54	899	81	918
Hospitalizations with diabetes as any diagnosis	Charleston	1,083	1,942	1,264	1,705	803	3,460	1,717	4,883
	Georgetown	398	3,260	420	2,866	212	4,058	385	4,882
Estimated prevalence***	4.3–12% and 13.5% in largely African American communities								

* Number and rate written as Charleston/Georgetown counties. Rates are used per 100,000 population and age-standardized to 1997 SC population. Prevalence is reported as per 100 population.

** 99% of non-Whites are African Americans.

*** Self-reported diagnosed diabetes among people aged >18 and number is weighted to reflect South Carolina population, according to the 1998 BRFSS and 1995 PRT Healthy Communities Survey (*n* = 1,700 persons).

Source: Charleston and Georgetown Countywide Data (1997).

groups, problems reported by inner-city participants from the Healthy South Carolina Initiative's Hypertension and Diabetes Management and Education Program (an inner-city screening and education program), and existing meeting minutes and reports from community programs participating in the Diabetes Initiative of South Carolina. Sources providing these data are shown in Table 9.1 as secondary data. Diabetes-related hospitalizations, ER visits, and deaths are shown in Table 9.2.

A random review of medical records in the partner health sites was completed annually using methods developed by the Professional Review Organizations (Med-QUEST). Training of reviewers was provided by Carolina Medical Review (now Carolinas Center for Medical Excellence). Results of the chart audit are shown in Table 9.3 and are used to document the coalition's progress in eliminating disparities related to health care and diabetes control. Except for influenza and pneumonia vaccines, African Americans received less care, as documented in their medical records, than did others in the sample, mainly non-Hispanic Whites, even when data were examined by number of visits and insurance status.

Focus groups, individual qualitative interviews, and mini-surveys were done with people with diabetes, health key providers, public health experts, and community leaders and key informants to collect information about their perceptions of diabetes in the two counties and their experiences with the health system and providers, and to further examine collected data and obtain community input for the community action plan. The list of disparities identified by the coalition is shown in Table 9.4.

Relationship between Social Determinants of Health and Diabetes Disparities

African Americans are proud people who are family- and community-oriented. However, they reported a lack of resources for quality diabetes care and management as a challenge for many, since African Americans report lower per capita incomes, less education, and larger families. Crime rates are highest in inner-city communities with large numbers of African Americans, and some communities reported unsafe areas for physical activities. Lack of resources for basic needs, transportation, care, medications, and assistance with lifestyle changes were particularly noted by all focus groups. Many individuals, groups, and organizations within communities volunteered to assist with decreasing disparities

Table 9.3

RESULTS OF MEDICAL RECORD AUDITS OF PEOPLE WITH DIABETES IN CHARLESTON AND GEORGETOWN COUNTIES FOR 1998–1999 (*N* = 136 CHARTS)

MEASURE (MODIFIED DQIP)	% OF ALL PERSONS 1999	% AFRICAN AMERICANS 1999	% OTHER NON-HISPANIC WHITES 1999	% DIFFERENCE FOR AFRICAN AMERICANS 1999
1 HbA1c test/year	80	81	94	−13
HbA1c <7.0%	33	31	41	−10
HbA1c >9.5%	18	22	6	−16
Nephropathy assessment	71	69	94	−25
Lipid profile	41	40	56	−16
LDL <130 mg/dL	55	53	58	−5
Blood pressure <130/85 mm Hg	66	59	88	−29
Blood pressure <140/90 mg/dL	78	72	94	−22
Referral for dilated eye exam	32	31	44	−13
Foot exam, including risk assessment	24	25	28	−3
Self-management education	63	64	78	−14
Aspirin therapy	16	11	18	−7
Influenza vaccine	28	33	17	+16
Pneumonia vaccine (ever)	21	24	17	+7

Table 9.4

IDENTIFIED DISPARITIES FOR AFRICAN AMERICANS WITH DIABETES IN CHARLESTON AND GEORGETOWN COUNTIES

Less	More/Greater
Per capita income	Prevalence of diabetes
Access to needed services	Complications
Funding and insurance	• Amputations
Care and education	• Renal failure (dialysis)
Satisfaction with care	• Cardiovascular disease
Medications and continuing care	Emergency medical services
Treatment	(transport) and ER use
Trust	Hospitalizations
	Costs of care
	Deaths, especially due to
	cardiovascular disease

related to diabetes. Quality diabetes care and education were identified as top priorities for action; however, no group identified the resources to address the top priorities. Funding was a major challenge and money from REACH 2010 and others was essential for action and obtained continuously from 1999 through 2007.

Additionally, some neighborhoods linked with other community agencies and the local, state, and federal government to improve neighborhood conditions. In both cities of Charleston and North Charleston, neighborhood leaders and the city policy departments worked together on a plan to improve safety and decrease crime by adding foot patrols and neighborhood policemen who attended community meetings and events and focused on building neighborhood relationships. One neighborhood even obtained police who participated in their walking groups. To increase access to transportation, bus routes were initially added (but later cut due to budget constraints), church vans were used to attend diabetes meetings and health care appointments, and the Health and Human Service Commission increased their transportation routes. In Choppee, one of the rural areas, community members and health providers lobbied the county council and legislators to obtain funding for converting an empty abandoned school into a "one-stop shop" with a community health center site, alcohol and drug services, public health department, youth services, Georgetown Diabetes CORE Group (the Georgetown County Diabetes Coalition), and other groups, and have recently added an exercise facility with a volunteer certified trainer working with members of the Georgetown Diabetes CORE Group to increase physical activity.

ORIGINS AND HISTORY OF CHARLESTON AND GEORGETOWN DIABETES COALITION

When the call for proposals for REACH 2010 was issued in 1999, community leaders, members, and local organizations asked the Diabetes Initiative of South Carolina to apply for funding on behalf of a newly organized coalition. Representatives from each group joined together, mobilized volunteers, identified available data, and developed a plan for assessing the assets and needs related to health disparities for African Americans with diabetes. Although no funding was specifically designated to the application process, many organizations donated staff, time, supplies, and data to engage the community in identifying the diabetes disparities and developing, implementing, and evaluating a plan of action to address those disparities. The group obtained a planning grant from the Centers for Disease Control and Prevention (CDC) in 1999 and has been continuously funded by the CDC, along with other government organizations and private foundations, since that time.

COMMUNITY AND INSTITUTIONAL PARTICIPANTS

The initial coalition partners listed in Table 9.5 have a long history of working to improve care for African Americans, and in 1999 the group formed the REACH Charleston and Georgetown Diabetes Coalition specifically to improve diabetes outcomes for African Americans in the two counties. Coalition assessments and activities include data from the two-county area of about 1,600 square miles of both urban and rural communities.

THEORETICAL FRAMEWORK

In accordance with Lewin's stages of planned change, we can clearly document a "process of progress" from unfreezing, moving process,

Table 9.5

REACH 2010: CHARLESTON AND GEORGETOWN DIABETES COALITION PARTNERS		
CENTRAL COORDINATION ORGANIZATION	**ORGANIZING PARTNERS**	**CONTRIBUTING PARTNERS**
MUSC College of Nursing Diabetes Initiative of South Carolina	Alpha Kappa Alpha Charleston County Library Commun-I-Care Franklin C. Fetter Health Center Georgetown County Diabetes CORE Group Harmony Gardening Project Project SUGAR SC DHEC Waccamaw and Trident districts St. James Santee Health Center Tri-County Black Nurses University of South Carolina School of Public Health	BI-LO Supermarkets and Pharmacies Carolina Medical Review Charleston's Enterprise Community City of Charleston City of North Charleston Diabetes Initiative of South Carolina Healthy South Carolina Initiative MUSC College of Nursing MUSC Medical Center and Clinics Pfizer Ralph H. Johnson VA Medical Center SC DHEC Diabetes Control Program SC DHEC Office of Minority Health

and refreezing in the implementation of the REACH diabetes program. Such strategic, systematic planning for change agents, individually and collectively, are necessary and dynamic and must be addressed in an open, honest, and gentle dialogue. At each step, putting the issues "on the table" and allowing collective permission to ask "What's in it for me (us)?" was essential for progress. This helped to keep everyone honest while facilitating open and direct communication and resolving conflicts of interest and resources. Notably, the most important influencer, internal and external, remains human capital that demonstrates and embraces passion and power of collective activism while welcoming diverse skills and knowledge to produce change.

PROGRAM COMPONENTS

REACH 2010 Charleston and Georgetown Programs

Specific programs conducted by the coalition were organized around (a) community-driven activities and healthy learning environments where people live, worship, work, play, and seek health care; (b) evidence-based health systems change using continuous quality improvement; and (c) coalition power built through collaboration, consultations, trust, and sound business planning. Many of these activities are listed below.

Community skill-building and neighborhood clinics were offered in community settings, such as community centers, faith-based groups and churches, service-oriented organizations, and health centers. More than 175 volunteer lay educators were trained, along with 5 salaried REACH community health advocates (CHAs). The volunteers and CHAs joined with the certified diabetes educator, nutritionist, and nurse to develop and offer more culturally appropriate diabetes self-management education, foot care training, and programs focused on taking care of our bodies (e.g., Wise Woman for African American women aged 40–70 years old, which is now transitioning into Wise Men helping Wise Women). These activities were supported by partner organizations and funding from REACH.

Community health professional training included programs for all health professionals with special emphasis on training 145 registered nurses in advanced foot and wound education, along with foot care education for 27 physicians. Annual updates on diabetes care, access to resources, working with culturally diverse populations, and literacy were provided to more than 250 health professionals each year. African Americans joined the REACH team and four who were supported by the coalition were certified as diabetes educators.

Outreach by professional and lay educators included a 30-minute taped television program that aired 34 times on cable, and tapes were provided to more than 30 community groups. REACH partnered with the National Network of Libraries of Medicine to develop, test, and now institutionalize a library-based program that teaches participants how to use diabetes information to learn about the Internet. The REACH 2010 Charleston and Georgetown Diabetes Coalition's Library Partnership won the 2006 Health Information Award for Libraries from the U.S. National Commission on Libraries and Information Science in May 2006.

Free diabetes self-management training classes and support groups were offered at eight sites throughout the area on a weekly basis. Although most area hospitals offer a similar program, the cost is around $400 for the series of 6–10 classes. Many of our participants continued to come to multiple series of classes to help develop needed skills and obtain ongoing self-management support for behavior change. Others did not want to attend classes, so walk-and-talk groups were led by lay educators and health professionals so others could learn needed skills while participating in organized physical activities.

After examining the evidence for changing health systems, each partner health care facility decided on their approach for systems change. Most decided to create a quality improvement team to guide their activities. Most of these teams created registries with reminder systems like diabetes flow sheets, whereas the academic health center sites switched to an electronic medical record. Most developed a systematic method for referring clients to diabetes self-management classes, whereas others created walk-and-talk about diabetes groups that were led by lay health care workers (i.e., REACH community health advocates and advisors).

Coalition building and policy change occurred through our work together, with the partners coalition deciding that each county needed their own coalition to facilitate local action. These coalitions obtained 501(c)(3) tax status and began generating small grants to support clients who were unable to pay for strips for monitoring blood glucose, raising money through community banquets, auctions, raffles, and other activities. The local county coalitions joined with the National Partnership to Fight Chronic Disease and other groups to expand their actions. Through working collaboratively with the Diabetes Initiative of South Carolina, the South Carolina Legislature passed a law requiring health insurance policies to cover diabetes education for persons who receive at least minimal standards of diabetes care (see South Carolina Code of Law 38-71-46).

COMMUNITY RESPONSE TO THE CHARLESTON AND GEORGETOWN DIABETES PROGRAM

Multiple groups that had previously worked together formed a partners coalition to initially apply for REACH funding in collaboration with the Diabetes Initiative of South Carolina. The community had identified diabetes activities as a priority need in several neighborhoods and were working together to address needs, then other organizations joined the efforts. The community response was very positive to improving diabetes and associated complications; however, there was some competition among the partners for needed funding. We agreed that the needed dollars to address the community needs related to diabetes and its complications far exceeded any one grant or program. Thus, each partner worked to meet the needs of their agency, organization, or local community and came together to share these actions and examine ways to collaborate and meet some of the needs of the larger African American community.

CHALLENGES TO PROGRAM IMPLEMENTATION

Initially, the challenge was to dispel reservations that this diabetes mellitus program was not another veiled attempt to create a project for researchers or political notoriety and/or gain, then leave the community; the other issue was true engagement of the community stakeholders and gatekeepers with university partners in collaborative ownership, decision making, and action, since the community was accustomed to being told by the university researchers about how a project would be managed after decisions were made and funding realized. Thus, program planners and implementers from the university needed to step back, roll up their sleeves, and listen to the overall needs through these powerful, passionate, and sometimes tense exchanges of information and learning; planners and implementers were given rights of passage to the information exchange network within the community by true collaboration with community leaders to integrate and disseminate epidemiological data with community information and evidence. The evidence included moving communities at risk, even stakeholders and gatekeepers, forward in realizing and espousing that diabetes mellitus is a killer, not "just a touch of sugar" or "oh, diabetes runs in the family." This strategic movement from diabetes being a generation-to-generation family history to an unwelcomed consequence of potentially preventable complications could be described as an epiphany. Clearly, this did not just happen. The REACH coalition achieved progress (wins and losses) through establishing relationships and openly addressing the diversity of people and the value of all, regardless of skin tone, gender, religious affiliation, and maybe most significantly socioeconomic status. Other challenges related to consensus building at times impeded progress because of both spoken and unspoken competing priorities.

We found that folks were accustomed to being autonomous. Thus, when presenting out-of-the-box notions like pooling resources to plan and implement joint ventures, such as a health education workshop or a more traditional health fair co-sponsored by multiple organizations (e.g., community centers and churches), within a walking radius of each other, sometimes these collaborations were not welcomed. Ownership and individual identity got in the way of collective ownership, capacity building, and identity. Again, starting where people are and valuing the individual identity (the person and the organization) became a seminal chain of events.

Together, we first focused on actions to meet some of the identified community needs and are currently engaged in increasing organization and structure for sustainability. Another ongoing issue that we faced is changes in partner leadership when different members representing some organizations moved to different positions and new people joined the coalitions. We developed Web site, marketing, and educational materials that included leaders and common folk who shared their stories about managing their diabetes, as well as a few who had major complications that they attributed to their lack of management. We worked together to meet some of the community and organization needs, and that work continues, and is even expanding, in many communities.

Although we have a set of initial operating guidelines that we added to over several years, we are now creating a more formalized process. We have passionate discussions, but remain committed to our goals. The challenges are many and the major driving forces include the devotion and loyalty of members of the coalition and the commitment to eliminating disparities for African Americans at risk and with diabetes, so that health equity is a reality for our communities and for other communities across the United States.

PROGRAM EVALUATION

Stories of improved health habits are plentiful and data from chart audits of care demonstrated improved care, improved control, and decreased ER visits. Health outcome data showed up to a 50% reduction in amputations in African American men, and our legislators know about our progress. Outcomes for hemoglobin A1c, the clinical test to track glucose control over 2–3 months, for 1999–2006 are shown in Figure 9.1, and decreased amputations in African American men with diabetes are shown in Figure 9.2.

Impact of Program on Social Determinants of Health

Institutional and organizational policy and environmental changes are broadly based. Through the community-academic partnerships and/or

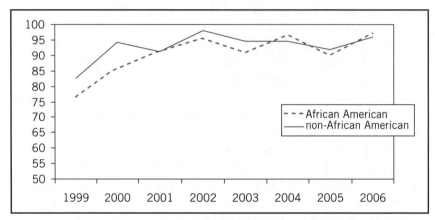

Figure 9.1 Percent with ≥ Annual A1c by Race (increased from 76.8% in 1999 to 97.1% in 2006)

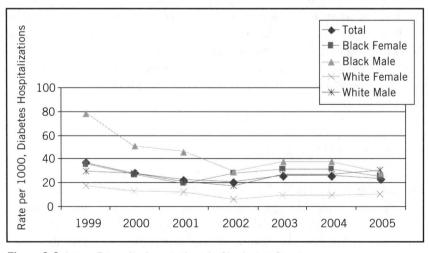

Figure 9.2 Lower Extremity Amputations in Charleston County

coalitions formations we have experienced internal and external policy and environmental changes related to social determinants of health (SDOH) and diabetes outcomes. SDOH encompass societal conditions of the social, economic, and physical environment.

Within local groups, we have seen community groups and policemen working together to improve neighborhood safety, so people feel they can walk in neighborhoods, and groups and organizations working together to improve transportation to health care facilities.

At the organizational level, Greater Saint Peters Church of Our Lord Jesus Christ, a relatively small church congregation, added food and a health education component to monthly health screenings, links those without a health care home to available resources, and provides a grocery bag full of healthy food to participants to help meet gaps in end-of-month budgets. Nazareth African Methodist Episcopal Church has trained its church kitchen committee on healthier food preparation to offer healthy meals.

At the policy level, the REACH Charleston and Georgetown Diabetes Coalition worked collaboratively with the Diabetes Initiative of South Carolina to bring about a law that mandates that insurance companies, other than those groups that are "self-insured", provide diabetes education coverage for clients who receive the minimum standards of diabetes care. If we want to reduce health disparities, our coalitions know that changes at the individual, group, system, and policy levels that involve changes in the SDOH are essential for progress.

LESSONS LEARNED

The lessons learned from our collective REACH experiences are many. Some of these lessons are:

- Continual reassessment of needs and resources is needed.
- The altruistic notion that you cannot assign value to everything is naive, allowing programs to develop and remain overcommitted and underfunded and perpetuating socioeconomic disparities.
- Negotiating for increased community control sooner than later facilitates community ownership.
- Explicit communication that partnerships can and do change over time is okay and to be expected.

■ Clear guidance and commitment that all are responsible for sustainability increases the possibility for success; thus, community-academic partner dyads should have written plans for answering the primary question of how to sustain program intervention. This involves funders, planners, and the community. No program intervention should be implemented without an evolving plan for sustainability.

Probably the most important lesson is that solutions for health disparities cannot occur in isolation. As health care agents of change, we cannot enjoy success or progress in improving health outcomes without understanding and working simultaneously for health equity through addressing SDOH. This is the true wheel in the middle of the change wheel of sustainability (community wheel of sustainability).

SUMMARY

The Charleston and Georgetown REACH program demonstrates that impressive reductions in health care disparities and diabetes-related complications can be realized among African Americans living in these communities. Community empowerment is the cornerstone of this program. Attending to improving neighborhood conditions, community education, and access to information resources, and sensitizing and reforming the health care system to eliminate disparities in care, all lend to the success of this community-based diabetes program. The collective efforts demonstrate that by working closely with a broad range of community and institutional partners, we can improve neighborhood safety, improve access to transportation services, and reduce the digital divide. Ultimately, the goal is to sustain these improvements as a matter of public and practice policy, rather than as a short-term achievement that goes away when "soft" grant monies end. The rich and compelling history of these communities reflects the cumulative health impact of an historical patterning of social and political inequality. The high burden of diabetes experienced by this community is not inevitable; it can be reversed through a comprehensive and sustained public health approach that incorporates strategies that address the SDOH.

REFERENCES

American Diabetes Association. (2008). Total prevalence of diabetes & pre-diabetes. Retrieved from http://www.diabetes.org/diabetes-statistics/prevalence.jsp, June 15, 2009.

Centers for Disease Control and Prevention. (2005). National diabetes fact sheets: United States. Retrieved from http://www.cdc.gov/diabetes/pubs/pdf/ndfs_2005.pdf, June 15, 2009.

Charleston and Georgetown Countywide Data. (1997). Retrieved from http://www.ors2.state.sc.us/, January 12, 2000.

Jenkins, C. (2003). REACH 2010 Charleston and Georgetown Diabetes Coalition: Approaches to reducing disparities for African Americans with diabetes. *South Carolina Nurse, 10(1),* 16–19.

U.S. Census Bureau. (2009). The 2000 population estimate for South Carolina. Retrieved from http://www.census.gov/, June 15, 2009.

World Health Organization. (2007). Diabetes. Retrieved from http://www.who.int/topics/diabetes_mellitus/en/, June 15, 2009.

10

American Indian Higher Education Consortium Honoring Our Health Grant Program

KELLY MOORE, CAROLEE DODGE-FRANCIS, AND LEMYRA DEBRUYN

Editor's Note: The prevalence of diabetes among American Indians is among the highest of any population group in the U.S. There are a number of different perspectives on what factors in the genetic, socioeconomic, and political environments that contributed to the rise in diabetes prevalence in tribal communities over the past 60 years. Many have attributed the incorporation of westernized lifestyles as a major factor in the recent development of diabetes among American Indians (AIs) and Alaska Natives, but the historical and sociological pathways to the current burden of diabetes among AIs is, by all indications in the literature, complex and not readily isolated into discrete, easily defined risk factors.

Honoring Our Health is one of two case studies representing community-based diabetes programs in AI communities. This program is based in the southwest U.S. and the second is underway in the southeastern region of the country. Although separated by thousands of miles and different terrains, there are shared historical and contemporary experiences related to diabetes, its risk factors, and associated complications.

In this case study, the developers of Honoring Our Health tap into community institutions for solutions in overcoming diabetes disparities. Building tribal capacity to eliminate diabetes disparities was closely tied to the education and professional development of the next generation of leaders, teachers, researchers, and so forth, enrolled in tribal colleges. Investing in their students would support the development of a workforce capable of designing culturally grounded health promotion and chronic disease prevention strategies practically nonexistent in some tribal communities in the Southwest. This program also focused on children and teens who are at a higher risk of developing serious complications associated with type 2 diabetes. The success of these programs required the involvement of the entire community, with families at the center of efforts to prevent and control diabetes among the youth. Families pass traditions and local knowledge from one generation to the next. When families are actively engaged, there is a positive impact on the entire community and healthier life choices are made to prevent diabetes.

As you read through this case study, consider the following questions:

- North American indigenous people often see diabetes as an "outside" or "unnatural" disorder. How can one learn more about indigenous beliefs about diabetes and other chronic diseases? How might trust factor into your ability to access this information? How would you use local knowledge that conflicts with western, biomedical knowledge?
- The American Indian Higher Education Consortium Honoring Our Health Grant Program experienced great success with many of the programs they implemented. Staff turnover, however, was a challenge. What suggestions would you make to decrease staff turnover in order to sustain the programs at current or higher levels?
- Community education was indicated as one key to preventing diabetes. Given the awareness to diabetes within the community, what methods would you use to promote making healthy choices given the economic and political challenges encountered by some tribal communities?

BACKGROUND

American Indians and Alaska Natives (AI/ANs) bear a disparate burden of type 2 diabetes (Centers for Disease Control and Prevention [CDC], 2003; Valway et al., 1993), with an increasing prevalence of diabetes noted among young people in many AI/AN populations (Dabelea et al.,

1998). From 1994 to 2004, the age-adjusted prevalence of diagnosed diabetes more than doubled among AI/ANs younger than 35 years of age who use Indian Health Service (IHS) health care services (CDC, 2006). Because young persons with type 2 diabetes develop the disease at such an early age, experience more years of disease burden, and have a higher probability of developing serious type 2 diabetes-related complications (Harris, 1995), effective diabetes prevention programs targeting younger age groups are a compelling priority for AI/AN communities.

Westernized lifestyles are commonly accepted as major contributors to the diabetes epidemic among AI/ANs, yet other factors, such as poverty, social injustice, trauma, and historical legacies of dispossession of their lands, culture, and language, also play a significant role (Joe & Young, 1993; Satterfield, Eagle Shield, Buckley, & Taken Alive, 2007). Diabetes is often seen by North American indigenous peoples as an "outside" (Huttlinger, Krefting, & Drevdahl, 1992) or "unnatural" (Joe & Young, 1993) disorder that is a "White man's sickness" (Garro & Lang, 1993; Lang, 1989) with both internal and external contributing influences (Morgan & Weedon, 1990; Wing, 1998). Holistic traditional native knowledge about health and other indigenous worldviews may be the source for an important framework in the development of community capacity in addressing the devastating epidemic of diabetes among tribal people (Chino & DeBruyn, 2006; Satterfield et al., 2007).

Community Needs Assessment

As part of the coalition building activity, community needs assessments were conducted to determine the types of programs requested by community members. These assessments varied from site to site in terms of the data collected. One grantee focused on the community need for paraprofessional education on diabetes through a survey conducted in schools, public health departments, and clinical diabetes programs of 10 Minnesota tribes. This same grantee also collected data on parental perceptions on the need for preventive education on diabetes at three local elementary schools. At another site, community and institutional participants assisted in the development of a health assessment administered to all tribal college students and faculty. One grantee designed a comprehensive tribal needs assessment by updating a previous community health survey that summarized diabetes incidence data. This same grantee also used their community health survey to identify what traditional foods and medicinal plants their community members utilized.

Areas to target for health education and prevention were identified. At one tribal college community, high cholesterol, hypertension, arthritis, and diabetes were the four major chronic diseases identified. At least one tribal health survey also collected data on the lack of health insurance among the tribal college population. Insurance status is a significant health care disparity for AI/ANs. Fronstin (as cited in Smedley, Stith, & Nelson, 2002) reported that nearly one-third of AI/ANs (32.8%) lack health insurance as compared with 17.5% in the general population.

A county youth health behaviors and attitude survey was collected twice in a 3-year time interval by a tribal college in collaboration with a regional inter-tribal epidemiology center. Of the 332 public middle school and high school students surveyed, 74 (22.3%) self-identified as AI. No significant gender or race differences were noted in the students' descriptions of their personal health (i.e., great, okay, or poor). No significant differences due to gender, grade, or race were noted for receipt of annual health exams (50.0%). Although no significant difference in exercise frequency due to race or grade was noted, AI females were more likely not to exercise than AI males.

Another tribal college's elementary school surveys indicated that almost 10% of all parental respondents used food stamps and 5% used commodity foods to stretch food dollars. For AI parental respondents, 13% reported they used food stamps and commodity foods, respectively. More than half (53%) of the parents disagreed or strongly disagreed to attending an education program on lifestyle factors that could help control their children's weight. Yet of the AI respondents, only 35% disagreed and none strongly disagreed, suggesting significant interest in learning more about lifestyle changes to prevent the development of diabetes. Whereas 72% of all parents agreed or strongly agreed that they would have their children attend a free program that taught healthy lifestyle choices, almost 95% of AI respondents agreed or strongly agreed. However, significant barriers to participation in any proposed educational programs raised by all parents included the children's lack of interest and busy schedules, as well as lack of transportation.

ORIGINS AND HISTORY OF HONORING OUR HEALTH

This culturally relevant initiative, Honoring Our Health: Tribal Colleges and Communities Working Together to Prevent Diabetes, was a partnership among the American Indian Higher Education Consortium (AIHEC), the CDC, and the Department of Health and Human Services Office of Minority Health to build capacity, establish and maintain a communication plan, promote health, and reduce the impact of diabetes in tribal colleges and universities (TCUs) and local communities. The AIHEC, in collaboration with the CDC, developed the proposal and review process and determined a distribution strategy for a competitive announcement. Proposals were accepted for either planning or implementation activities. TCUs that received a planning award were eligible to apply for an implementation award the following year. If the TCU initially received an implementation award, they were not eligible to compete for another competitive award the following year. These guidelines were set by the AIHEC Board to ensure that every TCU that wished to apply over the 3 years of competitive funding would have an equal chance to receive some money for at least 1 year.

TCUs that received awards included: Blackfeet Community College, Cankdeska Cikana Community College, College of Menominee Nation, Dine College, Fond du Lac Tribal College, Fort Belknap College, Fort Peck Community College, Haskell Indian Nations University, Keweenaw Bay Ojibwa Community College, Lac Courte Oreilles Ojibwe Community College, Leech Lake Tribal College, Northwest Indian College, Saginaw Chippewa Tribal College, Sinte Gleska University, Si Tanka-Huron University, Southwestern Indian Polytechnic Institute, Stone Child College, Tohono O'odham Community College, Turtle Mountain Community College, and United Tribes Technical College. (See Figure 10.1 for a map of the locations of these TCUs, the AIHEC central office, and the CDC Native Diabetes Wellness Program.)

FUNDING

In recognition of the need for community capacity building in addressing the epidemic of diabetes among AI/ANs, from 2002 to 2004 the AIHEC was awarded funding ($800,000, $850,000, and $1 million, respectively) from the CDC's Native Diabetes Wellness Program (formerly the National Diabetes Prevention Center). This funding sponsored cooperative agreements for TCUs to develop and evaluate diabetes prevention projects in tribal communities.

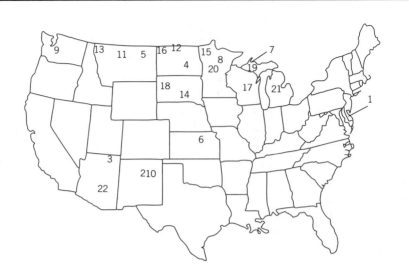

1. American Indian Higher Education Consortium, Central Office, Alexandria, VA
2. Centers for Disease Control and Prevention, Native Diabetes Wellness Program, Albuquerque, NM
3. Dine College, Tsaile, AZ
4. Cankdeska Cikana Community College, Fort Totten, ND
5. Fort Peck Community College, Poplar, MT
6. Haskell Indian Nations University, Lawrence, KS
7. Keweenaw Bay Ojibwa Community College, Baraga, MI
8. Leech Lake Tribal College, Cass Lake, MN
9. Northwest Indian College, Bellingham, WA
10. Southwestern Indian Polytechnic Institute, Albuquerque, NM
11. Stone Child College, Box Elder, MT
12. Fort Belknap, Harlem, MT
13. Blackfeet Community College, Browning, MT
14. Sinte Gleska University, Mission, SD
15. United Tribes Technical College, Bismarck, ND
16. Turtle Mountain Community College, Belcourt, ND
17. College of Menominee Nation, Keshena, WI
18. Si Tanka-Huron University, Huron, SD
19. Lac Courte Oreilles Ojibwe Community College, Hayward, WI
20. Fond du Lac Tribal College, Cloquet, MN
21. Saginaw Chippewa Tribal College, Mount Pleasant, MI
22. Tohono O'odham Community College, Sells, AZ

Figure 10.1 Honoring Our Health—Map of Tribal Colleges

COMMUNITY AND INSTITUTIONAL PARTICIPANTS

Community awareness about diabetes in AI/AN communities is already high, because diabetes is a pervasive problem. In addition, the implementation of the Special Diabetes Program for Indians (SDPI) by IHS in 1997 resulted in approximately 400 new or enhanced diabetes treatment and prevention programs in AI/AN communities (IHS, 2004). To build upon this existing community interest, many AIHEC grantees formed local advisory committees of prominent community members, such as respected tribal elders and elected tribal officials, as well as other key stakeholders, including physicians and nurses, tribal college students, tribal college administrators, health and nutrition educators, and school health personnel. Even where local advisory committees were not formed, the tribal college leadership and faculty, tribal college students, IHS, tribal health departments, SDPI and other existing diabetes programs, and community health representative (CHR) programs were the key community and institutional participants in mobilizing community efforts around diabetes.

To engage the tribal college population, some TCUs conducted tribal college community health assessments. Such assessments provided a synopsis of the current health status of the tribal college population, including faculty, staff, and students. This information was then used in the development of future course offerings and academic programs at the TCUs. The reports were also presented to the general community population.

Convening focus groups of community members ensured general community participation and empowerment. Other strategies for community engagement included community-wide forums on diabetes prevention and community outreach activities, such as health fairs and powwows. In order to demonstrate community involvement, activities were planned based on the analysis of the community health assessment results, reports from the focus groups and community-wide forums, and input from the advisory committees.

PROGRAM COMPONENTS

Data were also gathered to assess community customer satisfaction with the wide range of program activities. In 2003 the demographics of the Honoring Our Health AIHEC cooperative agreement indicated that over

5,700 people had been served by the projects, with 99% of the participants being AI/AN. In all projects, females showed a higher participation rate than males. Overall, for the final year of the project, 2005 implementation grantees reported that young adults (15–25 years of age) and adults (26–54 years of age) were the primary target populations for their program activities. However, despite the same high emphasis focused on the two age groups, the number of participants in the activities was significantly different, with adults averaging a 19.1% participation level versus young adult participation at 5.7%. Implementation grantees also reported that overweight adults with and without diabetes, tribal college students, and community nutrition programs were the primary target groups for their program activities. Greatest participation for the high-risk and special groups was reported for tribal college students at 32.8%. Specific activities of the AIHEC cooperative agreement are described below.

Nutrition Activities

In 2005 implementation grantee respondents indicated the methods or activities to provide nutrition information that they had emphasized and were able to develop or greatly improve through their AIHEC Honoring Our Health Implementation Grant. For the provision of nutrition information, their primary emphasis focused on the target groups of the whole community (67.1%) and their secondary emphasis on people with diabetes (58.1%). Training programs, group classes, grocery store tours, cooking classes, and individual sessions were the methods emphasized, developed, or greatly improved.

Tribal college students described changes made in their food choices as a result of program participation. Students reported eating fewer fried foods, foods with saturated fats, and sodas. One student stated, "What I've learned is like, in the cafeteria here we have hamburgers, fries, nuggets, stuff like that. So I've learned we have to stay away from that and eat regular food like chicken, steak, and vegetables." Another student commented that making changes in diet was a slow process, leading a third student to declare, "I haven't completely given up Cokes. I still have one a day right now."

Physical Activity Programs

These same grantees also indicated the methods or activities to increase physical activity that they had emphasized and were able to develop or greatly improve with this grant funding. The methods most emphasized, developed, or greatly improved were walking programs, traditional games, dances and other physical activities, and aerobics. TCU students and teachers had the highest participation level for walking programs (67.8%), followed by relatively equal participation from all other target groups of families (12.7%), elders (12.6%), elementary school children (12.9%), teens (12.5%), and the whole community (12.6%).

Several tribal college students related their experiences in getting their families involved in walking or other fitness activities. Students found this positive influence on their families to be one of the most rewarding aspects of their participation. A faculty participant described an especially enjoyable walking program: "[O]ur staff do a lot of walking in school, in fact a lot of them, and I don't know where they came from, but they have walking counters [pedometers] and we almost have a little competition of who can put on the most steps in a given day."

Traditional Approaches

Many grantees utilized traditional approaches in their program activities. Most often their programs utilized traditional foods (24.1%), stories and story-telling (17.2%), traditional games and activities (17.2%), talking circles (13.8%), traditional herbs or medicines and traditional practices such as sweats (a traditional practice used to elevate the temperature of the body and believed to purge the body of impurities), and other ceremonies (10.3%), and traditional healers (6.9%). A comprehensive grid-based inventory of traditional foods, medicinal plants, and mapping of indigenous plant species was accomplished in one community. Geographic information system-based software was customized and applied to this comprehensive inventory system for later protection, conservation, enhancement, and reintroduction efforts for these traditional foods and medicinal plants.

Diabetes Education

The methods for diabetes education were divided between four categories: community-based methods, education for people with diabetes, education for health professionals, and other education activities. The 2005 implementation grantees reported the major emphasis in community-based methods was placed equally (13.5%) on radio, newsletters, K–12 school-based curricula, tribal college school-based curricula, and community health fairs. Average emphasis (8.1%) was focused on traditional methods of stories and talking circles.

Other studies have shown that stories and talking circles are well-accepted and effective health communication tools for diabetes education in AI/AN communities (Carter, Perez & Gilliland, 1999; Hodge, Pasqua, Marquez, & Geishirt-Cantrell, 2002; Struthers, Hodge, Geishirt-Cantrell, & De Cora, 2003). Through the use of these traditional methods, participants can reconnect with traditional values that promote a healthier lifestyle. Also, since stories are often indirect and presented in a less threatening manner, the listener can reflect upon the lessons included in the story (Carter et al., 1999; Hodge et al., 2002). By sharing new knowledge that other people have faced diabetes successfully, stories can bring acceptance, rather than denial, and hope to assist AI/AN individuals with diabetes overcome the fatalism and hopelessness often associated with diabetes in their communities (Carter et al., 1999; Satterfield et al., 2007).

Within the education for people with diabetes category, the major emphasis (55.6%) was placed on group education, followed by average emphasis (33.3%) on clinic-based one-on-one education methods. In the education for health professionals category, only some emphasis (40%) was focused on Continuing Education Units (CEU) programs. CHRs and health aide training was included in the other education activities category. Average emphasis (37.5%) was reported.

Tribal College Courses

A three-credit course on the topic of diabetes awareness was developed at one tribal college. Diabetes awareness was also incorporated into existing courses. Another tribal college created a 2-year associate degree in applied sciences in fitness and health. A nutrition principles course was offered at a third tribal college. Through a partnership with the Expanded Food and Nutrition Education Program, this same college planned to permanently offer a 5-week series on nutrition each semester for all staff and students. This college also offered a physical fitness course called Native American Dance Forms. Gardening courses were offered at several tribal colleges. Moreover, a high level of success was reported in increasing diabetes knowledge and awareness for teachers. In addition to changes in course and program offerings, direction regarding learning styles, motivational strategies, and promotion of lifelong health and fitness habits for all community members resulted from Honoring Our Health project activities.

Finally, as in the Diabetes Education in Tribal Schools project, co-funded in 2000 by the National Institutes of Health's National Institute of Diabetes and Digestive and Kidney Diseases and Office of Science Education, the CDC, and the IHS to develop a diabetes prevention curriculum specifically designed for AI/AN school children, the changes in tribal college course and program offerings were linked to other community diabetes prevention efforts involving families and resulted in a more consistent, community-wide focus on diabetes prevention and education (Chino, Dodge-Francis, DeBruyn, Short, & Satterfield, 2007).

CHALLENGES TO PROGRAM IMPLEMENTATION

While grantees overwhelmingly reported success in working with organizations in their areas, there were a few problems. In one instance, an advisory committee and the tribal college had different goals for the project. Rather than successfully completing the original objective of a college curriculum on diabetes education and prevention, the grant director negotiated acceptance of options that were tailored more closely to college and community desires and existing programs. Grantees also reported other barriers, such as resistance to change at the tribal college level and difficulty at some sites in recruiting student participants. Resistance to change arose from inadequate administrative staffing and staff time, as well as bureaucratic tribal college departmental policies related to personnel, budgetary reporting, and procurement of supplies. One grantee also described boundary issues with the local clinical and public health staff on community-based diabetes prevention activities as an unexpected roadblock. Initially, some grant program activities were not well attended. But as community awareness increased, more and more community members participated.

Overall, the major barrier encountered was staff turnover. Hiring new staff, notably institutional policies on hiring consultants, was the second-most common barrier. This is not unexpected given the remote rural setting of many of these communities. Delay in the planning component of the grant, community buy-in, lack of administrative support, and lack of office or activity space were other important barriers. Presenting the least barriers overall were lack of cooperation from partners and lack of collaborative partners.

Examples of program successes included students' enrollment in new health courses with positive student evaluations. Scores on objective tests in a nutrition course indicated that student knowledge of nutrition increased, as well as their ability to apply that knowledge in their work and lives. Awareness and prevention activities continue as weekly, monthly, and yearly events. One planning grant recipient reported that following the needs assessment and development of a strategic plan, the following immediate results were noted: the commodity warehouse obtained refrigeration so that fresh fruit and vegetables could be offered, the elementary school menu changed to offer healthier choices and both staff and students started losing weight, community garden sites were developed, a farmers' market was organized, and the TCU began work with the U.S. Department of Agriculture Extension Service to develop a community organic garden at the college. In addition, intergenerational exercise programs were established. The involvement of elders in the projects and the students' increased awareness of their tribal and cultural histories were also very positive outcomes.

PROGRAM EVALUATION

The opportunity to be seen as a catalyst for social awareness elevated the TCUs' role in the community. The project also fostered the role of the AIHEC as a national organization in developing partnerships with federal agencies and tribal nations. This AIHEC grant opportunity allowed TCUs to both seek and actualize their vision as a TCU that in turn could raise the health status of the community. More importantly, this project began the emergent process of long-term capacity development with TCUs and Native community-based groups in the fight against diabetes.

Access to Care Increased

In collaboration with local Special Diabetes Program for Indians projects, blood glucose and blood pressure screenings were held at TCUs for staff and students, with referrals made for those needing follow-up testing. In addition, increase in access to nutrition information and promotion of physical activity for the entire community and clients with diabetes resulted from grant program activities. Grant activities also led to unexpected outcomes like the involvement in a state governor's summit on health care access for the uninsured.

Formation of New Partnerships

Increasing community collaborations was considered an impact of high importance and received the highest ranking for degree of success among both planning and implementation grantees. These collaborations resulted in partnerships that exceeded the duration of the grant period and should positively impact future health projects. Moreover, collaborations were formed that extended beyond diabetes prevention and control. One grantee also participated in a state policy forum on suicide prevention, which resulted in training for suicide prevention professionals at the local tribal college.

LESSONS LEARNED

Diabetes Prevention Program Translation

In 2003 grantee respondents participating in the initial evaluation of the project overwhelmingly saw community education as the key to preventing diabetes. Ignorance and fear were reported as the primary obstacles to diabetes prevention in AI/AN communities. Remarkably, the stigma associated with being labeled as a person with diabetes paradoxically resulted in behaviors that increase one's risk for the disease. Such behaviors noted by the grantee respondents included refusal of opportunities to receive diabetes-related information from health programs and ignoring recommended preventative measures. Respondents also emphasized the importance of relationships in educating a community about the results of the landmark National Institutes of Health randomized clinical trial, the Diabetes Prevention Program (DPP) (DPP Research Group, 2001). One respondent even stated that education begins in the home, meaning adults and all family members need to become involved.

Additionally, many respondents stressed the importance of reaching youth with the DPP results. However, without the commitment of their families, they noted that young people would have difficulty committing to the healthier life choices that prevent diabetes. Nonetheless, one respondent noted that their grant proposal, "Seeking Life: Preventing

Diabetes through Celebration of Native Wellness," was a direct response to the DPP findings and that they planned to use the DPP findings in other grant proposals as well. Another respondent reported that learned behaviors are very hard to change, but through creative information sharing activities and positive reinforcement, most individuals are more receptive to trying new approaches in practicing healthy lifestyle habits.

Respondents had suggestions for incorporating the results of the DPP into future projects for AI/AN communities, such as establishing wellness circles to promote family wellness in campus daycare sites. An agricultural program for the provision of more natural foods was also suggested. Greenhouses for natural foods and more programs to build capacity for community gardens were other ideas. Emphasizing cultural understanding and knowledge and including local tribal histories in physical education programs were mentioned as well.

Capitalizing upon this interest in agricultural programs, the CDC Native Diabetes Wellness Program has recently funded 11 cooperative agreements to support the use of traditional foods and sustainable ecological approaches to health promotion and diabetes prevention. This is based on a strong grassroots movement throughout the indigenous Americas that supports sovereignty and identity through the use of ancient seeds and traditional cultivation, horticultural, gathering, and hunting technologies.

Garden of Health is another innovative, intergenerational garden project funded by the CDC Native Diabetes Wellness Program after the project period of Honoring Our Health. Operated by United American Indian Involvement, an urban Indian health program serving the Los Angeles AI/AN community, this project aims to improve nutrition and introduce urban AI/AN youth to healthier eating alternatives through experiential gardening and cooking education.

Lessons Learned to Share with Other Tribal Colleges

In 2005 one respondent reported that tribal college students are often well-motivated and interested in helping their communities, especially when their own families are affected by a problem like diabetes. For more impressive student effort and participation, program design should offer tribal college students the opportunity to make a contribution to a solution. Video recording actual class sessions and guest speakers was also reported as helpful in developing a diabetes prevention education curriculum. Recommendations for new course development included flexibility and responsiveness to student and teacher needs.

Grant Planning

More than one grantee in 2005 indicated that limited staffing must be taken into consideration when a small grant is received. Completing a large number of objectives for a small team may not be feasible, practical, or realistic.

Working with Youth

Tribal college faculty noted the importance of following suggestions from elementary and secondary school teachers for grade-appropriate materials and making learning fun. Higher retention among youth programs to promote physical activity was more likely when activities were fun, obtainable by all fitness levels, and consisted of a wide range of activities, such as a locomotion egg hunt and jump rope relays. Incentives like small prizes and acknowledgments also promoted retention of youth in diabetes prevention activities.

Others

Successful administration of a health assessment required partnerships, advanced planning, careful development of an appropriate assessment tool, support of the community, and analysis of the data by knowledgeable evaluators. Achieving maximum results with minimal staff was especially difficult.

PROGRAM SUSTAINABILITY

Participants' plans to keep their projects going in the future are:

- work with tribal college administration to support continuation of health courses;
- continue campus activities through local student wellness programs;

- use ongoing efforts like diabetes talking circles for providing basic diabetes information to community members in a culturally appropriate manner and train tribal college students annually in this process;
- develop a strategic college vision on health education and diabetes prevention through community involvement, networking, and building infrastructure within the tribal college to create a holistic approach to wellness;
- work with other community programs to support dissemination and printing of program materials that were developed; and
- prioritize and select one successful program activity, such as a summer diabetes prevention program, for ongoing support to continue as long as possible.

SUMMARY

Honoring Our Health: Tribal Colleges and Communities Working Together to Prevent Diabetes enhanced community capacity building through the utilization of TCUs as the framework for program development and reinforced the need for culturally relevant diabetes programming based upon education and community involvement. However, much work remains to be done in the fight against diabetes in these communities. Effective diabetes prevention and management will require the development of new strategies that more effectively involve tribal communities in designing diabetes and other health programs in alliance with their own indigenous views. Lessons learned from other indigenous models, such as the Gathering of Native Americans (Substance Abuse and Mental Health Services Administration, 2008) and the Community Involvement to Renew Commitment, Leadership, and Effectiveness (Chino & DeBruyn, 2006), may one day allow the creation of a diabetes-free future for all tribal communities. Honoring Our Health brought hope that a vision of healthier tribal communities is possible, but long-term indigenous values-based interventions and funding will be necessary for ultimate change.

REFERENCES

Carter, J. S., Perez, G. E., & Gilliland, S. S. (1999). Communicating through stories: Experience of the Native American Diabetes Project. *Diabetes Educator, 25,* 179–188.

Centers for Disease Control and Prevention. (2003). Diabetes prevalence among American Indians and Alaska Natives and the overall population—United States, 1994–2002. *Morbidity and Mortality Weekly Report, 52,* 702–704.

Centers for Disease Control and Prevention. (2006). Diagnosed Diabetes Among American Indians and Alaska Natives Aged <35 Years—United States, 1994–2004. *Morbidity and Mortality Weekly Report, 55,* 1201–1203.

Chino, M., & DeBruyn, L. M. (2006). Building our capacity: Indigenous models for indigenous communities. *American Journal of Public Health, 96,* 596–599.

Chino, M., Dodge-Francis, C., DeBruyn, L., Short, L., & Satterfield, D. (2007). The convergence of science and culture: Developing a framework for diabetes education in tribal communities. *Journal of Health Disparities Research and Practice, 1(3).* Retrieved June 15, 2008, from http://chdr.unlv.edu/JHDRP.htm

Dabelea, D., Hanson, R. L., Bennett, P. H., Roumain, J., Knowler, W. C., & Pettitt, D. J. (1998). Increasing prevalence of type II diabetes in American Indian children. *Diabetologia, 41,* 904–910.

Diabetes Prevention Program Research Group. (2001). The Diabetes Prevention Program: Reduction in the incidence of type 2 diabetes. *New England Journal of Medicine, 346,* 393–403.

Garro, L. C., & Lang, G. C. (1993). Explanations of diabetes: Anishinaabeg and Dakota deliberate upon a new illness. In J. R. Joe & R. S. Young (Eds.), *Diabetes as a disease of civilization: The impact of cultural change on indigenous peoples* (pp. 293–328). New York: Mouton de Gruyter.

Harris, M. I. (1995). Chapter 1: Summary. In M. I. Harris, C. C. Cowie, M. P. Stern, E. J. Boyko, G. E. Reiber, & P. H. Bennett (Eds.), *Diabetes in America* (pp. 1–13). Washington, DC: U.S. Department of Health and Human Services, Public Health Service, National Institutes of Health. DHHS Publ. No. NIH 95-1468.

Hodge, F. S., Pasqua, A., Marquez, C. A., & Geishirt-Cantrell, B. (2002). Utilizing traditional storytelling to promote wellness in American Indian communities. *Journal of Transcultural Nursing, 13,* 6–11.

Huttlinger, K., Krefting, L., & Drevdahl, D. (1992). Doing battle: A metamorphical analysis of diabetes among Native people. *Journal of Personality and Social Psychology, 46,* 706–712.

Indian Health Service. (2004). *Special diabetes program for Indians: Interim report to Congress.* Retrieved June 6, 2008, from http://www.ihs.gov/medicalprograms/diabetes/resources/r_rtc2004index.asp

Joe, J. R., & Young, R. S. (1993). Introduction. In J. R. Joe & R. S. Young (Eds.), *Diabetes as a disease of civilization: The impact of culture change on indigenous peoples* (pp. 1–18). New York: Mouton de Gruyter.

Lang, G. C. (1989). Making sense about diabetes: Dakota narratives of illness. *Medical Anthropology, 11,* 305–327.

Morgan, G. R., & Weedon, R. R. (1990). Oglala Sioux use of medicinal herbs. *Great Plains Quarterly, Fall,* 18–35.

Satterfield, D., Eagle Shield, J., Buckley, J., & Taken Alive, S. (2007). So that the people may live *(Hecel Lena Oyate Ki Nipi Kte)*: Lakota and Dakota elder women as reservoirs of life and keepers of knowledge about health protection and diabetes prevention. *Journal of Health Disparities Research and Practice, 1(2).* Retrieved June 5, 2008, from http://chdr.unlv.edu/JHDRP.htm

Smedley, B. D., Stith, A. Y., & Nelson, A. R. (Eds.). (2002). *Unequal treatment: Confronting racial and ethnic disparities in health care* (pp. 84–85). Committee on Understanding and Eliminating Racial and Ethnic Disparities in Health Care, Board on Health Sciences Policy, Institute of Medicine, Washington, DC: The National Academies Press.

Struthers, R., Hodge, F. S., Geishirt-Cantrell, B., & De Cora, L. (2003). Participant experiences of Talking Circles on type 2 diabetes in two Northern Plains American Indian tribes. *Qualitative Health Research, 13,* 1094–1115.

Substance Abuse and Mental Health Services Administration. (2008). Center for Substance Abuse. Retrieved from http://preventiontraining.samhsa.gov/CTI05/Cti05ttl .htm, June 15, 2009.

Valway, S., Freeman, W., Kaufman, S., Welty, T., Helgerson, S. D., & Gohdes, D. (1993). Prevalence of diagnosed diabetes among American Indians and Alaska Natives, 1987: Estimates from a national outpatient database. *Diabetes Care, 16,* 271–276.

Wing, D. M. (1998). A comparison of traditional folk healing concepts with contemporary healing concepts. *Journal of Community Health Nursing, 15,* 143–154.

11 Cherokee Choices Diabetes Prevention Program: The Eastern Band of Cherokee Indians

JEFF BACHAR

Editor's Note: The alarming burden of diabetes among American Indians is a fairly recent phenomenon dating back only to the 1950s. In research conducted by Satterfield, Shield, Buckley, & Taken Alive (2007) with Lakota and Dakota elders, they found that there was a time when there was no word for diabetes in indigenous North American languages because it was an unknown condition. Until 1943 diabetes was undocumented among people native to the Plains, but by 1996 this same community was affected by diabetes at a rate four times higher than non-Hispanic Whites (Satterfield et al., 2007).

The emergence of diabetes in this population has been explained by some indigenous elders as an "outside" or "unnatural" disorder and a "White man's sickness" that requires "White man's medicine" (Satterfield et al., 2007). Native beliefs about health, for example, are not limited by biomedical knowledge, but is informed more holistically by traditional knowledge that understands the importance of harmony and balance in maintaining health and preventing disease. Traditional knowledge is defined as "a natural science grounded in lifetimes of intimate daily observation, habitation, and experience. . . . [it] is knowing the country (i.e., the environment and its interrelationships); it is holistic, rooted in spiritual health, culture, and language of the people. . . . [Yet] this local knowledge has been undervalued by conventional science" (Satterfield et al., 2007, p. 4).

Any program intending to eliminate diabetes disparities among American Indians must learn, respect, and incorporate into the program plans the meanings ascribed to this disease by the affected community. You are encouraged to read the full text by Satterfield and colleagues titled "So That the People May Live *(Hecel Lena Oyate Ki Nipi Kte)*: Lakota and Dakota Elder Women as Reservoirs of Life and Keepers of Knowledge about Health Protection and Diabetes Prevention."

There are over 500 recognized American Indian tribes in the United States. This case study describes the experience of the Eastern Band of Cherokee Indians (EBCI) in combating diabetes in the southeast region of the United States. Located in North Carolina, the EBCI Community Coalition was funded as one of the initial Racial and Ethnic Approaches to Community Health (REACH) 2010 programs, the flagship program of the Centers for Disease Control and Prevention (CDC) to eliminate health disparities. In planning this diabetes program, the community coalition fully appreciated the need to listen to the community, respect its history and traditions, and address perceptions associated with diabetes. Children were a central focus of this diabetes program, and systems and cultural changes were sought to insure the children had ample opportunity to pursue a healthier lifestyle. Key to eliminating diabetes disparities among the EBCI was deconstructing beliefs that communicated a fatalism and inevitability of diabetes. As you read this case study, consider the following questions:

- Considerable investment has been made in understanding the etiology of type 2 diabetes from the biomedical standpoint. How might we build a credible base of evidence that links the high prevalence of diabetes and other chronic illnesses to historical legacies of dispossession of lands, culture, and language in American Indians?
- Diabetes was described as a stigmatized condition in this community. What might cause a community to stigmatize one health condition but not another? Why might diabetes be counted among the stigmatized conditions?
- In addition to the strategies used in this program to reduce the prevalence of diabetes, what are some additional interventions you would propose? Pay particular attention to additional strategies that address the social determinants of health like racism.

BACKGROUND

The Eastern Band of Cherokee Indians (EBCI) resides on the Qualla Boundary, which is nestled within the Great Smoky Mountains of western North Carolina. There are more than 13,000 enrolled members of the EBCI, about two-thirds of whom reside on tribal land in four counties. With the advent of casino revenues in 1997, economic changes have affected the EBCI. Within the last decade, the poverty rate fell from 31% to 22%, and the median family household income increased 82% to almost $32,000; this amount is still less than the state median by nearly $14,500 (Martin, 2004). Although casino revenues have had a positive impact on family income, they may also have had a negative effect on family health behavior because families have more available funds to eat outside the home.

Sturm analyzed trends in childhood obesity nationally, including increases in soft drink consumption and carbohydrate intake, and noted that with increasing income, people are shifting toward eating food away from home because it is more convenient; these foods tend to be more energy-dense and contain more fats and sugars than foods prepared at home (Sturm, 2005). Likewise, as family income has increased on the Cherokee Boundary (the primary Cherokee district), the array of fast food choices has increased; more than 19 fast food restaurants are available within three miles of the district's center.

According to the National Center for Health Statistics (2004), rates for obesity and type 2 diabetes exceed those for the U.S. general population and the state of North Carolina. The age-adjusted prevalence for obesity among the U.S. general population in 2002 was 30%. According to the most recent data from the National Opinion Research Center (2005), the percentage of EBCI men who were obese was 53.4% compared with men from North Carolina at 25.1%. EBCI women had a prevalence of obesity of 56% compared with North Carolina women at 27%. In the U.S. general population for 2003, diabetes prevalence for males and females was 5.3% and 4.5%, respectively. In Cherokee type 2 diabetes prevalence is at 26.9% for EBCI men and 29.1% for EBCI women versus 9.4 % and 9.1%, respectively, for North Carolina men and women.

Eighteen percent of 85 children surveyed in the EBCI community reported eating at fast food restaurants five or more times per week, and 52% reported eating out at least twice a week (Cherokee Choices, 2004). Diet, along with sedentary lifestyle, may be contributing to the dramatic increase in childhood obesity among the EBCI. In 2003 61.9% of EBCI boys aged 6–11 years who received services at the local hospital were overweight or obese, and 58.6% of EBCI girls in the same age group who received services at the local hospital were overweight or obese (Indian Health Service, 2003). In addition, children as young as 10 years have been diagnosed with adult onset diabetes (A. Bullock, MD, EBCI, personal communication, 2003).

The combination of changes in the economic and food environments likely has a great influence on the prevalence of type 2 diabetes among the EBCI. In response, a multilevel community-based diabetes program was conceptualized and implemented in this community. In addition to the material culture and health data that informed the development of this project, indigenous meanings attached to diabetes were incorporated in the program plans.

Community Needs Assessment

Initial steps in program planning involved formative research to gauge the perception of diabetes among Cherokees; in other words, we needed to find out what Cherokee people thought about diabetes in terms of causality, prevention, and intervention. We found that diabetes for many in the community was a stigmatized condition and many felt powerless, or at worst hopeless, to reduce its prevalence among their families and community. A professional marketing group, the Goss Agency, was contracted to assist in conducting interviews related to diabetes and provided the following in an executive summary report:

> Because diabetes has touched so many Cherokee families, there is a broad awareness of diabetes throughout the Cherokee community accompanied by a general apathy. Because the disease is so rife, it has unfortunately created an almost fatalistic acceptance of diabetes as an "inevitable fact of Cherokee life" and a widespread belief that the disease is not preventable. (Goss, 2004, p. 3)

Some responses from their interviews that give insight to the meanings attached to type 2 diabetes in this community included:

- People believe that becoming diabetic is something that will happen, no matter what they do. For example, one respondent said "I know people who eat right and exercise and still get diabetes."

Statements like these perpetuate the belief that Cherokee people will develop diabetes in spite of any preventive actions they might take.

■ Another respondent stated, "It's (diabetes) like a car alarm. You hear it originally, but after a while you hear it so much that you don't pay attention anymore." If a condition becomes "silent" in the lived experience of the individual, it is difficult to attend to diabetes self-management and take actions to prevent complications of the disease.

■ "There's a fatalistic attitude. People say, 'I'm going to die some way anyway, so I'm going to eat what I want.'" This person is arguing "why make all of the prescribed behavioral changes, particularly denying oneself or restricting the joys of consuming certain foods if the ultimate end anyway is death by some means?" Privileging quality of life and simple pleasures, such as indulging in foods that are enjoyable if not necessarily in line with healthy eating for diabetes prevention and control, is not an uncommon choice that people with and at risk for diabetes make.

■ Overall, respondents feel that the broad acceptance of the disease and its inevitability is the key problem that must be overcome. Cherokee people must come to an understanding that diabetes is preventable and manageable.

The voice of our people is the heart and soul of our program. The concerns and perceptions of the community, voiced in either one-on-one interviews or larger venues, set our program priorities. Through talking with community members, agents of change, and partners who work together toward capacity building, a message is being voiced that through behavior change diabetes can be prevented and quality of life extended.

ORIGINS AND HISTORY OF CHEROKEE CHOICES

In 1999 the Centers for Disease Control and Prevention (CDC) provided REACH 2010 funds to the EBCI to develop a community-based intervention to improve health and prevent the rise in diabetes among this indigenous population. The REACH 2010 program is part of CDC's nationwide effort to reduce disparities in health among racial and ethnic minority populations. An important role of the Cherokee Choices program among the EBCI is to listen to the Cherokee community and respond. The role involves being aware of and facilitating environmental, organizational, and individual changes. Priorities also include addressing racism, historic grief and trauma, mental health, diabetes, and obesity and creating a supportive environment for developing positive policy changes. Diabetes and obesity were selected as the focus of the REACH 2010 program launched among the EBCI.

During the first year of the program, known locally as Cherokee Choices, grantees conducted formative research, formed coalitions, and developed a culturally appropriate community action plan to be implemented in subsequent years. The formative research, including in-depth interviews, focus groups, and reviews of existing epidemiological data, compelled an emphasis in the Cherokee community action plan on the prevention of type 2 diabetes with particular attention to children. Recognizing that successful interventions for children need to include parents, the elementary school, tribal worksites, and local churches were identified as key gateways for the intervention components.

THEORETICAL FRAMEWORK

The REACH 2010 logic model developed by staff at the CDC was the framework used to guide the development of the program (Tucker, Liao, Giles, & Liburd, 2006). A program logic model is defined as a picture of how an organization does its work, that is, the theory and assumptions underlying the program. The basic components of a logic model include factors (resources that potentially enable or limit program effectiveness), activities (techniques, tools, events, and actions of the planned program), outputs (the direct results of program activities), outcomes (changes in attitudes, behaviors, knowledge, skills, status, or level of functioning), impacts (organization-, community-, or system-level changes), and relevant external influences (Tucker et al., 2006).

The REACH 2010 logic model illustrates how a coalition could theoretically produce the desired local health disparity reductions and impacts in racial and ethnic groups. It focuses on the logical approaches of a community coalition that convenes to learn the context of, causes of, and solutions for local health disparities and is prepared to take actions to reduce and eliminate these disparities. For example, we paid particular attention to elements of the logic model focused on targeted action, community and systems change, and change among change agents. Targeted actions are all intervention activities believed to bring about a desired effect. Community and systems change refers to changing at-risk conditions by altering the environmental context within which individuals and groups behave. Change among change agents includes documented changes in knowledge, attitudes, beliefs, or behaviors among influential individuals or groups with the intent of diffusing similar changes to a broader community population (Tucker et al., 2006). The REACH 2010 logic model was also used to guide the evaluation of key components of our program.

PROGRAM COMPONENTS

The mission of Cherokee Choices is to delay the onset of type 2 diabetes and related complications by working with community and other organizations to develop and deliver community-based behavior change interventions. Cherokee Choices is committed to addressing this serious health problem and providing prevention education and services through garnering the input, perspective, and energy of the community. The "emic" or insider's understanding to this end is a critical element in the program's success. Through community coalition meetings, focus groups within each of the Cherokee communities, and one-on-one discussions, Cherokee Choices gains the guidance necessary to plan program services. The program also shares this information with others through a variety of media, including a video series entitled "Generations to Wellness," a series of advertisements on billboards and local television commercials, newspaper forums, and community outreach programs.

Many sociocultural factors were considered in designing and conducting a health promotion program among the EBCI. Although American Indian communities are not homogenous throughout North America, some traditional cultural values ring true for many. For example, many American Indians value the importance of spirituality for balance, the essential network of extended family systems, and the significance of intergenerational support. Consistent with the mission of the project and a keen sensitivity to the cultural values of this community, the following interventions were conducted.

Elementary School Mentoring

This program was conducted at Cherokee Elementary School. The school is the only elementary school in the community and is operated by the EBCI. It includes grades kindergarten through six and has approximately 600 students. Five adult mentors and a nutritionist work to alter the culture of the elementary school. The specific focus of the cultural changes they seek are increasing awareness of diabetes as a serious health issue through in-service training and during classes, increasing knowledge about good nutrition in class and as part of a weekly after-school program, increasing physical activity during the school day and after school, teaching stress management techniques and coping skills to children, and developing teachers as healthy role models through faculty fitness activities. In addition, the mentors developed lesson plans that they implemented in the classroom to enhance self-esteem, cultural pride, conflict resolution, emotional well-being, and health knowledge.

Worksite Wellness

During the community assessment phase, meetings were held with a host of tribal agencies and community groups to begin the process of planning and capacity building, leading to the development of a community action plan. This plan included a core program to target tribal employees and engage those interested in a worksite wellness program. Nutritionists, dietitians, and fitness workers help tribal workers participate in health challenges to reduce stress, eat healthier, and increase physical activity. Tribal offices compete for prizes earned by nutritional assessments, meeting physical activity and dietary change goals, and attendance at healthy cooking demomstrations, supermarket tours, and stress management workshops. Baseline clinical measurements are offered to participants through collaboration with the local diabetes clinic. This information gives them a baseline metabolic profile from which they can compare their progress over time as a result of participating in the worksite wellness programs. Measures include fasting blood glucose, blood pressure, and fasting lipid panel (total cholesterol, HDL, LDL, and triglycerides). Height, weight, and body fat percentage are taken within a week of participants' enrollment into the program. Body fat was measured with the Futrex 6100XL Near Infra-Red Interactance technique with a measuring range of 3–45%. Follow-up measures and interviews regarding goal attainment were conducted every 6 months of the program's cycle. Data was entered into an SPSS 13.0 statistical software program for analyses.

The Health Challenge

Friendly competition is a cultural value of the Cherokee Nation. To build upon this community norm, the program implemented a 16-week competition-based program that would reward decreases in weight and percentage of body fat, regular participation in activities sponsored by Cherokee Choices, and overall positive behavior changes. Nutritionists, dietitians, and fitness workers helped tribal workers participate in health challenges to reduce stress, eat healthier, and increase physical activity. Tribal offices competed for prizes earned by undergoing nutritional assessments, meeting physical activity and dietary change goals, and attending healthy cooking demonstrations, supermarket tours, and stress management workshops.

To stimulate physical activity, each participating tribal agency formed various teams that would challenge other teams to volleyball, racquetball, and basketball. Team members accrued points for participation and winning scheduled athletic events. Points could also be accrued by self-reported minutes of exercise per week and number of Cherokee Choices events attended. Each team selected a leader who acted as a liaison with Cherokee Choices, sent out regular emails encouraging members to continue the program, and solicited volunteers to attend wellness activities. The team leader also kept record of exercise minutes and scheduled competition in athletic events. Cherokee Choices staff stayed in touch with team leaders and visited each agency at least once a week for support, education, and encouragement. Follow-up measures and interviews regarding goal attainment were conducted every 6 months of the program's cycle.

The Life Challenge

To maintain the positive health outcomes achieved during the health challenge, an additional component was added to support the maintenance of weight loss, fat loss, increased physical activity, and any other health-promoting behaviors begun during the challenge. The life challenge was structured to be continuous during the year (2006) and offered in two 4-month program cycles. Participants from the health challenge could join at anytime during their involvement in the program. Staff were also available to provide support during this phase of the challenge. Wellness staff, for example, emphasized an open door policy, encouraging people to drop in for talks and one-on-one support. Wellness staff were comprised of a registered dietitian and licensed nutritionist, a certified fitness instructor who also has a B.S. in nutrition, a part-time staff member who is currently a B.S. candidate in nutrition, and an enrolled tribal member.

Church-Based Health Promotion

Nutritionists, dietitians, and fitness workers helped members of five churches participate in activities to improve diet and food preparation, raise awareness of tribal health-related services, and increase physical activity like walking. An interdenominational coordinators group was formed to represent the congregations and oversee the church-based efforts. One of the most exciting church-based programs was the "Walk to Jerusalem" community intervention. Groups from five churches participated in a Walk to Jerusalem project, in which congregations tracked with pedometers their progress toward walking the equivalent distance between Cherokee, NC, and Jerusalem. Each participant completed a pre- and post-intervention survey. Data collected included basic demographic information and queries regarding health, exercise time per week, and self-reports of daily water and fruits and vegetables intake. Over the course of the 5-month program, participants walked more than 31,600 miles, the equivalent of walking to Jersualem from Cherokee five times. Participation constituted 173 congregants, each averaging 183 miles walked. One respondent said, "It gave you an incentive to discipline yourself each day to walk more, which makes one feel better physically and mentally."

The incorporation of activities for extended family systems and churches are extremely important in promoting community support for any intervention project. The majority of EBCI identify themselves as Christian, even though there are some traditionalists who continue to practice without formal church attendance. The local Lutheran church infuses both Christian and traditional Native ideologies and rituals (i.e., going to water and sweats, a spiritualistic custom used to raise body temperature and believed to purge the body and their souls). There are at least 10 different denominations and more than 39 churches on the boundary.

The church-based activities included "Wellness Wednesdays," during which time they provided information about nutrition, cooking demonstrations, and physical activity programs for the children. There was also a gospel sing to kick off the Walk to Jerusalem program. The gospel sing promoted spirituality and health among the participants. According to one, the church-based program was "promoting education that good health can be spiritually divine."

Other Community-Based Interventions Sponsored by Cherokee Choices

Changing cultural beliefs and norms associated with type 2 diabetes in this community required a broad range of activities and targeted strategies. Following are key interventions that support the mission of Cherokee Choices:

- Monthly submissions were provided to the Cherokee newspaper, *One Feather*, of a "Living with Diabetes" page each month.
- Presentations were conducted at the Cherokee Youth Center on body image, weight training, and making wiser food choices.
- Presentations were conducted at locations visited by large numbers of community members, such as the Kidney Clinic, the Snowbird Senior Center, and the Unity Regional Healing Center.
- In addition to the schools, fitness classes were held at a variety of agencies like the Cherokee Life Center.
- Guided supermarket tours were provided and open to all community members.
- Health assessments were provided for participants.
- Stress management workshops were offered every 3 months.
- A health marketing campaign was designed and included:
  - "Generations to Wellness" video was produced and local televison aired the series that portrayed community members of all ages dealing with obstacles presented by diabetes and sharing visions of a healthy future.
  - Billboards were posted throughout the community to increase awareness about diabetes prevention and control.
  - Professional, culturally appropriate public service announcements were developed and aired on local television stations.

- Local libraries were given additional resources on health and wellness.
- Worksites allocated space and were equipped with exercise equipment and wellness information, such as recipes, motivational tools, and notices about upcoming events.
- Program managers allowed time off for employees to exercise and attend health challenge events.
- The tribal council called for a community-wide mandate for continued diabetes prevention programs to institutionalize community concern to eliminate type 2 diabetes in the Cherokee Nation.

PROGRAM EVALUATION

Impact of the Elementary School Mentoring Program

To monitor the effect of mentoring, students respond annually to surveys regarding issues of self-concept, perceived stress, cultural awareness, peer relations, and eating habits. Evaluation data is collected and analyzed using multiple methods. For example, mentors record their interactions and exchanges with students in daily logs. Quantitative survey data from this overlapping cohort design is collected and entered into SPSS for analysis. Qualitative data from daily logs are analyzed using ATLAS.ti to identify key themes and provide context for better understanding and interpreting data collected through the quantitative survey methodology. Qualitative data from the teachers and staff suggest there are changes in the school culture since Cherokee Choices has been implemented. For example:

- Teachers are requesting a fitness program at school.
- Teachers are now sending letters home to parents asking them to prepare healthy snacks from the "Healthy Party" handbook instead of having cake, sweets, and/or pizza as the usual school lunch fare.
- Teachers participated with the kids who qualified for an end-of-year swim party, particularly noteworthy given that this is the first class party ever to include physical activity and large participation of faculty.
- Teachers have commented on the increase in parent and teacher participation in school activities sponsored by Cherokee Choices.

- School menus were modified to include low-fat items.
- The program documented extensive community support and turn-out for the "Jumping against Diabetes" event, which raised more than $28,000.
- Local librarians provided space for new health books and have cooperated with the program in implementing the "Brain Food" project.

A comment from a librarian and 30-year veteran teacher at Cherokee Elementary School had this to say about the cultural changes taking place as a result of Cherokee Choices:

> At Cherokee Elementary, I've noticed that since we've had Cherokee Choices in our school, that the students are much more aware of the necessity of physical exercise and eating healthy and making food choices, and when they come to the library, they're looking for materials on cooking, they're looking for materials about their bodies and maturing, and we see them out walking on our track and ah, just that they're trying to be healthier overall. I feel that Cherokee Choices has made a good impact on the community as far as educating the parents, that how important it is that their child be eating healthy, making the right food decisions, and we see lots more parents in the school being involved with activities that have been sponsored by Cherokee Choices. We also see Cherokee Choices at every event and they're very cooperative and helpful when we have anything going on in the school.

Among the reasons for the positive changes observed with the children is that the project created a safe, non-threatening environment in which they could share their feelings with a responsible adult. With collaboration of the elementary school's guidance counselor, a "Walk and Talk" club was implemented, which also allowed children to increase their physical activity.

The heart of the program is being involved with Cherokee children and providing a safe and understanding person with whom they can talk. Even though most have a large, extended family with relatives who are willing to listen, sometimes the children needed another adult who was outside the family, yet knowledgeable of their world, to share their experiences and feelings.

An excerpt from a mentor's daily log is exemplary of how mentors' support is important for these children. The following log entry comes from a rafting trip with the Cherokee Elementary School after-school program participants:

> We stopped about three times on the river to swim. The water was freezing and the cool wind made it worse. All the kids jumped in like baby seals. We got to the place where there was a big rock and all the kids were jumping off of it. G. [age 12] climbed up to the top, but really was afraid to jump. I cheered her on because I knew she would regret it if she didn't jump. She looked right at me and I said YOU CAN DO IT!! And she jumped!! She did great. Then, I decided to climb up the rock and check it out. When you get to the top, you start to change your mind. Then I heard G. cheering for me. I felt like one good turn deserved another and I would really be letting her down if I didn't jump, so I jumped. It was freezing and it took my breath, but I did it and G. was cheering the whole time. It was a cool experience (no pun intended).

Impact of the Worksite Wellness Program

We are firefighters and first responders and we save lives, but these ladies save our lives. They are heroes too!

—*Worksite Wellness participant*

The total number of pounds lost during the first weight loss challenge was 399.5, which was an average of about 7 pounds per person. The group also lost 148% of their body fat, averaging 3% body fat loss per person. The worksite wellness program was effective in both recruiting and sustaining participation in the program among tribal workers. Some respondents indicated that they joined to "feel better," while others joined to "look better" and "improve their health." Still more participants joined to "support their coworkers" and "be a positive role model for their family and community." This program also was seen as "a start down a healthier path in life" for others.

When asked how they were able to be successful in achieving their personal goals, based on what was indicated in their initial assessment, some participants indicated that they made it a priority to lose weight even when juggling a marginal schedule (e.g., "even when soccer practice and a busy work schedule interfered"). It was a challenge for many to find time to exercise, avoid fast food, and replace their regular soft drinks with diet drinks and water, but they met those challenges. Working closely with the Cherokee Choices nutrition and fitness coordinator and her assistant, they received personal support and encouragement each week, learned how to be healthy shoppers, and learned smart ways to exercise. Also, during the 3-month program, the participants supported each other by exercising together and attending a monthly "Lunch and Learn" in-service education program that included a healthy catered lunch.

In evaluations of the program, participants identified a number of factors that helped sustain their involvement in the program. For example, participants were able to get managerial and specialized staff support for behavior change, information about how to eat well and improve health was provided, and help was provided that allowed them to exercise, lose weight, and feel better. They greatly appreciated activities being made available at their worksite and getting support from program staff, team leaders, program managers/supervisors, and coworkers. They also were appreciative of the large weekly fruit baskets delivered by the fitness and nutrition specialist to encourage healthy snacking and the wellness-related prizes awarded for accumulated exercise time reported. These prized included stress balls, jump ropes, yoga mats, hand weights, footballs, basketballs, tee shirts, and gift certificates to a local sports store.

As the worksite wellness and health challenge progressed from 2002 into 2004, over 100 employees from eight worksites participated. In the last 3-month challenge of 2004, three new and five continuing agencies requested the weekly contact and activities offered by the program.

Impact of Cherokee Choices on the Social Determinants of Health

In the final report of the World Health Organization's Commission on Social Determinants of Health (World Health Organization, 2008), the commissioners articulate three principles of action. The first of these is to "[i]mprove the conditions of daily life—the circumstances in which people are born, grow, live, work and age." Cherokee Choices/REACH 2010 primarily focused on the middle three conditions of daily life: circumstances in which people grow, live, and work.

Where We Grow

Teachers at Cherokee Elementary School have reported changes in the culture of the school and the learning environment toward more emphasis on health-promoting events and lessons beyond those implemented directly by Cherokee Choices. There seems to have been a ripple effect from the presence of Cherokee Choices in the classroom health lessons, offering teachers worksite wellness classes like aerobics and yoga and promoting health through after-school programs. Teachers are more conscious of utilizing more physical activity lessons and urging parents to supply healthy foods for classroom events. Parents who participate in Cherokee Choices' worksite wellness programs may also have been more willing to support improvements in the school menus and changes in policies regarding physical activity. The creation of the School Health Advisory Council also provided a means to alter the culture of the school in support of health-promoting changes. We have also observed greater readiness to learn. For example, our pre- and post-intervention surveys show that elementary school students participating in Cherokee Choices/REACH 2010 in-class and after-school activities have better attendance and look forward to being at school more so than students who do not participate in such activities.

Where We Live

Cherokee Choices/REACH 2010 began to collaborate with other tribal programs on initiatives to increase the number of greenways, sidewalks, and parks in Cherokee. This began later in the life of the program. There was already interest in this topic among the tourism and business development community here. Our participation underscored its importance and we were able to link health with economic development in a way that had not been done previously.

Where We Work

During the course of Cherokee Choices/REACH 2010, there were many improvements in working conditions for tribal employees. We achieved a major policy change that allows employees time off to participate in events sponsored by Cherokee Choices. We educated the tribal human resources program regarding best practices in worksite wellness, which contributed to the implementation of health risk appraisals, including lipid profiles and body mass index, for all tribal employees. Employees now demand the services of Cherokee Choices, such as exercise classes, lifestyle coaching, and cooking demonstrations.

LESSONS LEARNED

Below are selected lessons learned from the Cherokee Choices program, some of which relate to the day-to-day operation of the program, whereas others are broader in scope:

- Funding sources must be diversified. The precarious nature of federal funding makes it unreliable as the sole source. Local resources are essential to ensure sustainability and promote investment in the intervention.
- Regular feedback from community members is essential. Establishing a system to obtain input from those involved in the intervention is crucial. This system provides a means to allow the intervention to be sensitive and responsive to cultural needs, able to mitigate problems at the earliest possible point, and be an incubator for new ideas and solutions to problems.
- One-on-one support for community participants is important. Establishing relationships and sustaining them is essential.
- Being able to delve below the surface of the health issues is essential. Most physical health issues have a mental health component to them. Getting to the root of the problem is important (e.g., historical trauma, racism, and abuse). The intervention must be able to address these, if not directly, then through an effective referral system.
- Integrating and collaborating with other programs has been a key to success. Although this is a health program, we have to think of our partners as being relevant outside of the health system (e.g., the transit system, city planners, and businesses). Wellness as an economic issue resonates with the business community.
- Listening to community members in the design phase is essential. This generally takes more time than one might expect, especially in communities where input has not been sought regularly. People may not be accustomed to being truly involved in designing an intervention. Thus, initial input may be hard to obtain, and the quality of that input may not be at a useful level. Establishing a system to show people that their input will actually be used is crucial. Trust must be established in this regard and patience is required. Persistence is needed to dig deeper for more feedback and to be able to obtain information that may not come right away.

- At times you have to be fearless and willing to be seen as a rule breaker. You have to be willing to try things that have never been tried. Overcoming the mentality of "that's the way we've always done it" is a challenge that the program must be ready to meet.
- Establishing trust over years will enable the program to take more risks later. It may be prudent to hold back initially, while being watchful for opportunities to act more assertively later. Being politically astute is an essential skill. A particular policy change may be best approached in phases, building buy-in and acting in full force once a foundation of support has been laid.

Using multiple channels of communication has worked well for us. We use small groups, discussion groups, and celebrations of milestones with groups and church meetings to communicate health information and program details. This takes more time than some other methods, but allows for questions to be answered and feedback to be received. We also have used mass media with reasonable effect, although high costs have prohibited this type of communication from being used more extensively and for longer periods of time. We utilize email and phone calls to reinforce messages and maintain a link to clients. We have learned that even a minimal amount of contact can promote continuity in the program and lead to long-term sustainability.

SUMMARY

The Cherokee Choices community-based diabetes prevention and control program has proven worthwhile on multiple levels. It serves as a model for developing future interventions locally. We would advise others involved in funding and implementing similar work to allow an adequate amount of time for formative research. The use of a social network analysis is recommended as an initial step. In addition, we urge the use of social marketing in all phases of the intervention.

The community-based participatory approach of the program elicited high-quality community involvement and earned respect from community members. The approach adopted by Cherokee Choices is contrary to the history of top-down programs typically provided by social service agencies in Cherokee and has generated interest in using the same formative techniques for other health issues. The philosophy that underlies the Cherokee Choices interventions is that community and system changes can be effected through multiple, not necessarily linear, courses of action. It is essential to start with community members. For example, the success of participants in the worksite and church programs has inspired other worksites and churches to request an expansion of the Cherokee Choices program. Individuals have developed into role models who can help shift attitudes of coworkers, community members, and tribal leaders. There is a greater sense of hope among the community regarding diabetes prevention; however, there is still much work to be done.

REFERENCES

Cherokee Choices. (2004). *Daily eating habits questionnaire (Modified).*

Indian Health Service. (2003). Resource and Patient Management System (RPMS). Rockville, MD: Indian Health Service.

Martin, E. (2004). Reservations: Gambling has changed life for the Cherokee. *Business North Carolina, March,* 49.

National Center for Health Statistics. (2004). Prevalence of overweight and obesity among adults: United States, 1999–2002. Hyattsville, MD: National Center for Health Statistics. Retrieved from http://www.cdc.gov/nchs/products/pubs/pubd/hestats/obese/obse99.htm

National Opinion Research Center. (2005). National Opinion Research Center REACH 2010 Risk Factor Survey Year 3 Data Report for the Eastern Band of Cherokee Indians. Atlanta, GA: Centers for Disease Control and Prevention.

Satterfield, D. W., Shield, J. E., Buckley, J., & Taken Alive, S. (2007). So that the people may live (Hecel Lena Oyate Ki Nipi Kte): Lakota and Dakota elder women as reservoirs of life and keepers of knowledge about health protection and diabetes prevention. *Journal of Health Disparities Research and Practice, 1(2),* 1–28.

Sturm, R. (2005). Childhood obesity—what we can learn from existing data on societal trends, part 2. *Preventing Chronic Disease, 2(2),* A20. Retrieved from http://www.cdc.gov/pcd/issues/2005/apr/04_0039.htm

Tucker, P., Liao, Y., Giles, W., & Liburd, L. (2006). The REACH 2010 Logic Model: An illustration of expected performance. *Preventing Chronic Disease, January.* Retrieved from http://www.cdc.gov/pcd/issues/2006/jan/05_0131.htm

World Health Organization. (2008). *Closing the gap in a generation: Health equity through action on the social determinants of health.* Final Report of the Commission on Social Determinants of Health. Geneva: World Health Organization.

Making the Connection (*¡Conéctate!*): The Healthy Living Program[1]

12

LAURIE RUGGIERO AND EMILY E. ANDERSON

Editor's Note: This case study is one of two from the city of Chicago. As in other major cities in the U.S., racial and ethnic communities in Chicago bear a disproportionate burden of type 2 diabetes. Therefore, the engagement of many local institutions is desired in combating this public health problem. Researchers from the Illinois Prevention Research Center at the University of Illinois at Chicago built the Making the Connection initiative on existing collaborative partnerships between the university and other sectors within the city.

Public health partnerships that equitably involve community members, researchers, and organizations from various sectors in all facets of the research process are known as community-based participatory research (CBPR). Specifically, participation by community members affected by diabetes and entities that can facilitate a long-term and sustainable solution to the growing prevalence of diabetes in these communities is the key component of CBPR. Participatory approaches to research are intended to build community capacity and have social betterment

---

[1] This study is supported by cooperative agreement number 5-U48-DP-000048 from the Centers for Disease Control and Prevention. Supplemental funding was also provided by the Centers for Disease Control and Prevention's Division of Diabetes Translation. The findings and conclusions presented here are those of the authors and do not necessarily represent the official position of the Centers for Disease Control and Prevention.

295

as a driving force. The researchers in this case study describe how the characteristics of CBPR are put into practice in this program and how social determinants of diabetes are addressed in a medically underserved southwest Chicago community of Latino and African American residents living with or at risk of developing diabetes.

This case study also exemplifies how the landmark Diabetes Prevention Program, a randomized controlled trial conducted in centers across the U.S. and funded by the National Institutes of Health, was translated in a real world urban environment. In other words, the most effective arm of the Diabetes Prevention Program, an intensive lifestyle intervention, was tailored for implementation in southwest Chicago community settings by trained residents serving diverse community groups. Working together with a local board comprised of community residents and leaders from social service agencies, faith-based institutions, businesses, and community organizations, the researchers gathered qualitative and quantitative data to better understand the social determinants of diabetes in the community.

To integrate this knowledge into action, the assessment results were shared with the community and the partners' advisory board. Both the community partners and researchers used the results to develop shared goals for reducing the burden of diabetes and to establish common outcomes for improving access to health care. In reading this case study, you will discover the many lessons learned through the researchers and community partners' experiences; some lessons were more critical than others in the practice of CBPR. Despite the challenges of putting CBPR into practice, the authors repeatedly tout its worth in addressing diabetes in diverse community groups. As you read this case study, consider these questions:

- What are other societal conditions and psychosocial factors that affect access to health care? How might residents in southwest Chicago overcome those barriers to accessing health care in a medically underserved community?
- How might the community partnership be expanded to include partners from nontraditional organizations and sectors to address the societal conditions and psychosocial factors in this community?
- This case study indicated that annual health fairs served as a means for mobilizing community partners and an opportunity for recruiting participants, particularly those in need of health care.

What new policies and system changes might be implemented to improve the unmet health care needs of community members?
- In what ways might the researchers ensure collaborative partnerships among residents and organizations in all phases of the research?

BACKGROUND

Making the Connection (MTC) is the community-based participatory research (CBPR) initiative of the Illinois Prevention Research Center (IPRC) at the University of Illinois at Chicago. The MTC Healthy Living Program (HLP) is a community-based weight loss program based on the intensive lifestyle program of the Diabetes Prevention Program (DPP) and tailored for Latinos and African Americans living on the southwest side of Chicago, where the IPRC has collaborated to conduct research with community partners since 1999. Diabetes prevention was selected as a target for collaborative research efforts, because behavioral risk factor data demonstrated high rates of diabetes and obesity, low levels of physical activity, and insufficient fruit and vegetable intake. The HLP intervention translates the evidence-based DPP Intensive Lifestyle program (DPP Research Group, 2002) from the clinic to the community. The program, delivered in community settings by community residents, promotes healthy eating and physical activity to reduce the prevalence of overweight and obesity with a final goal of delaying or preventing diabetes, and ultimately other diseases. To enhance the public health impact, the program is delivered to a broad group of individuals at risk for diabetes based primarily on weight, ethnicity, and lifestyle habits. This case study will provide details on the background, implementation, and lessons learned from this CBPR initiative.

Learning from the Community: Community Needs Assessment

A comprehensive community health needs assessment included two community telephone surveys and quantitative and qualitative data from focus groups and key informant interviews.

The telephone surveys used items from the CDC Behavioral Risk Factor Surveillance Survey (BRFSS) core, diabetes, cardiovascular disease, and hypertension modules, as well as questions developed specifically to measure diabetes knowledge and preventive behaviors. Surveys were conducted in both Spanish and English. Over 400 surveys were completed in 2000 and over 500 were completed in 2003. In 2003 28.6% of community residents were obese (BMI >30) and an additional 43.2% were overweight (BMI 25–29.9). Over 50% of respondents reported fewer than three daily servings of fruits and vegetables. Almost 50% reported insufficient physical activity (defined as exercising less than five times per week for 20 minutes or less). Twenty-six percent of respondents did not have health care coverage, which is over twice the national rate of uninsured for the same year and significantly higher than rates of uninsured for Illinois and Chicago. Only 68% of respondents had been to the doctor for a routine checkup within the previous year. Although 22% of respondents had been told they had high blood pressure at the time of the survey, 38% of respondents have never had their cholesterol checked. As noted earlier, diabetes prevalence was also significantly higher in this community as compared with the U.S., Illinois, and Chicago. Despite these high rates of diabetes, only 58% of respondents had ever been tested for diabetes (Survey Research Laboratory, 2003).

Census data (U.S. Census Bureau, 2000) for our partner community, comprised of Chicago Lawn, West Lawn, and Gage Park, were also reviewed to collect information on social indicators related to diabetes. This is a very young community; almost 75% of the population is under the age of 45. Almost 16% of residents speak primarily Spanish in their homes; many are bilingual and a substantial proportion of residents are immigrants from Mexico. This is a stable, residential community that is diverse in terms of residents' socioeconomic status. Of approximately 20,000 families, about 12% have annual incomes below the poverty level, which is about the same as the city of Chicago overall. The unemployment rate for these three community areas was 12.8% in 2000, significantly higher than the rate of 7.8% for the city of Chicago in that same year. Only slightly more than 10% of community residents have a bachelor's degree and 34% of residents over the age of 25 have not completed high school (U.S. Census Bureau, 2000).

A variety of qualitative research methods were also used to conduct a comprehensive needs assessment, including focus groups, key informant interviews, community forums with residents and opinion leaders, and community surveys conducted at program events. Data from these activities have shed some light on the relationship between social determinants of health and diabetes in our target community. Surveys conducted at a 2002 health fair indicated high demand for community-based physical activity programs and nutrition classes. Focus groups echoed these suggestions and indicated an increased demand for medical care, due to improved awareness of health issues, and a preference for family-centered approaches to prevention. Frequently mentioned were the many logistical barriers to participation in health promotion programs, such as childcare, work schedules, and transportation. Community residents also expressed a desire for health promotion activities that include opportunities for community residents to assume leadership roles in both the educational and research components and receive training and skills development that could be applied to future community-based work. This suggestion arose from many sources.

ORIGINS AND HISTORY OF MAKING THE CONNECTION

The specific partner community is located in southwest Chicago and comprised of the three "Chicago community areas" of West Lawn, Chicago Lawn, and Gage Park. Our partner community has been rapidly changing and growing over the last 2 decades. Formerly a primarily Eastern European White ethnic community, Latinos and African Americans now comprise over 80% of the population (U.S. Census Bureau, 2000).

At the time the study was planned, community residents were more likely than other Chicago, Illinois, and U.S. residents to be overweight, obese, or have diabetes (Illinois Department of Public Health, 2001; Survey Research Laboratory, 1999). According to 2003 community-level behavioral risk factor data, 11.1% of community residents had diabetes as compared with 6.7% in Chicago, 6.1% in Illinois (Illinois Department of Public Health, 2001), and 6.5% in the U.S. (CDC, 2001). About 50% of community residents have or had a family member with diabetes (Survey Research Laboratory, 2003).

The CDC's Prevention Research Centers (PRC) program supports a network of academic researchers, public health agencies, and community members and conducts applied research in disease prevention and control (Centers for Disease Control and Prevention, 2009). The CDC-funded Illinois PRC (IPRC) has a primary mission to conduct research, translate research into practice, and measure the real world effectiveness and dissemination of health-promotion and disease prevention interventions. IPRC research focuses on community-based approaches to engage ethnic minority populations in the adoption of healthy behaviors for the prevention of chronic disease. MTC is funded by the CDC through the IPRC and supplemented by funds from the CDC Division of Diabetes Translation and generous contributions of staff time, meeting space, and other resources from multiple community partner organizations.

The IPRC has collaborated with community organizations in southwest Chicago to conduct CBPR projects since 1999. According to findings from initial focus groups and key informant interviews, community residents identified health as a priority, but felt the community lacked the infrastructure, resources, and organizing framework to address health issues, particularly diabetes. During 1999–2004, several community-based health promotion programs were designed and implemented through the IPRC's previous *¡Sí Se Puede!* (SSP) project, also funded through the CDC PRC program. SSP aimed to promote awareness of diabetes and activities primarily focused on health education, physical activity, and nutrition. Specific programs included school-based health for elementary-age children, parent walking clubs at schools, community cooking classes, and a community-wide media campaign. The success of SSP increased community interest in and support for diabetes education and prevention. The lessons learned from SSP informed the planning and implementation of MTC.

COMMUNITY AND INSTITUTIONAL PARTICIPANTS

Bringing the Community to the Research

Primary Partner Organization

MTC's primary community partner organization is the Latino Organization of the Southwest (LOS). LOS was founded in 1992 by a group of Latino immigrants who saw a need to work toward improving the lives and developing the leadership skills of Latino residents. The official mission of LOS is "to create the awareness of the social, political, economic, and cultural reality of Latinos on the Southwest side in order to enable Latinos to develop critical thinking and knowledge for further growth as individuals." LOS strives to complete its mission through a variety of educational, cultural, and social programs. LOS provides bilingual assistance to community residents applying for public benefit programs and navigating the immigration and citizenship process. Adult education programs include English classes, citizenship preparation, and GED and computer classes in Spanish. Youth programs include the Juvenile Justice Diversion Project, an alternative to prosecution and formal juvenile court action for minors referred by the State's Attorney's Juvenile Bureau that provides education and opportunities for recreation, cultural enrichment, leadership development, and community service. As a result of working with the IPRC and based on community input, LOS eventually added health as a priority to its overall mission.

Early in the partnership, a community advisory board (CAB) was created to guide the design, recruitment, implementation, and evaluation of community-based health promotion efforts. The CAB includes volunteer community residents, representatives of social service and community organizations, and religious, health care, business, and political leaders. Led by Hector Rico, the executive director and founder of LOS and an experienced community organizer, CAB membership has remained fairly stable since its inception. The CAB remains committed to collaborating with the IPRC to improve the health and health behaviors of community residents.

Qualitative and quantitative findings from the community needs assessments conducted when the MTC project was first planned were shared with the CAB. On the basis of these findings, the following shared health behavior and outcome priorities were identified: (a) increasing physical activity and (b) improving healthy eating in order to (c) decrease weight in overweight individuals and (d) lower the risk of diabetes in those at risk. With the support of the CAB, additional community partners were identified and recruited to assist with these shared goals.

Other Partners

As with any community-based program, community partners are needed to support and sustain MTC. Community partners are integral to efforts to promote awareness of MTC, assist with recruitment efforts, and provide space and other resources necessary for delivery of the HLP groups. Two other important long-term partners have been Holy Cross Hospital, a not-for-profit neighborhood health system serving residents of Chicago's southwest neighborhoods and suburbs, and Healthy Chicago Lawn, a community-based coalition started in 2004 to improve the overall quality of life and well-being of the Chicago Lawn community area.

STRATEGIES FOR COMMUNITY ENGAGEMENT

In addition to the ongoing activities of the CAB, several other strategies have been used to engage community partner organizations and groups. In preparation for initiating the translation study, a community forum was held to inform the community of MTC activities and recruit community partners to (a) serve as sites for conducting the HLP groups, (b) assist with participant recruitment by distributing brochures or allowing MTC staff to make presentations at their events, (c) donate items to serve as incentives for participants, and (d) provide other resources to support the delivery of the HLP groups. The forum was well attended with representation by a local alderman, businesses, schools, and social service organizations. This forum resulted in the recruitment of many new partners who have been instrumental in promoting MTC, assisting with recruitment efforts, and providing space and resources for conducting HLP groups.

Annual community wellness fairs have also served to mobilize community partners to provide health screenings and information about local health-related and social services. The partner community is in a medically underserved area with only one hospital, two hospital-affiliated health centers, one free health center, and one federally qualified health center within the geographic boundaries. For many residents with barriers to health care, health fairs provide a free, convenient, and accessible opportunity to obtain health screenings and information. The most recent community health fair was attended by over 1,000 adults and children. Health fairs have also been a great opportunity for recruiting program participants.

PROGRAM COMPONENTS

Learning from the Science: Sharing the Research Evidence with the Community

Once the community identified diabetes as a health priority, IPRC researchers searched the literature for the best evidence-based diabetes prevention interventions to share with the community partners. The DPP, a major clinical trial conducted at 27 sites around the country, had recently demonstrated that an intensive lifestyle intervention reduced the prevalence of type 2 diabetes by 58% in overweight people with impaired glucose tolerance as compared with 31% in the group receiving the medication metformin (Knowler et al., 2002). The lifestyle intervention group received intensive individual coaching from health care professionals on healthy eating, physical activity, and behavior modification (Knowler et al., 2002).

MTC was designed to translate the DPP's successful intensive lifestyle intervention from the clinic to the community. The intervention was tailored for this diverse community and delivered in community settings by community residents trained by project staff and multidisciplinary health professionals in a variety of areas, such as basic knowledge of research and diabetes, the group lifestyle program curriculum, and leadership skills. An additional aim was to take a public health approach by including a broader group of individuals at risk based on weight, ethnicity, and other diabetes risk factors.

Making the Connection Healthy Living Program

The DPP lifestyle intervention was very resource-intensive, conducted in a highly controlled clinic setting, and led by health professionals. MTC utilized a CBPR paradigm in which researchers partnered with the community to tailor, enhance, deliver, and evaluate a modified version of the DPP's intensive lifestyle intervention. The specific objectives of MTC are to (a) promote healthy eating, regular physical activity, and weight loss; (b) emphasize the prevention of diabetes; (c) use theory-driven and evidence-based approaches to diabetes prevention; and (d) tailor the lifestyle program for two priority groups, African Americans and Latinos, for example, by providing specific information on diabetes risk by group and providing culturally relevant and language-appropriate educational materials and session delivery. Other program goals included (e) identifying and training community residents to deliver the intervention program; (f) partnering with community groups and organizations to recruit participants and deliver the program; (g) minimizing the impact of barriers to participation, such as education and literacy levels, language, income, transportation, and lack of medical coverage; (h) planning for long-term sustainability; and (i) interpreting and sharing the findings of this research project with community residents, public health and health care professionals, and policy makers.

The program is delivered by community residents who serve as healthy life coaches. The coaches received intensive training and ongoing supervision and support in delivering the program. HLP program participants were recruited at community-based health screenings in partnership with the National Kidney Foundation of Illinois (NKFI). Participants who meet the following eligibility criteria are invited to join the HLP: (a) African American or Latino, (b) over 18 years old, (c) body mass index greater than 25 and less than 40, (d) low physical activity level, and (e) do not have diabetes. The curriculum included a 6-month core program and a 6-month after-core program delivered in a group format. The specific curriculum and content is based on the intensive lifestyle intervention used in the DPP (DPP, 1996; Knowler et al., 2002) and focuses on healthy eating practices like reducing fat intake, participating in regular physical activity like walking, and behavior change strategies. To overcome some of the barriers to participation described above, the program was held in convenient community settings, such as schools, social service agencies, and the local hospital, and written materials were chosen that were tailored for culture, language, and literacy level.

Program Support

As previously mentioned, financial support for MTC is provided through the CDC-funded IPRC with supplemental funding from the Division of Diabetes Translation. Many other partners provide technical, institutional, agency, and political support. The NKFI has provided invaluable assistance in recruitment by screening potential participants for diabetes. Two other key partners, LOS and Holy Cross Hospital, have provided significant support, including program promotion, space to conduct groups, staff time, and material support like program incentives. The Healthy Chicago Lawn Coalition has been very supportive in promoting the program and assisting in recruitment through their coalition member organizations and communication channels. Local schools have been very active in the recruitment of program participants and healthy life coaches. Many organizations have provided space and support for conducting groups in a variety of community settings, such as the local hospital, schools, LOS, and social service agencies. Local community leaders, including aldermen, have supported the project since its inception by writing letters of support to the funding agency and promoting the program with their constituents at community events.

PROGRAM EVALUATION

Qualitative data from the formative work on this project supports the feasibility and acceptability of the intervention delivered in community settings by community residents (Ruggiero, Rodriguez-Sanchez, & Oros, 2007). Quantitative data from multiple HLP groups are being collected to examine the impact of HLP on weight-related measures. Although the program was designed to be an individual-level intervention, feedback from our participants, CAB, and partners suggests that MTC has had a broader impact, extending beyond the program participants to family members, friends, and neighbors. For example, participants have reported that family members have also lost significant amounts of weight and neighbors and friends have joined them in walking groups. In addition, barriers to accessing diabetes prevention efforts were removed through providing this program in community settings by trained community residents. At the community level, responsibility for the annual health fair is being transitioned from the IPRC to the community to facilitate long-term sustainability. Efforts are also underway with current community partners to recruit and train healthy life coaches directly from the partner organization's members or constituency, so they can continue delivery of the program after completion of the grant to foster sustainability.

LESSONS LEARNED

The lessons learned have been many. Perhaps most importantly, conducting truly collaborative CBPR is a time- and labor-intensive process for all involved. The success of any community-based project is largely dependent on the choice of partners and the relationships established. Efforts need to focus on identifying shared goals, fostering trust, and developing mutually agreeable principles of partnership (Levy, Baldyga, & Jurkowski, 2003). Maintaining effective communication is an ongoing and important process. We have had the good fortune of recruiting many great community partners and identifying community champions from the leadership of our long-term community partner organizations and the CAB. These individuals and organizations have provided their time and dedication, as well as material support for the project.

In addition, one key strategy recommended by the CAB was the employment of community residents to fill many of the community outreach and research roles. This proved to be mutually beneficial for the community and research partners. In addition, the response of the community participants, coaches, gatekeepers, and stakeholders has been overwhelmingly positive. Lastly, a critical driving force in the success of the project has been the passion of the community and research partners for the overall mission of the project.

SUMMARY

Primary risk factors for the development of type 2 diabetes abound in our partner communities in southwest Chicago. Translating the lifestyle intervention from the landmark DPP in culturally and ethnically diverse communities is timely and necessary if we are to reduce the burden of type 2 diabetes. Effective translation of clinical trials like the DPP requires a close working relationship and true collaboration with the affected community and respected institutions and organizations serving that community. Beyond the focus on eliminating diabetes disparities, we must also attend to the social needs of the community, such as leadership development, improving literacy, and access to transportation, as well as planning for long-term sustainability of community members being able to deliver a lifestyle intervention that at a minimum delays the onset of type 2 diabetes. Engaging policy makers and politicians is also critical in bringing about change for improved health outcomes in large metropolitan areas like Chicago. Our experiences implementing Making the Connection (*¡Conéctate!*) demonstrates that we can build a bridge between science and the community that leads to better health.

REFERENCES

Centers for Disease Control and Prevention. (2009). Prevention Research Centers Program. Retrieved June 12, 2009, from www.cdc.gov/prc

Centers for Disease Control and Prevention. (2001). *Behavioral Risk Factor Surveillance System.* Retrieved October 22, 2008, from http://www.cdc.gov/BRFSS/

Diabetes Prevention Program. (1996). *Lifestyle manuals of operations.* Retrieved October 22, 2008, from http://www.bsc.gwu.edu/dpp/manuals.htmlvdoc

Diabetes Prevention Program Research Group. (2002). The Diabetes Prevention Program (DPP): Description of lifestyle intervention. *Diabetes Care, 25(12),* 2165–2171.

Illinois Department of Public Health. (2001). *Illinois Behavioral Risk Factor Surveillance System, Illinois and strata area prevalence data, 2001 state BRFSS data.* Retrieved October 22, 2008, from http://app.idph.state.il.us/brfss/default.asp

Knowler, W. C., Barrett-Connor, E., Fowler, S. E., Hamman, R. F., Lachin, J. M., Walker, E. A., Nathan, D. M., & the Diabetes Prevention Program Research Group. (2002). Reduction in the incidence of type 2 diabetes with lifestyle intervention or metformin. *New England Journal of Medicine, 346(6),* 393–403.

Levy, S. R., Baldyga, W., & Jurkowski, J. M. (2003). Developing community health promotion interventions: Selecting partners and fostering collaboration. *Health Promotion Practice, 4,* 314–322.

Ruggiero, L., Rodriguez-Sanchez, M., & Oros, S. (2007). Translating the Diabetes Prevention Program's (DPP) lifestyle intervention to the community: Making the Connection Latino pilot study. *Diabetes, 56(Suppl),* A226.

Survey Research Laboratory. (1999). *Greater Lawn Community Behavioral Risk Factor Surveillance System Survey.* University of Illinois at Chicago. Unpublished data.

Survey Research Laboratory. (2003). *Greater Lawn Community Behavioral Risk Factor Surveillance System Survey.* University of Illinois at Chicago. Unpublished data.

U.S. Census Bureau. (2000). *United States census 2000.* Retrieved October 22, 2008, from http://www.census.gov

Implementing Environmental Changes in San Luis Valley Colorado Elementary Schools: The School Environment Project[1]

ELAINE S. BELANSKY

Editor's Note: Two decades ago, type 2 diabetes in children was rare. Currently, there is an alarming rise in the prevalence of type 2 diabetes among children that coincides with growing rates of childhood obesity and physical inactivity. Children spend a significant part of the day in school. Recent concerns about improving academic performance and decreasing school budgets, among other things, have influenced decisions on the part of school administrators to reduce time spent at recess or in physical activity during the school day in exchange for more time spent on academics. As more families rely on two incomes, parents are often not home to supervise so-called free-range play after school, so physical activity outside of school has also declined. In addition, as our society has privileged in some instances technology over playgrounds, we see children spending more and more time watching television, interacting with the computer, and "playing" electronic games.

---

[1] The author wishes to thank the following individuals for their numerous direct and/or indirect contributions to the School Environment Project and this case study: Julie Marshall, Robert Chavez, Nick Cutforth, SEP Steering Committee, SEP School Taskforces, 5th graders participating in the focus groups, Emily Waters, Kandiss Horch, Lori Crane, John Brett, Terry Uyeki, Cathy Morin, Richard Hamman, Judy Baxter, and the RMPRC Community Advisory Board. The author wishes to thank Drs. Richard Hamman and Julie Marshall for permission to include portions of the partner community description originally written for a grant proposal submitted to the CDC.

Considerable research and program development is underway to reverse the public health problem of childhood obesity. Recommendations for combating obesity among children include eating five fruits and vegetables each day, watching television or playing video games for no more than 2 hours daily, and getting at least 60 minutes of physical activity every day. Meeting these recommendations is easier said than done. Yet, unless we can insure a healthy environment for the "whole child," that is, attending to the social, physical, and emotional needs of children, we will be limited in our ability to ward off chronic diseases in the future.

In this case study, the author describes a university, elementary school, and community partnership to improve the school environment by increasing access to healthy foods and time for physical activity. This university-led project utilized community-based participatory research (CBPR) to engage the community, school staff, and the children. They describe in detail the strategies used to mobilize key stakeholders, answer key planning questions, and bring about positive changes in the school curriculum and environment that would reinforce healthy behaviors in a small rural community. As you read this case study, consider the following questions:

- When children are affected by a health issue, schools are often thought of first as the most promising site for health promotion interventions. What are some of the limitations of relying so heavily on schools to achieve improved health outcomes for children? What other community settings influence the knowledge and health-related behaviors of children?
- In some communities, school policymakers have eliminated or greatly reduced time spent in health and physical education classes in exchange for more time devoted to the academic subjects. What are some of the fallacies inherent in this thinking? What is the role of public health in changing this thinking and undoing such policies?
- This case study is largely qualitative in its orientation and reports mostly qualitative data. In fact, early on in the CBPR process, members of the task force are instructed to take pictures documenting what is going on in the school that is contributing to poor nutrition and physical inactivity. What are some of the strengths and weaknesses of photographing as a data collection method? What other data collected through participant observation would be helpful in developing a policy and environmental change program for this elementary school?

- Sometimes our biggest obstacle to change involves the people who must implement the change. In this case study, we see instances where the school leadership is very directive and change is achieved in spite of some teacher resistance. We also see instances where teachers refuse to implement the recommended changes, and children feel "pushed around" by food policies that restrict sugary foods. What leadership styles might be more effective in achieving and sustaining healthy school environments and policies? In a free and democratic society, how can we foster healthy eating among children who prefer to eat less healthy options?
- One of the respondents indicated that they had avoided the "bigger battles" like seeking change in the school lunch menu and what was sold in vending machines at the schools. What are some strategies to build confidence in the community to take on these issues, as well as move their emphasis on children's health outside the bounds of the school system?

BACKGROUND

The University of Colorado's Rocky Mountain Prevention Research Center (RMPRC), funded by the Centers for Disease Control and Prevention (CDC), in partnership with its San Luis Valley (SLV) Community Advisory Board, School Environment Project (SEP) Steering Committee, and 10 schools across the SLV, implemented the School Environment Project to increase student opportunities for physical activity and healthy eating while at school.

The University of Colorado has a long-standing, strong partnership with the SLV community dating back to 1983 when university researchers conducted epidemiologic studies of the natural history and etiology of type 2 diabetes and related conditions. In 1998 the CDC funded the establishment of the RMPRC. The center's mission was to "promote healthy lifestyles in rural communities." (Rocky Mountain Prevention Research Center, 2009) While epidemiologic studies continue in the region, the RMPRC uses a community-based participatory research (CBPR) approach to translate research into practice. Since 1998 an array of family, school, and community-based interventions have been implemented to increase physical activity and healthy eating in hopes of lowering risk for obesity and type 2 diabetes (Belansky et al., 2006; Brett,

Heimendinger, Boender, Marshall, & Morin, 2002; Heimendinger et al., 2006).

ORIGINS AND HISTORY OF THE SCHOOL ENVIRONMENT PROJECT

The SLV is located in the southern, central part of Colorado on the upper Rio Grande River. At an elevation of 7,500 feet, this rural intermountain valley has the Sangre de Cristo mountain range running north to south along the eastern border and the San Juan Mountains along the western side. There are 46,190 people living in the six counties and 4,000 square miles that comprise the SLV. The valley floor is mostly flat with numerous potato farms. Throughout the region there are natural hot springs, wildlife refuges, and the Great Sand Dunes National Park and Preserve. Most towns are quite small with only a post office and a handful of buildings, such as a general store, gas station, and perhaps a public health facility. The largest city in the area, Alamosa, has 8,682 residents. It has several stores, markets, repair shops, restaurants, and a small airport. The city also has two small colleges. People living in the northern and southern parts of the valley travel approximately 45 minutes to reach this commerce center.

The area has a rich Hispanic heritage, and residents are both Hispanic and non-Hispanic White. Many families remain in the valley from generation to generation. In fact, it is quite common for grandparents to live next door to their grandchildren. The partner communities are medically underserved and have some of the lowest per-capita income levels of any region of Colorado and the nation. Despite these lower socioeconomic indices, the people of the SLV have a strong history of working together to improve health. Yet, like other communities across the country, SLV residents are facing increasing rates of obesity and high rates of type 2 diabetes.

In the 2005–2006 school year, the RMPRC collected height and weight data on 591 first and fifth graders in 10 SLV schools. Approximately one out of every three children was overweight or at risk for overweight: 16% were obese (body mass index at or above the 95th percentile) and 14% overweight (body mass index in the 85th to 94th percentile). Through the earlier CDC-funded Parents, Advisors, Children Together program, the RMPRC collected 24-hour diet recalls and accelerometer data annually for 3 years in a cohort who started second grade in fall 2000. On average these second graders were only eating half of the recommended daily servings of fruits and vegetables and their level of physical activity dropped by 25 minutes per day from second to third grade and by 53 minutes per day from third to fourth grade.

When asked about health problems facing children in their community, fifth grade students from elementary schools across Colorado's SLV often mentioned obesity and diabetes. The following comments exemplify themes raised by students in focus groups conducted in the fall of 2007:

> Some kids are diabetic. Like when you eat too much candy, you have to check your blood. If it's too high, you have to go to the doctor and get a shot.

> I think kids have health problems because they are getting too fat. I think we should get an hour recess. When my dad went to this school, he only got one recess a day. But he got a whole hour a day. We only get a half hour. [Recess is important] because you get to run. If you don't [run], you could get diabetes. [I know this] 'cause my brother tells me and my mother tells me.

> Since we're on farms, we have to go outside a lot [to do chores]. But some kids don't. They just sit on the couch and play video games and keep eating.

In response to concerns about childhood obesity and implementing interventions difficult to sustain over time, the RMPRC's Community Advisory Board, in partnership with faculty and staff from the RMPRC, decided to focus its core research project on creating opportunities for students to be physically active and eat healthy foods via permanent, sustainable enhancements to school environments and policies.

STAFFING

The SEP was the RMPRC's core research project for the 2004–2009 CDC funding cycle. Embracing a CBPR approach (Israel, Eng, Shulz, & Parker, 2005), the project leader (and author of this case study) convened a steering committee comprised of three RMPRC faculty and staff, as well as 10 community members including three principals, a school nurse, a physical education teacher, two food service managers, a school counselor, a director of superintendents, and a public health nurse. This committee was responsible for overseeing the research project and deciding on issues such as study design, evaluation, and communication of findings.

COMMUNITY AND INSTITUTIONAL PARTICIPANTS

The School Environment Project: A Community-Based Participatory Research Approach

The overall goal of this project was two-fold: (a) to facilitate environment and policy changes aimed at increasing physical activity and healthy eating in the school setting and (b) to adapt a comprehensive planning process called intervention mapping (Bartholomew, Parcel, Kok, & Gottlieb, 2001) to be used as a CBPR tool. A steering committee (described earlier) was formed approximately 18 months before the intervention. The group's purpose was to oversee the design, implementation, evaluation, and dissemination activities of this 5-year study. The group met for 2 hours once a month to discuss topics like research design, study hypotheses, evaluation plans, school recruitment strategies, and communication plans. However, prior to discussing those research issues, the group first created meeting norms (e.g., listen with the intent to fully understand), decision-making rules (e.g., group consensus), and a vision statement: "The School Environment Project Steering Committee will celebrate healthy active children living in environments where the entire community creates a cycle of lifelong physical activity and healthy eating." Annual day-long retreats were held to create goals and timelines and make important decisions about the SEP.

At the first retreat, held a full year before the intervention was scheduled to begin, the steering committee reviewed and discussed the study design originally proposed in the grant application: an early/late randomization design with schools assigned to the late condition serving as comparisons to the early schools during the first 2 years of the study. Community members of the steering committee were not in favor of this design because of ethical concerns related to making five school communities wait 2–3 years before making important school environment changes. Thus, the study design was changed so that all schools started the intervention in the fall of 2005: half were randomized to the adapted version of intervention mapping (AIM) and the other half to the CDC's School Health Index, a self-assessment and planning guide (Centers for Disease Control and Prevention, 2009). To overcome the loss of the control group in the new design, a random sample of 45 elementary schools throughout low-income parts of Colorado was established to serve as a comparison group.

The remainder of this case study will focus on the five schools using AIM to create environment and policy changes aimed at increasing student opportunities for physical activity and healthy eating. Each AIM school was asked to form a task force comprised of at least seven individuals with at least one representative from administration (i.e., principal [the preferred choice], counselor, or secretary), physical education, food service, classroom teachers, and at least two parents. For the classroom teachers, we suggested kindergarten, first, or second grade teachers, because they do not have to administer state-required academic assessments.

Three members from the RMPRC—a social psychologist based in Denver and two professional research assistants based in the partner community—comprised the university partners working with the five schools. These individuals are referred to as AIM facilitators. All three RMPRC members received intervention mapping training through the University of Texas. The main roles of the AIM facilitators were to lead the task force through the AIM process by conducting each meeting and bringing research, information, and resources to the task force, such as data on the childhood obesity problem, an analysis of local school data in terms of how the school environment and policy features met or fell short of evidence-based practices and national recommendations for daily eating and physical activity, school success stories, evidence-based practices for increasing physical activity and healthy eating in schools, and methods and strategies to implement those practices.

In using AIM, the AIM facilitators and community members (in this case, school task force members) joined forces to systematically identify problems and pose evidence-based solutions aimed at improving the health of the school environment. Task forces met 10 times in the first school year (approximately once a month) and twice in the fall of the next school year. (For more information about these 12 meetings and the AIM process, please see Belansky, Cutforth, Chavez, Waters, & Horch [2008].)

It is important to point out that CBPR was happening at two levels in this project. The steering committee, comprised of RMPRC faculty and staff and community representatives, provided oversight and direction to the project. In addition, each of the five school task forces, comprised of the seven individuals listed above, participated in the AIM process and held the decision making power to select and implement environment and policy changes that made sense for their respective schools.

STRATEGIES FOR COMMUNITY ENGAGEMENT

After the initial AIM task force meeting, which focused on introductions, overview of project goals, creating meeting norms, decision making processes, and other ground rules to create healthy group functioning, the task force's first task was to conduct an assets and needs assessment of how the school environment and policies facilitated and/or hindered student opportunities for physical activity and healthy eating. Several approaches were used. At the end of AIM meeting 1, task forces were given a disposable camera and asked to photograph the school environment. In taking pictures, members were asked to consider the following: What do you notice about the school environment and students' eating and activity behaviors when they are at school? What is being served for lunch? What do students bring from home for snacks or lunch? What foods are in the staff lounge, main office, and vending machines? What do students eat in the classroom? How are students getting to school in the morning? What do they tend to do during recess and physical education class?

Then, at AIM meeting 2, AIM facilitators shared the photographs and presented the task force with a partially completed PRECEDE (Predisposing, Reinforcing, and Enabling Constructs in Educational Diagnosis and Evaluation) model (Green & Kreuter, 1999) (see Figure 13.1). The childhood obesity and quality of life outcomes boxes of the model were completed ahead of time by the facilitators. In a brainstorming session, task force members completed these boxes: What student behaviors may be contributing to childhood obesity at your school? and What aspects about your school environment and policies contribute to inactivity and poor eating?

Next, schools were given tailored reports that compared information about their school to national recommendations and evidence-based

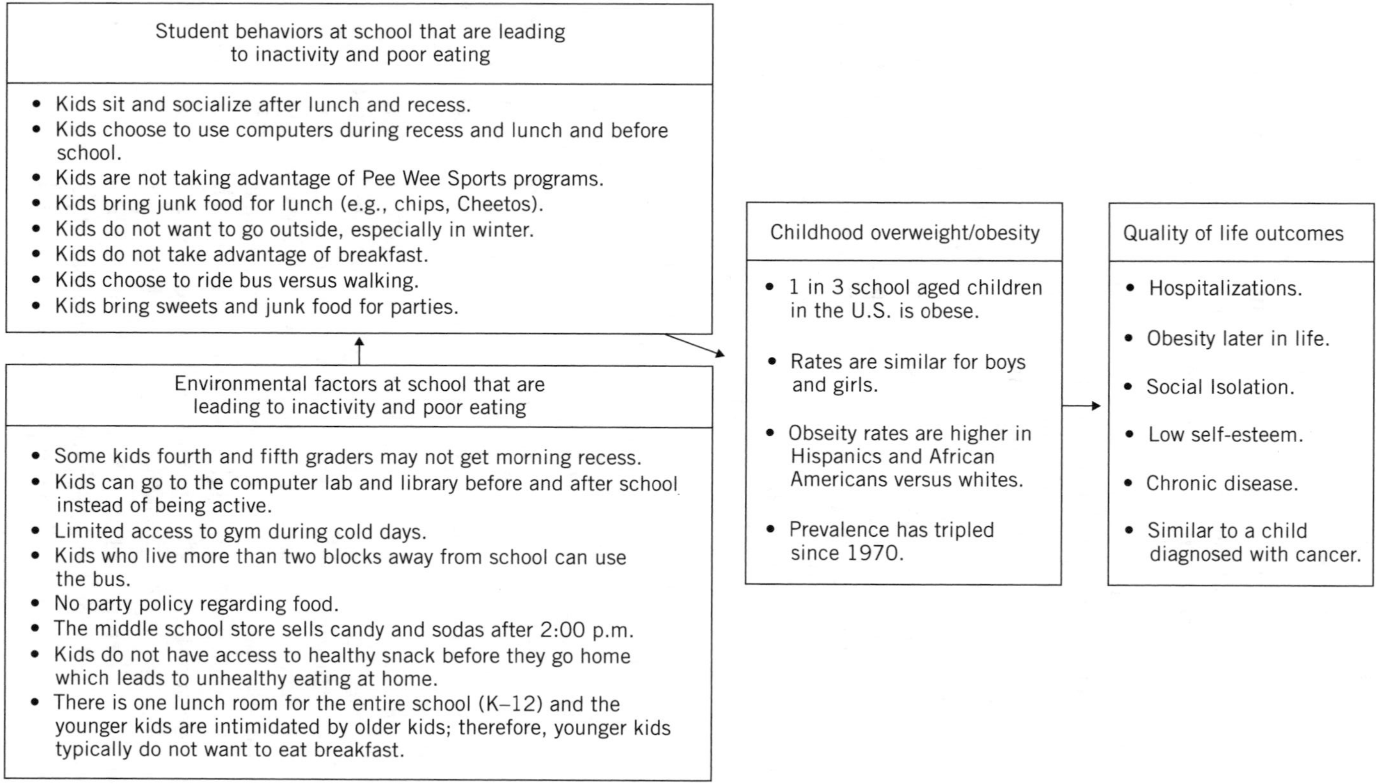

Student behaviors at school that are leading to inactivity and poor eating

- Kids sit and socialize after lunch and recess.
- Kids choose to use computers during recess and lunch and before school.
- Kids are not taking advantage of Pee Wee Sports programs.
- Kids bring junk food for lunch (e.g., chips, Cheetos).
- Kids do not want to go outside, especially in winter.
- Kids do not take advantage of breakfast.
- Kids choose to ride bus versus walking.
- Kids bring sweets and junk food for parties.

Childhood overweight/obesity

- 1 in 3 school aged children in the U.S. is obese.
- Rates are similar for boys and girls.
- Obesity rates are higher in Hispanics and African Americans versus whites.
- Prevalence has tripled since 1970.

Quality of life outcomes

- Hospitalizations.
- Obesity later in life.
- Social Isolation.
- Low self-esteem.
- Chronic disease.
- Similar to a child diagnosed with cancer.

Environmental factors at school that are leading to inactivity and poor eating

- Some kids fourth and fifth graders may not get morning recess.
- Kids can go to the computer lab and library before and after school instead of being active.
- Limited access to gym during cold days.
- Kids who live more than two blocks away from school can use the bus.
- No party policy regarding food.
- The middle school store sells candy and sodas after 2:00 p.m.
- Kids do not have access to healthy snack before they go home which leads to unhealthy eating at home.
- There is one lunch room for the entire school (K–12) and the younger kids are intimidated by older kids; therefore, younger kids typically do not want to eat breakfast.

Figure 13.1 PRECEDE Model for an AIM School

practices related to school environment and policy features correlated with physical activity and healthy eating. At the beginning of the school year, principals, physical education teachers, and food service managers completed the RMPRC's School Environment and Policy Survey. This three-module questionnaire was designed to assess and track changes in physical activity and nutrition features of a school (e.g., number of minutes of recess per week, number of minutes of physical education per week, playground features, total number of fruit and vegetable offerings at breakfast and lunch, presence and enforcement of policies regarding the nutrition content of items sold in schools, presence of a school health team, and familiarity with LWP and other state and federal mandates).

The RMPRC used the school's survey responses to generate a report for the task forces to see how aspects of their school environment related to national recommendations and/or best practices. For example, if fifth graders had 90 minutes of physical education per week, the report said, "5th graders at your school get 90 minutes of PE per week. The national recommendation is 150 minutes per week. Consider increasing PE minutes if possible." Task force members used the tailored survey report to add, delete, and modify ideas generated during the brainstorming session.

Finally, task force members were asked to consider whether they were missing certain types of information to build a comprehensive picture of ways the school environment was or was not supporting healthy behaviors. In several cases, task force members collected additional information. For example, a classroom teacher in one school conducted an informal survey of the number of students who had eaten breakfast that morning. A nurse at another school calculated body mass index for a subsample of students.

In summary, the assets and needs assessment phase of this project involved drawing from the different and complementary sets of knowledge and expertise held by community members and university researchers. School task force members brought a keen sense of which aspects of the school day and school environment made it difficult or easy for students to be engaged in healthy behaviors. They also shared a deep understanding of student and staff attitudes and behaviors related to nutrition and activity in various settings, such as the lunchroom, playground, gym, before and after school, and home. The AIM facilitators contributed to the process by sharing evidence-based practices, national recommendations, and tailored reports of school-level data.

PROGRAM COMPONENTS

School Environment and Policy Changes

After going through a comprehensive decision making process, task forces typically selected up to three physical activity and three nutrition-related changes to make. The AIM decision making process consisted of the following steps: (a) AIM facilitators shared national dietary and physical activity guidelines and recommendations highlighting the types and quantities of foods and activity needed during the school day; (b) task force members used information generated during the needs assessment phase regarding student behaviors and environmental factors related to poor eating and inactivity and brainstormed ideas about changes to make to their schools to help children achieve daily recommendations for nutrition and activity; (c) AIM facilitators shared best practices information from the literature (e.g., the key environment and policy changes shown to increase fruit and vegetable consumption and/or physical activity); and (d) task force members individually completed an Importance by Changeability worksheet where they rated each of the possible changes according to importance factors, including evidence the change will lead to increased activity and/or healthy eating, how often the change would impact student behaviors, and whether the change would affect all or only some of the students, as well as changeability factors such as potential barriers to implementing the change, difficulty of implementation, people who would need to be involved in implementation, and financial implications. Each task force member then voted on their top three physical activity and top three nutrition changes. The changes with the most votes were adopted by the task force for implementation.

Table 13.1 shows the list of environment and policy changes that schools decided to make as a result of the AIM process. Each school typically chose two or three changes in each area. Reversing recess and lunch and establishing some type of "healthy food zone" were the most common nutrition interventions. Schools varied with respect to the type of physical activity interventions selected.

Once the changes were identified, task force members answered the following questions for each environment and policy change: Who needs to be involved to make this change happen? What are the steps to implementing this change? and What are the possible barriers that might

Table 13.1

SCHOOL ENVIRONMENT AND POLICY CHANGES MADE DURING AIM PROCESS

NUTRITION

Breakfast/Lunch/Snack Program
- Provide free breakfast and lunch for all kids.
- Serve breakfast in elementary school classrooms.
- Offer more healthy choices as part of school lunch program.
- Provide children with a daily healthy snack.
- Teachers verbally encourage kids to eat healthy.
- Create a reward system for kids that make healthy choices at lunch.

Policies
- Create a "Healthy Food Zone" that would include guidelines, such as 100% fruit juice only, for foods sold at school (e.g., in vending machines, à la carte, in the school store and third grade café, and as concessions at sporting events), as well as for foods brought from home for snacks or parties in the classroom.
- Remove soda machines.

Rewarding Students
- Staff rewards students with non-food items.

Scheduling
- Reverse the order of recess and lunch, so recess comes first.

Nutrition Education
- Provide health and nutrition classes for elementary kids.

PHYSICAL ACTIVITY

Physical Education (PE)
- Provide daily PE classes for all elementary students.
- Increase amount of PE time.
- Schedule smaller PE classes.
- Provide additional PE equipment.
- Use an evidence-based curriculum, such as Catch or Spark, that has been shown through research to increase kids' physical activity levels during PE class.

Recess
- Provide additional equipment for students to use during recess (e.g., balls).
- Encourage or require students to be active at recess.
- Provide organized activities at recess (e.g. car races, four-square, walking program, and indoor activities on cold days).
- PE teacher provides structured and intramural activities during daily lunch recess, including a pedometer contest.
- Paint courses, hopscotch, and a walking track on the playground
- Add new playground equipment and facilities, including more cement surface and a track for walking.

After-School
- Provide noncompetitive physical activity options for kids after school (e.g., mountain biking, yoga, golf, gymnastics, dance, martial arts, tai chi, and skiing).

Policies
- Create a policy that states that staff and teachers cannot use recess removal as a punishment.

Other
- Build an additional gym and a swimming pool.

be encountered? Based on literature searches and knowledge of other schools' success stories, the AIM facilitators also provided information to help answer these questions.

By and large, task force members, and in some cases a few additional key people in the school building (e.g., janitor, secretary, or teacher), were the change implementers. AIM facilitators presented the social cognitive theory (Bandura, 1977) to task force members as a way to help them identify personal and environmental determinants needed to implement change. Task force members considered this question: What would it take—inside a task force member and in that member's environment—to accomplish the steps to implement the change?

This discussion generated ideas such as members needing to establish nutrition guidelines for foods allowed on campus and have the skills to assess whether foods comply with those guidelines; members needing the skills and knowledge to advocate for increased financial resources to hire additional physical education teachers; and resources needed to implement change such as concrete for a new basketball court. After identifying these determinants of change, the AIM facilitators created matrices with determinants along the top of the table and steps to success along the side. The body of the table included change objectives. These were specific tasks that needed to be accomplished in order for the determinant (e.g., knowledge) to be addressed in completing a particular step (e.g., share benefits of recess before lunch with faculty).

After the planning was mapped out, task force members broke into subcommittees with at least two members overseeing each environment and policy change. Timelines were set and subcommittees reported on their progress to the larger task force at the AIM meetings. AIM facilitators volunteered to meet with subcommittees in between larger task force meetings to provide resources and any help needed. In some cases, subcommittees conducted pilot tests before full implementation (e.g., reversing recess and lunch for one grade only during the last month of school).

COMMUNITY RESPONSES TO THE SCHOOL ENVIRONMENT PROJECT

The RMPRC conducted key informant interviews with task force members directly after schools first implemented changes (roughly the same time the AIM process was concluding at the beginning of the second school year) and 1 year later. The majority of task force members were quite pleased with the type and amount of changes the school made as a result of AIM. A nurse at one school said that if another school was considering using AIM, she would tell them, "Definitely do it; it's a great opportunity to effect some change in your school." However, a few people said they wished their task force had taken on bigger battles like lunchroom and vending machine offerings. As one parent said, "One thing we didn't really hit on a whole lot was the cafeteria and what they serve there. I wanted to, but I sensed that it was a sensitive area because there are so many restrictions." A secretary at another school said her task force was never able to change the contents of the vending machine because members could not agree on nutrition standards.

Task force members talked about how the rest of the school community responded to the environment and policy changes. These responses varied by school. Recess before lunch is a good example of this. Three schools chose to rearrange schedules so that recess occurred before lunch: two were successful and one ran into some problems. In one of the successful schools, the principal described it as:

> It's working really well. At first teachers were complaining about it. But I said, "This is how it is and this is what we're doing. So make it work." Now it's the second year and it's working good. The teachers are enjoying it. The kids are eating more. Parents don't worry about that part of the day.

This top-down, somewhat heavy-handed approach led to school-wide implementation of the change and teacher acceptance. At the less successful school, the principal used a more democratic and phased-in approach to implementing recess before lunch. He said,

> We switched our recess and lunch last year with the third, fourth, and fifth graders. We did try that with our K, 1, 2 . . . and we ended up going back to recess after lunch. That was against my better judgment. But teachers were very upset about the time issue. The little kids don't eat as fast or as consistently as the bigger kids, so coming back after lunch we had down time where there was a 10-minute chunk when some were done and they'd come back and others weren't.

When we visited the school a year later to learn how recess before lunch was going with grades 3–5, a classroom teacher who served on the task force said,

> We went back to recess after lunch. We have two teachers who wanted it this way; the rest of us aren't happy about it and I think at some point this

will be addressed again and we'll probably go back to recess before lunch. I know [students] aren't eating enough lunch. The minute they can go out, they raise their hands to rush out.

A year after changes had been implemented at the schools, our team conducted focus groups with fifth grade students and asked them to share their opinions. Responses to the nutrition changes were both positive and negative. One school decided to establish and enforce stricter guidelines about foods allowed from home. A student talked about what happened to her during snack time: "Today I was eating a cupcake and [my teacher] told me to put it away because it wasn't healthy. I felt okay but sort of mad, too, because it was the only thing I had for snack and I was hungry." At another school, a student talked about changes made to the lunchroom: "We used to have dessert every day, but now we hardly ever do except for healthy things like fruits. Now they are serving more healthy foods." When asked how that felt, the student responded, "It's bad. It feels like teachers are bossing us around." Several others in the focus group disagreed, however. One student said, "Some kids think it's good; some kids are trying not to eat unhealthy food." Students at another school talked about more fruits and vegetables in the lunchroom. The response was generally positive. One student said, "I started eating more fruits and vegetables because I don't want to be big and I [want to] have a good life when I get older."

Responses to changes made to physical education programs were also mixed. One school was able to increase the frequency of physical education by allocating resources to hire an additional physical education teacher. Students reported that the majority, if not all, of the students were quite pleased with having more physical education. While task forces at other schools sought to make improvements to physical education programs by either increasing the quantity or implementing a new curriculum, the students did not always appreciate the change. Most complaints pertained to doing similar activities over and over (e.g., capture the flag and basketball). Concerns about repetitive, unchallenging, and innovative activities point to the importance of advocating for increased quality physical education time and the need for further research on improving the quality of physical education in rural communities.

Changes made to the playground generally received positive response. One group of students talked about having fun on the playground: "They have more playground equipment, so you have a variety of choices. They put in tires [referring to recycled tires for the surface] so that you can play on the bars and not get hurt. Instead of wall time [used for punishment], they make you run, and you have to run around the playground." At another school, the principal and janitor worked together to lay concrete for a new basketball court. According to children in the focus group, the court was being used by fourth graders.

PROGRAM EVALUATION

The AIM process led to many school-level environment and policy changes aimed at increasing opportunities for physical activity and healthy eating. Baseline and follow-up data were collected on physical activity levels during recess and physical education class. Those data are being analyzed to identify whether the school level changes led to increased activity.

The AIM process led to other important changes in the social environment that have been documented. For example, several task force members reported increased communication and conversations happening throughout the school community related to health issues. In the week prior to being interviewed, one principal described four separate conversations he had with task force members about the various changes their school decided to make. Understanding correlations between the school environment and the development of risk factors for diabetes is a critical first step in mobilizing action for change.

At another school, the student council president had a conversation with the school secretary about snack foods he wanted to make available at an upcoming winter holiday party. Anticipating possible resistance to his choices, he was able to justify his proposed snack choices by studying the nutrition labels before seeking the secretary's permission. AIM also led to an increased awareness throughout the broader school community about the importance of healthy foods. A nurse described how their healthy snack program not only led to healthier food choices at school but also increased teacher awareness and knowledge about healthy foods. Perhaps most importantly, the AIM task force experience built capacity among some task force members to effect change in their community. The strongest example of this comes from a school secretary. Throughout the interview, she mentioned that she now uses the Internet to find nutrition resources for a newsletter she sends home to families. She also talked about how much she appreciated being treated as an individual during the AIM meetings as opposed to being "pigeonholed" as the secretary who only knows about certain types of things. As a result of the AIM process, she says,

> I think I'm more knowledgeable. I'm willing to go out there and look for the knowledge that I'm passing on to the students and what our expectations are for healthier classroom parties. I feel like I have the courage to know that there is something out there that I can look for. Before the process I was like, "Well, whatever you say," but now I can take it on myself, I know what I'm looking for.

LESSONS LEARNED

Key informant interviews were helpful in identifying strengths and weaknesses of the AIM process. Strengths included brainstorming sessions, listening to other people's ideas, having a forum to express concerns about the school environment, information collected and discussed for the needs assessment, and the decision making process used for narrowing down the list of environment and policy changes to make.

Task force members also identified weaknesses to the AIM process. These included a feeling that the process stagnated in the spring of the first year, frustration that certain key changes were not considered perhaps due to feasibility issues, a perception that the AIM facilitators' conclusion of the planning process and withdrawal from the task force felt abrupt, and that preparations for sustaining changes occurred too late in the process. All of these issues will be addressed in the next iteration of the AIM process.

Overall, the AIM process led to many school-level environment and policy changes. In part this was due to a strong planning process that included several important stakeholders along the way: principals, teachers, food service, physical education teachers, nurses, and parents. It is important to note that certain changes either never came to fruition or were not sustained due to a variety of reasons, such as competing priorities, lack of time for implementation, lack of buy-in from the community, and lack of financial resources. For example, one school chose to build a new gym. While small steps have been taken toward reaching this goal, the school has not yet succeeded in building the new gym, because it will require substantial financial resources, zoning ordinances, and community support. In another school, a healthy snack program was established and implemented the year after the AIM process was completed. The school requested each household contribute money toward the snack program; however, not all families were able to afford this. After 1 year, the school had to discontinue the program due to lack of funds. In yet another school, the task force decided to reverse lunch and recess. However, the principal left the decision to teachers in each grade level and only a few teachers agreed to make the switch. These examples suggest that even more careful planning and/or stronger principal leadership is needed for certain types of changes to succeed.

SUMMARY

The San Luis Valley School Environment Project details the processes and benefits of changing an environment where children spend a considerable portion of their day to foster healthy eating and daily physical activity using community-based participatory research. This project demonstrates that building knowledge and awareness of the relationship between obesity, physical inactivity, and type 2 diabetes is an essential first step in achieving community engagement and commitment to working for long-term health goals. Even in a small rural community with a relatively small commerce center, removing barriers that "make the healthy choice the easy choice" is challenging. Changing the school environment by restructuring the school day to add more time for physical activity and reinforcing healthy eating at school, school-sponsored events, and home builds the foundation for systems and inter-generational behavior change that will contribute to reversing the growing tide of childhood obesity and type 2 diabetes in a community.

REFERENCES

Bandura, A. (1977). *Social learning theory.* Englewood Cliffs, NJ: Prentice Hall.
Bartholomew, L. K., Parcel, G. S., Kok, G., & Gottlieb, N. (2001). *Planning health promotion programs: An intervention mapping approach* (1st ed.). San Francisco: John Wiley & Sons.
Belansky, E. S., Cutforth, N., Chavez, R. A., Waters, E., & Horch, K. (July 2008). *An adapted version of intervention mapping (AIM) is a tool for conducting community-based participatory research.* Manuscript submitted for publication.
Belansky, E. S., Romaniello, C., Morin, C., Uyeki, T., Sawyer, R. L., Scarbro, S., Auld, G. W., Crane, L., Reynolds, K., Hamman, R. F., & Marshall, J. A. (2006). Adapting and implementing a long-term nutrition and physical activity curriculum to a rural, low income, biethnic community. *Journal of Nutrition Education and Behavior, 38(2),* 106–113.

Brett, J., Heimendinger, J., Boender, C., Marshall, J., & Morin, C. (2002). Using ethnography to improve intervention design. *American Journal of Health Promotion, 16(6),* 331–340.

Centers for Disease Control and Prevention. (2009). School Health Index. Retrieved June 12, 2009, from https://apps.nccd.cdc.gov/shi/default.aspx

Green, L., & Kreuter, M. (1999). *Health promotion planning: An educational and ecological approach* (3rd ed.). Mountain View, CA: Mayfield Publishing.

Heimendinger, J., Uyeki, T., Andhara, A., Marshall, J. A., Scarbro, S., Belansky, E. S., & Crane, L. (2006). Coaching process outcomes of a family visit nutrition and physical activity intervention. *Health Education & Behavior, 34(1),* 71–89.

Israel, B. A., Eng, E., Shulz, A. J., & Parker, E. A. (2005). *Methods in community-based participatory research for health.* San Francisco: Jossey-Bass.

Rocky Mountain Prevention Research Center. (2009). Rocky Mountain Prevention Research Center Mission. Retrieved June 12, 2009, from http://www.uchsc.edu/rmprc/mission.htm

14

Pacific Diabetes Today: Cultivating Community Partnerships for Successful and Sustainable Diabetes Programs in Hawaii and the U.S.-Associated Pacific

NIA AITAOTO, JOANN U. TSARK, AND KATHRYN L. BRAUN

Editor's Note: In 2000 I spent two weeks traveling to Hawaii, Guam, and the Federated States of Micronesia to learn more about their diabetes prevention and control programs. Looking back I was first of all struck by the time it took to get to these destinations: a 10-hour flight from Atlanta to Honolulu, a 7-hour flight from Honolulu to Guam, and a 3-hour flight from Guam to Chuuk, one of dozens of islands that make of the Federated States of Micronesia (FSM). I was charmed by the breadth and depth of the Pacific Ocean: a scuba diver's paradise, the pace of life, the beaches, the artistry and craftsmanship of the local merchants, and the breathtaking sunsets that hovered over Pohnepei in the FSM each evening. I recall the banana trees growing outside my hotel balcony and the people napping while fishing in canoes.

There were relatively few cars on the islands of Pohnepei and Chuuk but a lot of travel by boat to neighboring islands and atolls. Much of the local economy of the Pacific jurisdictions receives funding from the U.S. government. There were military bases on some of the islands. In addition to English, many indigenous languages are spoken. People were friendly to visitors, and there were indicators of strong social cohesion. For example, neighbors helped each other build their homes. Parents, grandparents, children, aunts, and uncles often lived in one home together or in close proximity to each other. Churches of many denominations dotted the hills of Pohnepei. I met expatriots who had discovered this part of the world during their time in the Peace Corps or while fulfilling some other mission and had adopted the FSM as home.

In the midst of the beauty of the region, I was challenged to expand my thinking to imagine strategies for diabetes prevention and control when the physical, political, and economic environments shaped many of the possibilities. For example, at that time it was difficult to meet the national objectives for preventive care practices like periodic hemoglobin A1c screening, because the moisture in this tropical climate was damaging to hemoglobin A1c machines. When specialty and tertiary care was needed, people had to travel by plane to Hawaii which was costly for the modest incomes of most people living in Pacific jurisdictions.

The warm, tropical climate also influenced how people dressed, such as wearing flip-flops that did not protect the diabetic foot from injury. In spite of the ready access to fresh foods that grew naturally on the islands like bananas and the ocean full of fresh fish, local stores stocked and sold processed, pre-packaged foods like canned meat, commercial cookies and crackers, and other foods associated with American culture. Effective community-based approaches to eliminating diabetes disparities in the Pacific must be positioned to reclaim that which is health-promoting in their indigenous cultures and physical environment and through economic development.

In this case study, you will discover how the Centers for Disease Control and Prevention's Diabetes Today program was translated for implementation in the Pacific region. With leadership and technical assistance from Papa Ola Lōkahi in Hawaii, the jurisdictions modified the training curriculum to fit the unique needs and resources of the islands. In reading this case study, consider the following questions:

- What is the relationship between a history of colonization and the current burden of diabetes in the Pacific Rim?
- How might the political relationship between the Pacific jurisdictions and the U.S. government be (re)negotiated to garner support for strategies that would facilitate the elimination of diabetes disparities in this region?
- How might the local jurisdiction governments minimize the importing of processed foods to the region and establish commercial food ventures that reclaim a more health-promoting indigenous diet?

- What gaps are there in the Diabetes Today curriculum if the objective is to address the social determinants of health?

BACKGROUND

The United States-associated Pacific Islands (USAPI) refers to six separate and distinct island-based jurisdictions in the Pacific that have formal relationships with the U.S. government: American Samoa; the Commonwealth of the Northern Mariana Islands (CNMI); the Federated States of Micronesia (FSM), inclusive of the four states of Chuuk, Kosrae, Pohnpei, and Yap; Guam; the Republic of the Marshall Islands (RMI); and the Republic of Belau (also known as Palau). There are unique and distinct cultures and languages in the jurisdictions, but they all share a history of colonization. The islands first were claimed by various European nations starting in the 16th century. Hawaii was an independent monarchy that was illegally overthrown in 1897 by the U.S. The U.S. won American Samoa in an 1898 treaty with Germany, obtained Guam after the Spanish-American war in 1898, and gained control of the remaining jurisdictions, which had been under Japanese control, following World War II. All areas have been used by the U.S. for military purposes and some were also used for nuclear weapons testing (Tsark, Cancer Council of the Pacific Islands, & Braun, 2007). Native Hawaiians refers to a distinct people who can trace their ancestry to the original inhabitants of the Hawaiian archipelago prior to Western contact in 1778. (U.S. Congress, PL102-396: Native Hawaiian Health Care Improvement Act of 1992).

Today, all six Pacific jurisdictions have strong economic and political relationships with the U.S. American Samoa and Guam are unincorporated U.S. territories and Hawaii is a state. The CNMI is a U.S. commonwealth. The FSM, the RMI, and Palau are independent Pacific nations with compacts of free association. All are eligible to compete for many U.S. government programs. In the area of health, for example, all jurisdictions may apply for grants from the Centers for Disease Control and Prevention (CDC), the Health Resources and Services Administration, and the National Institutes of Health. American Samoa, CNMI, and Guam have Medicare and Medicaid programs (Tsark et al., 2007). Despite economic aid, most jurisdictions are economically unstable with only marginal health and educational systems. They have experienced rapid cultural upheaval and are heavily dependent on the U.S. and other foreign aid. Most jurisdictions are burdened with health conditions found in developing countries (e.g., malnutrition, filariasis, and dengue fever) and diseases associated with developed countries (e.g., diabetes, heart disease, and cancer) (Tsark et al., 2007).

According to the World Health Organization (WHO) statistics, the USAPI have some of the highest diabetes prevalence rates in the world and Native Hawaiians have the highest diabetes mortality rates as compared with the other major ethnic groups in the State of Hawaii, their own homeland (Hirokawa et al., 2004; WHO, 2007). Although published prevalence data for specific USAPI jurisdictions are difficult to find, diabetes specialists from these jurisdictions who are often affiliated with health department programs, many of which are CDC funded, have reported prevalence and burden of diabetes data at regional meetings.

American Samoa has reported an estimated prevalence of diabetes at 47.3% and has reported that 93.5% of the population is either overweight or obese. In the RMI, the prevalence of type 2 diabetes is estimated at 29.8%, and the amputation rates increased by 28% between 2000 and 2001. In the CNMI, a survey of tenth graders suggested that 78% of students had family members with diabetes and 64% of the students had three or more risk factors for diabetes (e.g., family history, high body mass index, elevated cholesterol, high blood pressure, and tobacco use). The prevalence of diabetes in Guam was estimated at 10.3% in 2003, double the prevalence reported in 1996. A door-to-door survey in Palau yielded a diabetes prevalence of 2.2% in the 30–49 age group, 13.8% in the 50–64 age group, and 23.5% in the 65+ group (Pacific Diabetes Education Program, 2007).

Community Needs Assessment

In the Pacific, increased mortality and morbidity from diabetes are attributed to drastic changes in lifestyle over the past 50 years. Traditional Native Hawaiian and Pacific Islander lifestyles were active, and diets consisted primarily of low-fat, high-fiber foods from the land and sea (Englberger et al., 2003). Today, most islanders have sedentary lifestyles and their diets are high in calories, salt, fat, and refined foods (Hezel, 2001). As the incidence and prevalence of chronic diseases like diabetes have increased, island governments have spent increasingly larger portions of their health budgets on secondary and tertiary care, leaving increasingly limited resources for chronic disease prevention and control (Tsark et al., 2007).

During a 1998 community assessment conducted in Hawaii and the USAPI, Pacific Islanders identified several contributors to the high prevalence of diabetes, including lack of awareness and knowledge about health and diabetes, poor lifestyle behaviors, and lack of health services and healthy lifestyle infrastructures. At the same time, informants recognized that many diabetes programs tried in Hawaii and the Pacific had been developed by outsiders who are unfamiliar with Pacific cultures, health beliefs, infrastructures, and local politics. Programs developed elsewhere were difficult to implement due to cultural mismatch and difficult to maintain because most were supported by short-term (1–3 years) funding sources. Thus, by the time people became familiar with the program, it was discontinued, and communities started over when a new funding source introduced a new diabetes program (Braun et al., 2002).

Geographic isolation and language diversities are additional barriers to program implementation in the Pacific. Geographically, the six USAPI jurisdictions consist of more than 2,100 islands spread over three million square miles in the Pacific Ocean with a total landmass of 919 square miles. Only a small number of islands are inhabited, making this one of the most dispersed populations in the world. Within jurisdictions most have outer island populations, defined as areas that require more than 1 day of travel to and from the national or state center. For example, in the RMI, medical evacuation from an outer atoll to the urban center of Majuro by ship can take up to 2 days and the option of evacuation by plane can only be done on the larger atolls with airstrips. Residents within the atolls must travel either by foot or boat to reach the airstrips.

Living conditions vary widely throughout the USAPI, with the variation being between the main, more developed islands and the outer island settings. The developed island "centers" have built modern power plants in recent years, providing a variable supply of electricity. There are public sewer systems and water supply, but the infrastructure is frequently inadequate for the growing population and limited water and power hours are not unusual throughout the region.

The more developed areas have access to a wide variety of imported foods from the U.S., Asia, Australia, and New Zealand, resulting in a major dependence on processed and less nutritious foods and a move away from healthier subsistence food sources of fish and locally grown fruits and vegetables. In contrast, the outer islands, with few exceptions, have no electricity, running water, sewer systems, or telephones. Families cook on an open fire or small kerosene stoves. Largely imported, food supplies are primarily sent to the outer island residents by field trip ships that visit the individual communities every 2–3 months.

Throughout the Pacific region, each island group has one or more distinct cultures and languages. In the FSM alone, nine different native languages are spoken as primary languages, although English is taught in the schools and is the official language for the national government. The educational system in the Pacific varies from jurisdiction to jurisdiction. For example, in the FSM and the RMI, education is compulsory of youth up to 14 years old; in American Samoa and Palau compulsory education age for children is up to 18 years old. Educational attainment also varies: of persons over the age of 25, 36% of the FSM population and 58% of Palau residents held a high school degree in 2004 (Micronesian Seminar, 2008).

ORIGINS AND HISTORY OF THE PROJECT

Pacific Diabetes Today Resource Center

A comprehensive approach to address all of the determinants that contribute to the high prevalence of diabetes in the USAPI was beyond the capacity of the Pacific Diabetes Today Resource Center (PDTRC) alone. With intensive community input, we prioritized the spectrum of influences on diabetes prevalence in the Pacific and focused on increasing community participation in reducing the burden of diabetes. To respond to the need for community-planned programs and capacity building in Hawaii and the USAPI, PDTRC was established by Papa Ola Lōkahi, a Native Hawaiian health organization in Hawaii, in 1998 through a contract with the CDC. PDTRC provided training and small training grants to community groups in each jurisdiction and five major Hawaiian islands to conduct an assessment and plan, implement, and evaluate a diabetes prevention and control program (Braun et al., 2003).

In the first year of this 5-year initiative, we listened to the community by conducting discussion groups, convening a Pacific-wide advisory council, and gathering data from informants throughout the region that led to the tailoring of CDC's Diabetes Today curriculum for the Pacific (see Figure 14.1).

The PDTRC curriculum was field tested in the second year and modifications were made based on participant feedback. In program years 3–5, the curriculum was used to train 11 community groups, and

Pacific Islanders: Who We Are
Diabetes in the Pacific
  o Diabetes, signs and symptoms of diabetes, types of diabetes, risk
     factors for diabetes, complications of diabetes, and control of
     diabetes
  o Diabetes statistics for the Pacific, the United States, and the world
  o Community assessment findings
Module 1: Assessing Your Community
Module 2: Planning Your Diabetes Program
Module 3: Monitoring and Evaluating Your Diabetes Program
Module 4: Implementing Your Diabetes Program
Getting Help: Obtaining Technical Assistance
Resources
Glossary

Figure 14.1 Contents of the Pacific Diabetes Today curriculum.

PDTRC staff provided technical assistance to facilitate group development, planning, resource identification, and project implementation and
evaluation (Aitaoto, Braun, Ichiho, & Kuhaulua, 2005). Unlike other
Diabetes Today programs that held regional training meetings, PDTRC
trainings were held in each participating jurisdiction and island in villages, churches, and municipalities. This allowed the training to be tailored for each group, utilizing the local resources, cultural and medical
expertise, and cultural framework (Aitaoto, Tsark, & Braun, in press).

COMMUNITY AND INSTITUTIONAL PARTICIPANTS

PDTRC staff obtained permission from leaders at the various levels in
the community and villages, including political, traditional, local health,
church, and community leaders. It was important to gain the trust of
community leaders by demonstrating respect for their cultural protocols. Commitment from these leaders gave legitimacy to our program,
thereby allowing our program to be conducted in their community.
PDTRC also involved participation from different segments of the community, such as:

■ individuals with diabetes and their family members who shared
  their challenges and successes with diabetes control;

- community elders, youth, clergy, business owners, and local government officials who actively supported planned activities in the community;
- women's groups and other community-based organizations that served as fiscal agents for the newly formed groups; and
- local physicians and health care providers who participated in the training as faculty and provided medical support to groups on an ongoing basis.

In keeping with community-based participatory principles, the involvement at multiple levels reinforced collaboration, provided a broader perspective and knowledge base, created an open dialogue, and fostered community support and acceptability (Aitaoto et al., in press).

When CDC's Diabetes Today funding ended in 2004, PDTRC had successfully trained and facilitated the development of 11 PDTRC coalitions that established community-relevant programs to address diabetes in their respective communities. PDTRC hypothesized from this experience that coalitions needed three factors for sustainability: (a) a supportive host agency for the coalition-developed program, (b) a leader or champion for the program, and (c) continued access to technical assistance (Ichiho, Aitaoto, Kuhaulua, & Tsark, 2004). Our observations mirrored a similar set of sustainability factors identified by Scheirer (2005). In a review of literature on program sustainability, Scheirer identified a similar set of sustainability factors: a champion, program-organization fit, ability to adapt the program, perceived program benefits, and assistance (Scheirer, 2005). A program monograph was produced in the final PDTRC program year that reported on how these sustainability factors impacted the development and sustainability of each coalition, as well as lessons learned in the process (Ichiho et al., 2004).

Despite the discontinuation of Diabetes Today funding, Papa Ola Lōkahi maintained relationships and contact with the 11 established coalitions and provided technical assistance to the extent possible with support from other program funds. With the support and encouragement of our Pacific partners, Papa Ola Lōkahi successfully competed for a 5-year National Diabetes Education Program (NDEP) cooperative agreement from CDC in 2005, which we named Pacific Diabetes Education Program (PDEP). PDEP was enriched by the relationships and momentum from our PDTRC partners and each group was invited to participate in PDEP to provide support in the development and distribution of culturally and linguistically appropriate diabetes education materials.

THEORETICAL FRAMEWORK

PDTRC's work was guided by the principles of community development and the goal of empowering coalitions to take action around diabetes. Activities like working with community members to assess their community, develop program goals and objectives, and identify resources were aimed at strengthening individual competence and community capacity to identify and resolve their own problems (Israel, Schulz, Parker, & Becker, 1998; Minkler & Wallerstein, 2003). In accordance with capacity-building principles, PDTRC employed culturally appropriate strategies to gain access to communities, transfer knowledge and skills to individuals, strengthen community coalitions, and provide technical assistance (Braun et al., 2003; Ichiho et al., 2004).

PROGRAM COMPONENTS

Four case studies are shared to show the diversity and similarities of groups and programs.

Chuuk Women's Council

The Chuuk Women's Council (CWC) is a non-government organization in Chuuk, FSM. It was chartered in 1980 to assist women to become more productive and self-sufficient members of society. Women's groups from the 40 inhabited islands within Chuuk State are part of the CWC, with membership ranging between 40 to 120 women per island. When PDTRC entered Chuuk State, CWC was identified by community leaders as a potential host agency for training to plan, implement, and evaluate diabetes programming. Although the CWC's focus was not on health, PDTRC saw benefit in working with an existing, well-networked organization. PDTRC approached two leaders of CWC to consider including health and diabetes in their mission. CWC accepted the offer, because diabetes was a recognized health problem in their community and among their membership.

The PDTRC training was held in-country in 2002, and CWC embarked on diabetes programming soon thereafter. The two CWC leaders continue to champion diabetes awareness and prevention education, including projects to promote diabetes prevention, nutrition, and physical activity. CWC also implemented numerous faith-based diabetes initiatives and sponsors diabetes screenings in the communities and referrals to the Chuuk Diabetes Clinic. In addition, CWC members have supported people with diabetes by visiting them at home and in the hospital to provide encouragement and assistance. Currently, CWC has expanded their capacity as a working partner of the PDEP to develop culturally and linguistically appropriate educational materials in Chuukese language and as a member of a newly formed regional Pacific diabetes coalition. CWC has since expanded their health focus beyond diabetes, providing community education on sexually transmitted diseases, tuberculosis, and breast and cervical cancer.

Kosrae Diabetes Today Coalition

In 2000 there were no community groups or organizations in the state of Kosrae focusing on diabetes. PDTRC worked with the Kosrae Department of Health to coordinate training and provide fiscal management of the subcontract to conduct Diabetes Today. After receiving training, PDTRC training participants decided to form the Kosrae Diabetes Today Coalition (Kosrae DTC) to plan and implement activities to increase diabetes awareness and prevent the onset of diabetes and its complications. The founding membership included people with diabetes, policy makers, church leaders, and health care providers. The champion for the Kosrae DTC is a political and church leader whose energy and enthusiasm have not waned since the PDTRC training. He and the majority of the founding members are still engaged in leading the coalition and sponsoring diabetes-related activities. He successfully sponsored a workplace wellness bill that allowed employees of the government, the largest employer in Kosrae, to participate in physical activities during work hours.

One year after the training, the Kosrae DTC became independently chartered as a nonprofit organization. A major focus of Kosrae DTC has been physical activity. The group, for example, has successfully influenced the mayors and traditional leaders to improve street lights and sidewalks to encourage physical activity, equipped villages with physical activity equipment like volleyballs and volleyball nets, sponsored island-wide sporting events, and effectively lobbied the government to allocate part of the workday to exercise for all employees. Volleyball games are underway regularly in all four municipalities. One primary care physician has utilized the volleyball game site to promote weight loss, helping players track their weight loss over time.

Guam Diabetes Association

The Guam Diabetes Association (GDA) was the only existing diabetes coalition in the Pacific before the PDTRC training. Established in 1982, GDA's mission is to help people with diabetes stay healthy. The champions, the president of the Guam Diabetes Association who has diabetes and his wife, have grown the coalition to nearly 200 members since its inception. PDTRC trained GDA leaders and members on program assessment, planning, and evaluation in 2002. Training and technical assistance planned and supported GDA's expansion of their community programs in diabetes education and screening outreach to more rural areas. Their annual diabetes conference, the largest in Micronesia, now attracts an average of 500 attendees, and their annual 5K run/walk averages 4,000 participants. As a result of the training, GDA applied for and received CDC Diabetes Today funds in 2005 to provide outreach and establish diabetes coalitions in other villages in Guam in addition to their other activities.

Kaua'i Diabetes Today Coalition

On Kaua'i, a county in Hawaii, PDTRC partnered with the health department to offer training in 2002. The Kaua'i Diabetes Today Coalition (KDTC) was established by the trainees, and within a year the group became a 501(c)(3) tax status organization with a membership of 40 people. The group's two champions are civic leaders: one is the president of the Kaua'i Filipino Association, which is a community organization that provides a lot of community services, and both are members of the Kaua'i Lions Club.

During the PDTRC training, the Kaua'i group identified several community needs; the main priority was to provide diabetes supplies, such as glucometers and strips, to low-income residents who are uninsured or underinsured. KDTC held several fundraising events, including a "Valentine's Day Sweetheart Ball." The ball has since become a popular annual event, raising about $10,000 each year. To increase diabetes awareness, KDTC supports and hosts multiple community education events, including an annual picnic, and participates in health fairs on Kaua'i.

CHALLENGES TO PROGRAM IMPLEMENTATION

Initially there was resistance from several Diabetes Prevention and Control Programs (DPCP) in Hawaii and across the Pacific. DPCP administrators and staff feared that funding for Diabetes Today coalition projects would mean competition with their program funding. DPCP staff were also concerned about additional work and responsibilities, since many of the initial trainings and meetings needed to be coordinated by the DPCP. To address this, PDTRC held several meetings to answer questions and concerns and included DPCP coordinators in the PDTRC advisory council to maintain ongoing communication and discussion. PDTRC also provided a lot of technical assistance and support to the staff to minimize additional workload.

At the end of the 5-year project, DPCP administrators became coalition advisors and champions. Pacific DPCP programs also reported an increase in the amount of funding and resources available to their jurisdictions. Additionally, diabetes awareness and prevention activities increased with the assistance and support of the coalitions and their local partners. In American Samoa, the American Samoa Diabetes Association works very closely with the schools to provide diabetes prevention education to primary school students, and in 2004 the American Samoan government budgeted $25,000 from local funds to supplement the DPCP program resources.

The challenge PDTRC staff faced was working with diverse cultures, languages, political entities, and resources. To address this, PDTRC sought the advice, support, and assistance of local champions, such as faith-based leaders, traditional leaders, political leaders, health care professionals, and people with diabetes. These local champions and facilitators helped with the PDTRC trainings conducted in the villages.

PROGRAM EVALUATION

In 2008, 4 years after PDTRC funding discontinued, Papa Ola Lōkahi conducted a survey to assess the status of the PDTRC coalitions. Nine of the 11 PDTRC coalitions were still active and implementing successful diabetes activities in their community. Activities included outreach to increase diabetes screening and provide prevention education in American Samoa and the RMI, sponsoring diabetes conferences for health care providers in American Samoa and Guam, fundraising for medical supplies for diabetes to aid Guam, Kaua'i, the RMI, and Kosrae, expanded partnerships with other chronic disease programs to develop an integrated chronic disease prevention campaign among all nine active coalitions, and community action to influence village, church, local and national policies on diabetes and health in the CNMI, the RMI, Chuuk, Kosrae, and Palau; Palau's coalition successfully advocated for increased funding for diabetes programs. In the CNMI, the coalition assisted the Catholic church to adopt a policy on nutrition and the types of food served during funerals and other events (Aitaoto et al., in press).

All nine active coalitions had champions, supportive umbrella organizations to house and/or manage their programs, and available technical assistance from contacts made through affiliations with PDTRC. Umbrella agencies include non-government community agencies and organizations already in existence before Diabetes Today training (i.e., Chuuk Women's Association and the GDA), new community agencies and organizations founded by the PDTRC coalition (i.e., Kaua'i Diabetes Today and the Kosrae DTC), and the health departments of Marshall Island and Palau. Supporting a diabetes coalition appealed to the agencies and health departments that already existed, because they share a common mission (Aitaoto et al., in press).

The two inactive coalitions experienced the loss of a key component for sustainability. The champion of the American Samoa Diabetes Coalition passed away in 2003 and the group is currently reorganizing itself. Also, the Yap Diabetes Group's champion, a local primary care physician, passed away in 2007. This death left a big gap in the coalition, because its champion had been influential in getting and maintaining agency commitment, resources, and technical assistance (Aitaoto et al., in press).

LESSONS LEARNED

Pacific Diabetes Today coalitions confirm the importance to program sustainability of a champion, a supportive host agency, and access to technical assistance and resources.

The Importance of Champions

Each of the 11 coalitions stressed the importance of a champion. The two inactive coalitions cited "loss of champion" as the key reason for their inactivity. The nine active coalitions all identified champions, which included people with diabetes, family members of people with diabetes, health care providers, politicians, pastors, and traditional leaders. Among the four coalitions featured in the case studies above, seven champions were recognized. All had attended PDTRC training and continued to lead activities, because they were personally affected by diabetes and recognized the need for community people to get involved. As volunteers they provide 60–160 hours per month for diabetes activities that include recruiting new volunteers, providing encouragement to members, providing diabetes education to individuals and groups, coordinating large community events, educating policy makers, and raising funds.

Supportive Host Agency

A supportive host agency is critical to the sustainability of activities. A host agency needs to provide a place to meet, office space, and other logistical support. The agency needs to be able to secure and manage funds raised through grants, contracts, and activities. In our experience, it does not matter if the host agency already existed like CWC and GDA, was founded by the local PDTRC coalition like the Kosrae and Kaua'i Diabetes Today organizations, or was a health department that adopted the coalition as an advisory group like in the RMI and Palau. The important thing is that the diabetes programming fits the mission of the host agency, which justified its support. As for local businesses, they were willing to support diabetes programs because of their relationship with coalition members and because the coalitions were very clear and specific in their request for the type of support businesses can provide.

Access to Technical Assistance and Resources

The third essential principle that all 11 coalition interviewees mentioned was access to technical assistance and resources. In addition to the technical assistance that they received from their host agencies, coalitions also received resources from other local organizations, including churches, women's groups, and businesses. The coalitions received monetary support, incentives and prizes, volunteer time, technical assistance, and free advertisements. The coalitions also accessed ongoing technical assistance from Papa Ola Lōkahi through the PDEP program.

PROGRAM SUSTAINABILITY

Scheirer (2005), in her literature review of program sustainability, identified two other important factors. Specifically, she found evidence to suggest that programs that could be modified by the participating agency and showed benefits were more easily sustained than those that did not. We also found support for these factors with PDPRC. All 11 coalitions gained skills to develop and implement their own programs. They had 100% control over their programs and modified them at will. PDTRC (and later PDEP) helped coalitions actualize their plans, rather than forcing packaged programs on them. PDTRC coalitions have reviewed three NDEP campaigns (i.e., Small Steps Big Rewards, Control Your Diabetes for Life, and Be Smart about Your Heart), adapted and developed 28 in-language materials, distributed over 100,000 materials, and implemented over 50 diabetes initiatives reaching over 50,000 people. The coalitions also influenced nine policies on diabetes and health. Seven coalitions expanded their memberships or started new chapters in other areas and nine integrated cancer, cardiovascular disease, and tobacco activities in their initiatives.

Because of the success of these coalitions, Papa Ola Lōkahi feels confident that this approach and process can be used to address other community health concerns. Papa Ola Lōkahi also applies this approach in our work in cancer and tobacco control in Hawaii and the Pacific. Additionally, we enhanced diabetes programs in the Pacific using the lessons that we learned from the coalitions. Our current initiative, PDEP, builds on the priorities and plans from the PDTRC community coalitions.

SUMMARY

The USAPI is challenged by a number of political, economic, and environmental issues that bear on the problem of diabetes in this region. As the region achieves greater stabilization in the larger political economy, we expect to see positive influences on the social determinants of health that characterize the Pacific. In the interim, it is apparent that community-driven diabetes coalitions in the Pacific provide a needed infrastructure for community members to plan, implement, and evaluate their own diabetes initiatives. The PDTRC experience and our lessons learned from evaluating the PDTRC coalitions support our hypotheses that community diabetes coalitions can be developed and sustained with the support of a host agency, the leadership of a champion, and continuous access to technical assistance and resources.

REFERENCES

Aitaoto, N., Braun, K. L., Ichiho, H. M., & Kuhaulua, R. (2005). Pacific Diabetes Today: Reports from the field. *Pacific Health Dialog, 12,* 124–132.

Aitaoto, N., Tsark, J. U., & Braun, K. L. (in press). Sustainability of Pacific Diabetes Today coalitions. *Preventing Chronic Disease.*

Braun, K., Kuhaulua, R., Ichiho, H. M., & Aitaoto, N. (2002). Listening to the community: A first step in adapting Diabetes Today to the Pacific. *Pacific Health Dialog, 9,* 321–328.

Braun, K., Kuhaulua, R., Ichiho, H. M., Aitaoto, N., Tsark, J. U., Spegal, R., & Lamb, B. (2003). Empowerment through community building: Diabetes Today in the Pacific. *Journal of Public Health Management and Practice, 9(Suppl),* S19–S25.

Englberger, L., et al. (2003). Insights on food and nutrition in the Federated States of Micronesia: A review of the literature. *Public Health Nutrition, 6,* 5–17.

Hezel, F. X. (2001). *The new shape of old island cultures.* Honolulu: University of Hawaii Press.

Hirokawa, R., Huang, T., Pobutsky, A., Noguès, M., Salvail, F., & Nguyen, H. D. (2004). *Hawaii diabetes report, 2004.* Honolulu: Hawaii State Department of Health.

Ichiho, H., Aitaoto, N. T., Kuhaulua, R. I., & Tsark, J. U. (2004). *Pacific Diabetes Today: Lessons learned.* Honolulu: Papa Ola Lōkahi.

Israel, B. A., Schulz, A. J., Parker, E. A., & Becker, A. B. (1998). Review of community-based research: Assessing partnership approaches to improve public health. *Annual Review of Public Health, 19,* 173–202.

Minkler, M., & Wallerstein, N. (Eds.). (2003). *Community-based participatory research for health.* San Francisco: Jossey-Bass.

Pacific Diabetes Education Program. (2007). *Pacific Advisory Council meeting minutes.*

Scheirer, M. A. (2005). Is sustainability possible? A review and commentary on empirical studies of program sustainability. *American Journal of Evaluation, 26,* 320–347.

Tsark, J. U., Cancer Council of the Pacific Islands, & Braun, K. L. (2007). Reducing cancer health disparities in the US-associated Pacific. *Journal of Public Health Management Practice, 13(1),* 49–58.

World Health Organization. (2007). *Diabetes facts.* Retrieved November 6, 2007, from http:www.who.int/diabetes/facts/world_figures

15

A Multilevel Intervention Approach for Reducing Racial and Ethnic Disparities in Diabetes: The Bronx Health REACH Nutrition Evaluation Project[1]

AMANDA M. NAVARRO

Editor's Note: African Americans and Hispanics/Latinos account for the majority of the population in the South Bronx neighborhood of New York City, yet are more likely to be diagnosed and die of diabetes than non-Hispanic Whites. Mounting evidence shows that interventions must move beyond individual lifestyle changes to instead examine sociocultural, economic, political, and broad environmental conditions that impact health in order to effectively eliminate racial and ethnic health disparities.

Although the public health community is beginning to recognize the need to develop and implement interventions that address these health determinants, limited information is available on multilevel strategies that can be used to address these determinants impacting racial and ethnic disparities in diabetes. The Bronx Health Racial and Ethnic Approaches to Community Health (REACH) program works to eliminate disparities in diabetes among African Americans and Hispanics/Latinos living in the South Bronx by providing information and tools to promote

[1] This project was a collaboration between the Division of Adult and Community Health, National Center for Chronic Disease Prevention and Health Promotion, Centers for Disease Control and Prevention, and the Institute for Family Health's Bronx Health REACH 2010 program.

lifestyle changes and addressing environmental barriers that prevent people from maintaining healthy behaviors.

This case study provides a brief overview of the Bronx Health REACH Nutrition Evaluation Project, a qualitative assessment examining the development and implementation of multilevel nutrition activities that the Bronx Health REACH program initiated to improve nutrition as a way to reduce disparities in diabetes in the South Bronx. Nine in-depth interviews and four focus groups, each consisting of six to eight participants, were conducted with key partners and staff from the Bronx Health REACH program. Audio recordings of the focus groups and interviews were transcribed, and select program records were reviewed to provide information regarding the history and characteristics of the activities being examined. A team of three Centers for Disease Control and Prevention and two Bronx Health REACH program staff members analyzed the data. Triangulation of the focus group and interview transcripts and program records was conducted to determine reliability and validity of the data.

Findings from this evaluation suggest that broadening the focus on traditional lifestyle interventions to address the broader underlying social and economic determinants, adopting community-based participatory approaches to develop and implement interventions, incorporating nontraditional public health partners, seeking multiple sources of financial and human support, adapting to the changing community needs and realities, and building the capacity of community members is critical in eliminating racial and ethnic health disparities across our nation's communities.

As you read this case study, ask yourself the following questions:

- What are the various social and economic determinants impacting the health of African Americans and Hispanics/Latinos in the South Bronx? What are the program and policy implications of these determinants for eliminating diabetes disparities?
- What is the role of public health professionals in helping to transform power imbalances between communities and the corporations and institutions that affect their health?
- How can community-based participatory approaches more effectively help to eliminate diabetes disparities? What are other ways not described in the case study that can promote engagement of community members in political and institutional decision making processes?

BACKGROUND

African Americans and Hispanics/Latinos make up the two largest racial and ethnic groups in the United States, representing more than 80 million people, or almost two-thirds of the U.S. population (U.S. Census Bureau, 2006). In the Bronx neighborhood of New York City, Hispanics/Latinos and African Americans account for the majority of the population (i.e., 51% and 43%, respectively) (U.S. Census Bureau, 2008). Non-Hispanic Whites make up only 13% of the Bronx population.

Despite their numbers, African Americans and Hispanics/Latinos are facing significant barriers in accessing fundamental resources or social determinants (e.g., food supply, housing, economic and social opportunities, transportation, health care, and education) that support health. For example, the New York City Department of Health and Mental Hygiene reported that in the South Bronx, one of the poorest neighborhoods of New York City, more than one in three residents live in poverty (Karpati et al., 2004). Residents living in the South Bronx are more likely to seek routine health care in the emergency department, be uninsured, and lack a usual source of care compared to their counterparts in wealthier Manhattan communities (Olsen, Van Wye, Kerker, Thorpe, & Frieden, 2006a, 2006b). Primary care doctors are less common in the Bronx than in Manhattan (Jasek, Van Wye, Kerker, Thorpe, & Frieden, 2007). During 2001–2005, the Bronx experienced a shortage of physicians, with an 8% decrease in physician supply during this time (Center for Health Workforce Studies, 2006).

African Americans and Hispanics/Latinos are also disproportionately burdened by diabetes-related mortality and morbidity compared to non-Hispanic Whites (National Center for Health Statistics, 2007). For example, diabetes-related prevalence and hospitalization rates were significantly higher in South Bronx neighborhoods compared with Manhattan neighborhoods (Kim, Berger, & Matte, 2006). According to recent findings from the Racial and Ethnic Approaches to Community Health (REACH) Risk Factor Survey, African American and Hispanic/Latino adults in the South Bronx were more likely to report being overweight or obese, having hypertension, being physically inactive, and having high cholesterol compared with the state averages (Centers for Disease Control and Prevention, 2006).

Additionally, many current urban environments across the nation, including the South Bronx, are poorly designed to promote health behaviors. For example, many urban neighborhoods lack easily accessible nutritious food and safe open spaces like parks and playgrounds for exercise. Instead, they are inundated by stores that sell alcohol and targeted by advertisers that promote the use of alcohol and tobacco products (Perdue, Stone, & Gostin, 2003). The promotion of unhealthy eating habits in these primarily minority neighborhoods is influenced by the proliferation of fast food restaurants, a deficiency of supermarkets providing fresh produce, and the higher cost and poorer quality of healthy foods (i.e., low-fat dairy products, fruits, and vegetables). All of these factors may account for diabetes-related disparities among racial and ethnic groups (Glanz, Sallis, Saelens, & Frank, 2005; Glanz & Yaroch, 2004; Moore & Diez Roux, 2006). Changes in the nutrition environment, such as the increasing popularity of eating out, larger portion sizes, social norms, policies, and advertising also seem to contribute to the diabetes epidemic (Glanz et al., 1995, 2005).

Disparities in diabetes among African Americans and Hispanics/Latinos continue to persist. Mounting evidence shows that individual risk-reduction interventions are having a limited effect on reducing these disparities; thus, the need to further examine and address environmental conditions that are negatively impacting the health of affected populations is paramount.

Community Needs Assessment

A qualitative assessment, known as the Bronx Health REACH Nutrition Evaluation Project, was conducted to gain a greater understanding of the factors contributing to disparities in diabetes in the South Bronx, as well as capture detailed information on the multilevel nutrition interventions that the Bronx Health REACH program developed and implemented from 1999 to 2006. A broad socioecological model, such as the one presented in chapter 3, was deemed appropriate in guiding the design of this assessment, because it allowed for a more general examination of factors contributing to disparities in diabetes and more appropriately corresponded with the approach that the Bronx Health REACH program utilized in targeting program and policy interventions at multiple levels (i.e., individual, interpersonal, institutional/organizational, community, and broader environmental conditions) to address racial and ethnic disparities in diabetes. A total of nine in-depth interviews and four focus groups were conducted among key partners from the Bronx Health REACH program, including program staff, coalition members, and other external partners (e.g., government agency representatives and restaurant managers). A select number of program records (i.e., progress reports, meeting minutes, budget records, and other summary reports) were also reviewed. Participants were asked questions on racial and ethnic health disparities affecting their community, factors contributing to these disparities, and key characteristics of the program's nutrition interventions.

Contributing Factors to Racial and Ethnic Health Disparities

Participants reported several factors contributing to disparities in diabetes among residents in their community. These factors extended across the multiple levels of the socioecological model (i.e., individual, interpersonal, institutional, community, and broad environment). They included lack of power and control in seeking health care; economic barriers to healthy eating; racism and discrimination in the health care system; relationships between culture and food; real-life conditions of community nutrition environments, such as residential segregation and perceptions of the South Bronx as a "food desert"; corporate power; and the social production of diabetes. Qualitative findings elucidating how these factors impact disparities in diabetes are highlighted below.

Economic and Cultural Influences on Healthy Eating

Some participants reported that economic barriers often prevent people from buying healthy foods, which tend to be more expensive. Because of limited incomes, families are often unable to buy healthy foods like fruits and vegetables and, in turn, are forced to buy less nutritious foods to stay within their budgets.

People's food choices are very much affected by even their own personal economics like their household economics—when they're trying to stretch their dollar, so the biggest expense—I've found that they go shopping infrequently, and they're buying for a long period of time. So it's usually not fresh fruits or perishable produce.   *—focus group 3 participant*

Participants explained the challenges that many families experience in their ability to obtain healthy foods through government-assisted programs (i.e., the Women, Infants, and Children program and food stamps). Due to limited support provided by these government programs, many families are economically strained and often forced to negotiate the purchase of non-eligible, less-nutritious food items, which compromises their ability to maintain a healthy diet. Further, the stress of poverty—the economic burden that residents face in purchasing healthy foods—impacts their mental health. For example, families often experience anxiety and frustration, because they are forced to make trade-offs (e.g., paying electric bill vs. buying fruits or vegetables) given their limited income.

The fruits and vegetables and regular groceries that are sold in the stores in our communities . . . it's more expensive, which contributes to the anxiety that a lot of our folk experience . . . So they have limited resources, but they're paying more for an inferior product. That's frustrating. That generates a lot of tension, a lot of anxiety and pressure, and it's probably one of the reasons why a lot of the folks in our community come down with this heart disease. It's real, I mean the burden. *—interview 2 participant*

Participants had opposing views about the role culture plays in nutrition and diabetes. Although some believed that the dominant "American" culture led to the deterioration of health among racial, ethnic, and immigrant populations, many participants felt that traditional cultural dishes contributed to the diabetes and obesity epidemic. For example, many participants identified Southern cooking ("soul food") as a major contributor to the prevalence of diabetes and obesity among African Americans.

A lot of people in our congregation are from the South. Love Southern cooking, and you grew up on it, and you've been doing it, been living off it for so many years, and all your family, your family, all of your relatives been living off this. And they introduced it to you, from the time you was a baby, it have been continuing and continuing. It's hard to just get away from that but we must understand, what we must realize is that these foods come from waaaaay back to the time of slavery. That's what we have to realize. And those foods that we were eating was the food that Master didn't want . . . That's what he didn't want. It was the bad food. We got the scraps. What's no good, that's what we got. And you get people talking about fatback and all this kind of thing. That's not something for anybody to eat. But you got people talking about they make fatback sandwiches. It's ridiculous. [T]hat's why you have especially black people dying from diseases like heart disease and diabetes and blood pressure more so than anybody else, it's because of the food that we eat. It's not that we don't eat better food, but we love that stuff, okay? And it's not good.

—focus group 2 participant

A couple of participants were cautious about labeling native cultural traditions as a "risk," but rather recognized that the interplay between acculturating to the "modernization" of the dominant culture and the traditions of native cultures may explain the disparities in diabetes.

I think part of what it makes it not healthy in a nutritional sense is just also the environment that we're in, where there's TV and computers and fast food, in cars, so that in combination with the traditional dish, it can make you unhealthy. But maybe in their own culture, wherever they originated from, if they were actually still living there, the combination wouldn't necessarily be unhealthy.   *—focus group 4 participant*

Participants expressed difficulties in persuading community members to undo centuries of tradition by modifying their diet or to recognize the importance of having community members access fruits and vegetables that are of their native culture to promote healthy eating.

[W]e deal with churches and organizations where, in fact, the thought has always been "meet, eat, and greet." And so, therefore, food has been a real part of the culture of the churches, be it Latino or African or African-American or Caribbean or whatever. In our community, food is a big piece, a fellowship, a piece of family, a piece of our ethnicity. So when we tell people that you are eating food that is not beneficial to you, unhealthy, I think it takes a minute for them to want to accept that. Like anybody else, it's just hard to change a habit or change something that is inherent in your being. You know, your mama did it and her mama before, that kind of thing.   *—interview 5 participant*

Racism and Discrimination in the Health Care System

Many participants felt they were not receiving the same quality of care as compared with others (e.g., not getting referrals and limited medication or treatment options) and believed people experienced different levels of care because of discrimination. Institutional racism was perceived as a primary contributing factor to the different treatment experienced by community members, as well as to the perpetuation of health disparities.

Because of your color that you're not getting the health care that you're supposed to get. So it's just like racism in the past all over again. But it's undercover. It's in the health care system. So, because I'm black that don't mean that I can get the same—I'm supposed to get the same health care as a Caucasian person.   *—focus group 2 participant*

Participants explained how discrimination and stereotyping is manifested through their interaction with providers. Some participants presumed that providers were racist and claimed that providers' discrimination contributed to the poor quality of care and health outcomes that they experienced. Others further challenged this behavior by asking whether it is a provider's duty to help a person get better regardless of who they are or what they know.

I mean I think that most of us don't look at a treatment physician as being capable of—not seeing us as being whole, and deserving, and not receiving the same information and treatment as the person who's next to us.

—interview 4 participant

Residential Segregation

Most participants discussed the current state of their community's nutrition environment in relation to the limited availability of healthy foods in their neighborhoods. One participant specifically articulated the negative impact of racially and economically segregated neighborhoods on access to healthy foods.

When you have a large supermarket, you're more likely to have [a] certain product in that supermarket as opposed to a small bodega owner. So it's an economic issue, and it's an environmental—as far as what is available in the neighborhoods.   *—focus group 3 participant*

I think that in areas where people have been labeled "ghetto" or whatever else they might choose to . . . or when people are considered a different class or a poverty level . . . I think there clearly is not the same services. So therefore the stores and the—I think that the stores and other places where food is purchased do not have the same kind of quality of food.

—interview 5 participant

Many participants reported that the inability to obtain high-quality, healthy foods (e.g., fresh wheat bread, fruits and vegetables, and low-fat milk) in the South Bronx is due in large part to the excessive number of local small bodegas or food stores and the lack of large supermarkets in the area. In addition, the proliferation of fast food restaurants in primarily low-income, minority neighborhoods like the South Bronx was perceived to perpetuate racial and ethnic health disparities in the community. The inability to get healthy foods within close proximity has led community residents to migrate into other neighborhoods in search of such foods. Further, people having to "go out of their way" (e.g., additional travel, time, and money) to find healthy foods became overwhelming and caused them to settle for what was available in their own neighborhood.

And when we're in the schools and we're working with the parents and we're saying, "Make sure you get this and that," then they're coming back and saying, "We can't find it. Nobody has it." So this doesn't make any sense. And then you can't say, "Well, go to Pathmark," because then you're talking taking three buses, and how do you carry it? You can't get your shopping cart up on the bus . . . But if we're saying to families, "This is what you should have," and our Office of School Food is also preparing and providing these things, but then when you go out to the store, it's not there, then there's the contradiction, and then the parent says, "Well, this is my reality. Outside of those four walls is my reality. That's what I'm going to go for." —*interview 5 participant*

A few participants discussed the difficulties in obtaining bodega owner support for providing healthy foods, particularly if the owner believes it is not economically viable. Some participants discussed market forces (i.e., supply and demand) as underlying factors influencing the allocation of healthy foods in the community.

So it's interesting to look at supply and demand. The bodegas have no fresh fruits and vegetables available. You could get a banana. You could get onions. You could probably get platano—just kind of the ones that are less perishable—potatoes. But you can't get apples, oranges, pears, strawberries—forget it—even lettuce, tomato—maybe at the deli counter, but not so readily available. Well, which is the chicken and which is the egg? For a merchant, there's a financial question. —*focus group 3 participant*

Corporate Power

Participants recognized the significant resource and power imbalance experienced by communities having to compete with marketing giants, such as Coca-Cola® and Frito-Lay®, to create environmental change to improve nutrition. For example, the power imbalances between local bodega owners and large food and drink distributors greatly limits the owners' control over what types of foods are provided in their stores and where healthy food items can be shelved.

Well, the bodegas don't control a lot of things that happen in their bodega. For example, the milk is essentially controlled by the distributor it turns out. So if the distributor wants to put the whole milk at eye level, that's where they're going to place it when they stock the case. The bodega owner, actually, it turns out, has very little say in that. So they're providing the space for the distributor to put their stuff. I don't know whether the other things are in bodegas work that way, but I have hunch that that's the case also. So if something's on sale, the bodega owner's not putting that thing on sale; the distributor is putting that thing on sale. So the bodega is a bit player in the way the food gets put out . . . You go in there; they have things that are very nonperishable: onions, lemons, potatoes, other root vegetables, and not very much fresh produce anyhow; it's mostly the canned stuff. So I think that's going to be hard to change because the market has to help change that. People have to [want] that thing before— you can't just change people's desires by changing what's in the store. They have to go hand in hand.   —*interview 7 participant*

Also, the amount of public health funding to market healthy foods is noticeably inadequate when compared with the millions of marketing dollars that large corporations use to advertise unhealthy "junk" foods.

So I think that's going to be rough without the . . . we don't have the dollars that Coca-Cola has or Frito-Lay have, or whatever the big companies are that when they decide to put something on sale, like Doritos, they can say it's on sale in the city, have a big campaign around it. That costs hundreds of thousands of dollars, if not millions of dollars. And the public health dollars for that kind of marketing are not as big unless the CDC wants to take on major companies. Well, doing distribution and marketing to the tune that major companies do it to promote their stuff. There's nobody out there promoting fresh apples. So apples have a relatively good shelf life for produce, but they're not going to sell if people don't—part of what they have to see is the marketing around it. And we can't compete right yet with the marketing that's done for unhealthy foods. So that's going to be tough.   —*interview 7 participant*

Further, the power imbalance that disparate communities like the South Bronx face in garnering political support for creating community-wide changes is apparent. Participants believed that the lack of political power to regulate markets to improve access to healthy foods requires government intervention (e.g., government regulation of tobacco) in order to more effectively improve population health.

THEORETICAL FRAMEWORK

Social Production of Diabetes[2]

Participants cited modern political, cultural, and economic changes that are potentially influencing disparities in diabetes in their community. For example, families experiencing difficulties in preparing healthy meals, because they work long hours or multiple jobs, have resigned themselves to eating outside the home. This broader economic pressure has resulted in a social shift that has eroded traditional family norms of cooking and eating at home and now favors, and even promotes, a "quick and easy" approach to eating.

I think that a lot have to do with external things that impact on the family because you have two parents now that have to actually work to keep the family going. So you have less food being cooked at home and more food being eaten outside. And when they eat food in restaurants, the restaurants tend to now give everything super-size, or "bigger is better." So we end up with people eating double portions, gaining more weight, and it's a vicious cycle because you now have a generation of young people growing up eating out.

—focus group 2 participant

As a result of this social and economic shift, many families are no longer skilled in selecting healthy foods or preparing them, and cooking at home is now considered a "lost art." In addition, some participants said

---

[2] The phrase *social production of diabetes* refers to the correlation between the burden of diabetes and the changing patterns of subsistence, loss of political and economic autonomy, and the subsequent cultural evolution that accompanies these dramatic changes in a population (Liburd & Vinicor, 2003).

that eating outside of the home has resulted in people being socialized to believe that a "burger and fries" is more filling and satisfying than fruits and vegetables.

ORIGINS AND HISTORY OF BRONX HEALTH REACH

In 1999 the Centers for Disease Control and Prevention (CDC) launched the REACH 2010 program, a federal initiative to help affected communities eliminate racial and ethnic health disparities. REACH 2010 was a 7-year demonstration program project (fiscal years 1999–2007) that supported community coalitions to design, implement, and evaluate community-driven strategies to eliminate racial and ethnic health disparities (CDC, 2006).

COMMUNITY AND INSTITUTIONAL PARTICIPANTS

The Bronx Health REACH program, one of 40 REACH 2010 communities, was created in 1999 by a coalition coordinated by the Institute for Family Health. It included the Center for Health and Public Services Research of New York University and three community-based organizations: Mount Hope Housing Company, the Women's Housing and Economic Development Corporation, and St. Edmund Episcopal Church. The institute was awarded over $6.5 million over 7 years to launch the Bronx Health REACH program to eliminate disparities in diabetes among African Americans and Hispanics/Latinos who live within four zip codes in the South Bronx and make up 95% of the area's population.

A number of factors influenced the institute's and Bronx Health REACH Coalition's involvement in eliminating diabetes-related disparities in the South Bronx. The significant disease burden and a majority-minority population in the neighborhood were leading indicators of a high-risk population for diabetes. Equally important, the institute and its original community- and faith-based organizational partners had a history of being involved in social, economic, and health care reform in the Bronx (i.e., neighborhood housing, economic and educational regeneration, and health center development) and thus felt that addressing disparities in diabetes was a natural extension of their work. The importance and urgency of addressing diabetes disparities in the South Bronx was reinforced by community residents who reported five key issues that concerned them about the health care services provided in the community: (a) distrust of the health care system, (b) lack of quality and caring in the health care system, (c) a sense that the health care system undervalued and disrespected them, (d) difficulty in communicating with doctors, and (e) inadequate and insufficient health education and information.

The Bronx Health REACH program oversees several general community initiatives, including a faith-based outreach initiative, a community health advocacy program, a nutrition and fitness initiative, a training curriculum for health care providers, a legal and regulatory committee, and a public health education campaign. The nutrition and fitness initiative works to educate community residents, health professionals, and local leaders on the role of nutrition and fitness in preventing the onset of diabetes and the importance of effective management of the disease. The goal is to raise awareness and provide the necessary information and tools to help people make lifestyle changes and improve their behavior and to address environmental barriers that make it difficult for community residents to maintain healthy behaviors. Activities in this initiative include nutrition programs in elementary schools and after-school programs, grocer and restaurant outreach initiatives, a church-based culinary initiative, and a faith-based nutrition and fitness program.

PROGRAM COMPONENTS

Nutrition Interventions of Bronx Health REACH

The qualitative findings presented in the previous section provide a rich depiction of the realities confronted by community leaders and members in addressing disparities in diabetes and the deep impact that these health inequalities have on their daily lives. Participants noted significant environmental barriers (e.g., no large supermarkets, bodegas not supplying fruits and vegetables, and schools with only heating cafeterias) that impede residents' ability to access healthy foods in the community. Participants also described broader political and economic influences (e.g., large food corporations, institutional and local policies, and mass marketing) that perpetuate racial and ethnic health disparities in the South Bronx. In addition, participants felt that individual determinants, such as income, employment, culture, and lack of nutrition education, have negatively affected the health of community members.

Based on its initial community assessments, the Bronx Health REACH program developed nutrition activities to address some of these determinants. The program developed seven initiatives targeted at the various levels of the socioecological model: individual, interpersonal, institutional/organizational, community, and broader societal/public policy (see Figure 15.1).

The client-based fitness and nutrition activity was aimed at providing fitness and nutrition education to increase knowledge and skills to community members on proper nutrition, physical activity, and diabetes management. Two faith-based nutrition activities were initiated to increase nutrition and diabetes knowledge and skills. The community members also were able to change organizational policy to increase access and availability of healthy foods at church events. The primary aim of the school-based nutrition activities was to change institutional policies to increase access to healthy meals and snacks for schoolchildren. These programs also included an educational component for parents, school staff, and children.

In addition, the school-based nutrition activities spawned the creation of the bodega/grocer initiative, as program staff and partners recognized that the diet of schoolchildren is influenced by the schools'

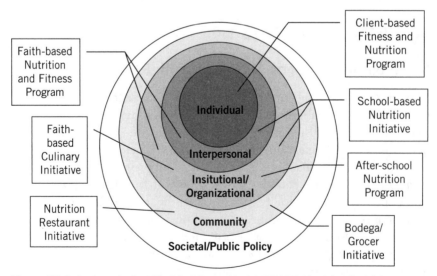

Figure 15.1 Socioecological Model of Bronx Health REACH Nutrition Activities

surrounding businesses. Therefore, this initiative was aimed at creating community-wide change by attempting to increase the supply of healthy food items and prominently display those items to encourage healthy food purchases. The restaurant initiative also was initiated to create community-wide change by providing healthy menu options for diners.

In order to capture detailed information on the Bronx Health REACH program's multilevel nutrition interventions, focus group and interview participants were asked specific questions on various characteristics of the interventions and the participants' experiences in developing and implementing the interventions. Themes that emerged from the responses included descriptions of cross-cutting elements of the program, such as the use of participatory and ecological approaches, the need to adapt interventions to local cultures and traditions, factors that helped or hindered the interventions (i.e., programs, enablers, and barriers), and the perceived impact of the nutrition interventions. Below is a more detailed description of these qualitative findings.

Incorporating Participatory and Ecological Approaches in Nutrition Interventions

The Bronx Health REACH program used community-based participatory approaches (CBPA) to develop and implement its interventions. To support these efforts, the program conducted qualitative and quantitative community assessments and created a community coalition Nutrition and Fitness Work Group to participate in and have ownership of the various nutrition interventions. The program also used current community assets to build community ownership and capacity within the targeted intervention settings, such as churches and schools.

All participants felt that the nutrition activities initiated by the Bronx Health REACH program were driven by the needs of the community. Participants cited the initial assessments conducted by the program as efforts made to allow community voices express such needs. Furthermore, some participants felt that as leaders in the community, their participation in the program's coalition allowed for that voice to be heard. Other participants believed that community members may not "know what it needs, because they do not know any better"; therefore, it was the community members' responsibility to "help them see the need and identify the need." More importantly, as part of using CBPA, participants recognized the importance of engaging in colearning between program staff, community members, and partners.

[I]t's been really important to be sort of open and humble and kind of understanding of the fact that I'm learning as much from them as they are from me. Because it's true, you know. I'm not going to walk in and tell them that this is what you need to know, this is the way that you're going to do it. But I think the only way that we're going to be successful is for all of us to sort of work together. —*focus group 4 participant*

Another way the program promoted community participation and ensured representation of the communities' interests in its health disparities agenda was to provide opportunities for community members to engage in civic and democratic practices. For example, participants cited local action rallies and trips to the state capital of Albany to educate legislators on health disparities issues in the Bronx. When community members engage in such activities, it empowers them to voice concerns or questions in other aspects of their lives (e.g., regarding equal and fair treatment received by their health care providers) and increases their self-efficacy to choose alternatives if they are not satisfied with their current options.

Many of the participants reported the need for community residents to empower themselves by gaining knowledge and taking action, such as complaining when mistreated, switching doctors, engaging in the political process, and simply "speaking up." Participants expressed the importance not only of "empowering ourselves" but also of changing the providers' perceptions of the patient to increase communication. The participants also felt they had a right to demand equal, affordable health care and acknowledged the importance of being "your own advocate" and training community members to do the same.

So my message is that you now know not only is it in terms of the nutrition piece and that you must exercise and you must do all of these things, but if somebody's not supporting this for you then you need to go someplace else and do something else. So to have a voice, to use your voice. —*interview 5 participant*

Tailoring Interventions to Cultural and Spiritual Identities

Participants described some approaches to adapting the nutrition interventions to fit the particular religious or cultural beliefs and traditions of the community members. Strategies included modifying traditional cultural dishes; promoting snacks, fruits, and vegetables familiar to community members' native cultures; tailoring messages to coincide with religious beliefs; and providing educational materials in both English and Spanish. Participants noted that although resources may be limited, they realized the importance of tailoring the activities to reflect the cultural and spiritual beliefs and traditions of the affected populations.

Participants reported several modification strategies within their faith-based and restaurant nutrition interventions. For example, restaurant owners were not receptive initially to implementing major changes to their cooking methods. The program had to modify its approach by suggesting more incremental changes, such as increasing healthy options on menus. Although a few restaurants have made significant changes, the implementation of such changes has not been consistent. Two other tailoring approaches identified by participants included modifying traditional Southern dishes offered at church events and providing nutrition and diabetes information to community members in English and Spanish. Participants felt that the nutrition interventions would be more effective if they were adapted to reflect and respect the community members' native cultures.

Although participants reported a range of messages that have been conveyed through the various nutrition activities, some messages were tailored to incorporate cultural or spiritual beliefs and values. Participants overwhelmingly expressed the importance of integrating health-related information with spiritual messages, such as "the body is God's temple." Health-related messages also were synchronized with spiritual callings for individual and social responsibility. For example, one of the faith-based nutrition interventions emphasized "choices, decisions, and consequences" as the primary motivating message for changing behavior.

And one of the things that's taught from the pulpit, preach from the pulpit, is love. And you must start with yourself, and you can't love me if you're going to kill me while you cooking for me . . . And that's what I have—and I mean, now, that's what's being done. People, you may not want to look at it that way, but that's what is being done . . . People come off, "Baby, look what I got for you," and you did it with all the wrong things, and that's what's happening, not intentionally, but that's what's happening. So if—the more we talk about it, the more we'll be about it and the longer we'll be here.

—focus group 2 participant

Participants reported messages of good health being preached from the pulpit, and they felt their pastors played a critical role as "messenger" and "visionary." Pastors have great influence on individuals' actions and attitudes and act as change agents within their churches because of their position in the community. Obtaining pastoral leadership and support in advocating and promoting healthy changes among congregants was considered essential. Many believed that both the church and the Bronx Health REACH program were spreading "the good news."

[My role as a pastor is] to help my people understand that there is a direct connection between my spirituality and my physical health and well-being, and that there is a direct correlation between their spirituality and the care that they give to themselves and to their families.   *—interview 1 participant*

I [as a pastor] try to evidence to the people that it's important to me, and that translates into them wanting it to be important to them. They're saying, "Well, Pastor likes what we're doing, so it must be something to it." That's how I help.
—interview 2 participant

Participants also explained that "consciousness raising" efforts went beyond conveying healthy messages, but were believed to be an integral part of one's worship of God and a ministry of the church. As such, messages urging "faith in action" helped to motivate community members to take active steps in leading healthy lives.

It has to become for us a serious discipleship issue . . . For us, there needs to be Biblical and theological foundations for what we do. It's best, if we want to relate this to faith and if we're going to talk about these as things that the people of faith need to take responsibility for, we must make it relevant from a Biblical and a theological perspective. And I think that's the reason why we've seen such success in our communities here in the South Bronx is we have made an all-out effort to help people to understand that this is just as much a spiritual matter as it is a physical matter. And if it's a spiritual matter, if this is something that we're able to guide them to some Scripture reference to understand—that we're directly responsible for the steps we take to ensure our health or the health of our family and the health of our community—it would serve to galvanize our community and to help each one of us to take another look at how we look at what we do . . . Helping people to understand that the very act of cooking and preparing a meal can be an act of worship in and of itself; and the act of preparing and serving, and eating a healthy meal can be a worship experience itself.   —*interview 1 participant*

COMMUNITY RESPONSE TO THE BRONX HEALTH REACH PROGRAM

Program Leadership

Program champions were individuals considered to be leaders or advocates of the nutrition activities. All participants identified program staff as program champions. Pastors, the faith-based program coordinator, and senior staff of the New York City's departments of health and education also were believed to be program champions. Some participants expressed their reliance on program leadership and the program staff's support and resources as critical elements in the churches' continued participation in the program activities. Key characteristics of a program champion identified by participants included passion and conviction.

Participants felt that the Bronx Health REACH program's leadership and consistent efforts in building partnerships with various entities positively influenced the success of the nutrition interventions. The program's ability to show leadership through its commitment and loyalty to maintaining partnerships and the nutrition activities also played a key role in organizations' willingness to partner with the program. Participants also identified the lack of a "bureaucratic mindset" as a key element of leadership. They defined this as a refusal by individuals to be confined by administrative procedures or rules in their attempts to address racial and ethnic health disparities.

[There] is an absence of a bureaucratic mindset. It's the folks who, when you think of any sort of revolution or struggle, it's always the folks that are not going to be bound necessarily by the rules and regulations or their ambitions but are the folks that are willing to step out and then tell their organization—you know, make a case why they think their organization needs to be involved and why they got their organization involved . . . I think that is what has made this partnership and collaboration and coalition really unique, the fact that we're sort of not looking over our shoulder as to who has had the sword that's going to chop us down and say you can't do it. We have to do this and we are doing this, and then we'll go back and explain to the others who maybe don't quite understand why this must be the public policy agenda.   —*focus group 4 participant*

Institutional History

The Institute for Family Health's history within the Bronx community provided a strong collaborative foundation by which to expand the REACH program. Because of this history in the community, the institute was viewed as a trusted convener and advocate. A few participants felt that working within stable, trusted institutions like faith-based organizations facilitated behavior change among congregants, particularly because it provided a "captive audience" who "made a commitment to change."

Unified Vision and Goals

Participants acknowledged that the most significant enablers in continuing their work are the partnerships that have been built, the shared vision among all partners, and the "universal recognition of how bad the health problems are here in our community" that has increased the sense of urgency to provide and create change.

You're not an island by yourself. We're all trying to reach the same goal, and we're all coming together to help each other to reach their goals. We all have the same problem . . . So we're working at it . . . We're an army.
—*focus group 2 participant*

Program Support and Capacity Building

Participants were able to continue the nutrition activities because of the consistent support and resources they received from Bronx Health REACH. The program initiated several capacity building efforts, including workshops and presentations on nutrition and health disparities and trainings for congregants who wanted to become faith-based nutrition coordinators or fitness instructors.

Although some participants did not seek external funding for their nutrition activities, others did explore or obtain additional funding. Participants were less likely to assert that the activities would continue if they no longer received funding or other resources from Bronx Health REACH. Others believed that continuing their work in addressing racial and ethnic health disparities was critical and would not cease even without funding and support from the program.

So we're the resource that Bronx Health REACH has invested in . . . I don't think we could stop if we wanted to. They wouldn't let us.

—focus group 2 participant

Partnership Building

Participants felt that creating diverse collaborations with various individuals and organizations would increase the ability to pool and leverage resources, as well as create a more powerful influence to address racial and ethnic health disparities.

So the intent is not this program out here, sort of trying to find its way, it's not this program here, but meeting together, our efforts . . . [T]here was also sort of a recognition that we needed to partner, or be involved, with others in order to address it . . . So it's not just individually programs struggling with their own issues, but now there are more resources added that they know of and are partnered and collaborating with. *—focus group 4 participant*

The beauty of this is this blossoming that has happened is this creation of partnerships that really is a meshing of one with the other, has created some concerted efforts. And borough-wide and, in some cases, probably citywide, in effect, a great coordinated effort to really achieve something. You think that we all work together, but the reality is we don't, generally. I mean, there's different funding sources from all over the place—local, city, state, federal—and everyone's doing their own thing, and they want to do it best. It's not about credit, it's about us all working together to get there. So by partnering together, including health centers and everyone that has been created, you created a healthy cycle instead of a destructive cycle. And I think it's a great model.

—focus group 4 participant

Participants recognized the considerable value that partnerships have in continuing the work of improving community nutrition and having a greater impact on environmental changes, as well as acknowledged the need for community organizations and entities to communicate openly about their programs and activities to find areas of agreement and avoid opposing priorities or agendas. Some participants also discussed changes in partnerships and the challenge in adapting and maintaining the partnerships in the face of change. In addition, expecting local businesses like restaurants to participate in the nutrition initiatives meant taking time to establish and build those partnerships and acknowledge community realities by modifying action steps to meet those needs.

I think this whole business of change and the different cultures and different languages, and the changing community. I mean, that's the hardest thing. That is incredibly difficult to do, and no one wants anyone telling them what to do. So you have to work from within the community to branch out. . . . I think that our willingness as an organization to be flexible, as you said, and to really listen to the community. I think, as an organization we show that we care about the community. That we're coming in with our own agenda, but we really need their help in order to move it forward so we want to know what the challenges are actually from the people who experience them. And I think, hopefully, that makes us able to do our job a little bit better.   *—focus group 4 participant*

CHALLENGES TO PROGRAM IMPLEMENTATION

Conflicts and Limitations

Some participants believed that competing priorities with partnering organizations like local schools led to difficulties in conducting nutrition activities. Participants discussed the challenge of garnering support in schools to set nutrition-related priorities, such as serving healthy foods, and also felt a need to help school staff recognize the important link between health and academic success.

I think also trying to connect to the school administration and the staff's minds that health is related to academic . . . Because at this point they're stressed about just passing the tests and all of that. That definitely takes priority, but trying to connect is like, "Well, they get their exercises. If they go out during lunch and get their energy out they'll be able to focus better." If they eat less sugar, they'll be able to sit still and learn.   *—focus group 3 participant*

Participants also expressed limited time, other obligations, and limited resources as major barriers to doing the work in some program settings (i.e., churches, schools, and community-based fitness centers). Specifically, participants discussed resource limitations within the local school system (e.g., heating-only cafeterias and overwhelmed teachers and staff), which was perceived to create "cyclic dysfunction." These limitations created challenges in implementing the nutrition interventions and were believed to significantly hinder the ability to create a supportive environment that promotes healthy eating.

Participants asserted that limited resources are also a major barrier to implementing and maintaining their activities, as well as in their battle to eliminate disparities.

Let us not ignore the obstacle that lack of resources presents in terms of achieving even some of the successes. The resources, I don't know why we think that poor communities somehow can do a better work around lack of resources than anybody else. Why we think we can conjure magic out of limited resources, it's ridiculous . . . But the fact is that things don't happen unless there are resources to make it happen. We are so creative and adept at creating magic to have things happen. But we keep slamming up against that brick wall that says there is just so much you can do without resources, and that's the real critical piece. Resources are extremely important and have been real obstacles in terms of all that we can achieve.   *—focus group 4 participant*

A few participants expressed frustration at the constant pressure to demonstrate impact and create community change, particularly within a limited timeframe.

Why are we being judged about impact and change over activities that have either taken place within the last year or even the last 6 years? Why are we being asked to reverse trends that have taken years to lead us to this crisis point? Something, to me, is wrong with that picture. And I am not worrying for anybody to back us into a corner and say, "Where's your data?" "Well, we don't know about the data. We understand that it's an important thing for us. We're paying attention and trying to gather." But we have multiple stories to talk about changes that have been made on multiple levels. And so individually we think there's a reduction in disparity.   *—focus group 4 participant*

PROGRAM EVALUATION

Participants' responses to whether disparities have been reduced as a result of the Bronx Health REACH program's nutrition interventions were mixed. Although some participants believed that disparities were being reduced as a result of their work, others were more hesitant to conclude that disparities had been reduced. However, they did acknowledge that incremental changes have been made among community members and, cumulatively, have influenced policy and environmental change.

> But I think also Bronx REACH, by going into the communities and going into the churches and bodegas, to go where the people are and to educate and make them aware of what's available, hopefully it's one chain in that big link that helps to reduce it. I don't think we're anywhere near there yet . . . I think a picture is emerging. We have many of those stories, and I think individually, yes, those are indicators that we are eliminating it. [B]ut I don't think we need to be ashamed of these individual stories of changes that have been made that we feel—where, as you said, 20 years down the road when we look back, we're like—it's a combination of all these actions and activities that have led us to this point.   *—focus group 4 participant*

Participants perceived that some of the nutrition activities initiated by Bronx Health REACH have created change, particularly in "raising the consciousness" of community members. Other changes included increased screening and diagnosis, understanding the importance of healthy eating, skills and knowledge for modifying recipes, and willingness to try healthier versions of traditional dishes. There were also many testimonies among the participants on the weight loss they experienced or witnessed among fellow residents. As a result of increased knowledge and skills, participants feel empowered and connected to their fellow community members, and this knowledge has helped them to become change agents among their church and family networks.

Participants offered several examples on the informal policy changes that occurred with organizations and businesses. For example, faith-based organizations changed their Sunday service menus to include healthier versions of traditional cultural dishes (e.g., baked vs. fried chicken), offer new healthy dishes, and change the presentation of foods to promote the healthy dishes. One faith-based organization reported re-engineering its entire kitchen to ensure greater availability and provision of healthy meals during all church events.

Participants also reported changes in informal policies within local businesses, such as restaurants and bodegas. For example, restaurants modified their regular cooking methods (e.g., using olive oil or products free of trans fat) and added a few healthier items to their menus (e.g., baked vs. fried fish or chicken). Local bodegas promoted healthy snacks by placing them in more prominent areas (e.g., a basket with bananas and apples by the cash register) and began offering more healthy products (e.g., low-fat milk). Fruit purchases increased as a result of these strategies; however, because low-fat milk did not sell as well, some bodegas stopped offering it. Participants also reported success in creating policy change by banning whole milk in elementary schools, which also became a city-wide policy.

LESSONS LEARNED AND PROGRAM SUSTAINABILITY

Findings from the qualitative evaluation suggest that broadening the focus on traditional lifestyle interventions to address broader institutional and community changes may be more effective in influencing the reduction of disparities in diabetes. Therefore, an ecological approach should be used to examine the relationships between these various factors, and multilevel strategies are encouraged. Incorporating an ecological perspective into the development and implementation of interventions that target various levels and settings of influence will allow for greater impact and sustainability of behaviors. Moreover, such ecological approaches may better address the broader, underlying determinants of disparities in risk and burden of diabetes among affected communities.

Local communities are facing considerable barriers in their efforts to eliminate racial and ethnic health disparities. The findings from this evaluation clearly demonstrate the challenges that the Bronx Health REACH program confronted when implementing nutrition interventions within local businesses. In addition, the current state of schools in the South Bronx may preclude their ability to support disparities-related initiatives. Therefore, public health professionals and community leaders must find innovative ways to encourage and support local businesses and schools to collaborate in efforts to address health disparities. This approach may include using a "business" model in education campaigns and program/policy interventions, as well as providing stipends to small local businesses to provide and promote healthy food items. Community and program leaders also should work closely with local and state education agencies, school boards and staff, and parents to address institutional barriers within schools by initiating strategies that target policy change.

Adopting a CBPA to develop and implement nutrition interventions is critical to successfully eliminating racial and ethnic health disparities across our nation's communities. CBPA not only encourages a deeper understanding of the sociocultural, geographical, and historical contexts of a program or intervention, it also promotes the importance of community participation in all aspects of a program and its evaluation. CBPA is also a valuable way to increase community empowerment and capacity for social action by ensuring alignment of intervention goals with community needs and promoting civic engagement among community members. Faith-based organizations like African American and Latino churches can serve as powerful advocates and mobilizers that can reach beyond their walls to raise community consciousness and foster community and civic engagement through civil rights and social justice ideology.

Incorporating nontraditional public health partners who represent multiple sectors and settings can help to leverage resources and better address the various individual and environmental health determinants that effect disparities in the community. Therefore, community-based organizations should consider reaching out to a range of "grassroots" (e.g., community organizations) and "grass tops" (e.g., government, business leaders, and other institutional leaders) as possible partners to help mitigate institutional barriers, foster program sustainability, and create greater public health impact. In addition, conducting assessments of the potential partners' assets, resources, and weaknesses will help program staff to organize the partnership best and leverage additional resources to develop, implement, and sustain interventions.

Encouraging partners to seek and obtain multiple sources of funding, as well as offering leadership and skills-based trainings, will help increase community capacity and sustainability. For example, integrating a competitive process for mini-grants or a "ramping down" approach (i.e., gradual decrease in amount per year) may not only help to provide initial support for the activities but also maximize opportunities for learning through shared leadership and accountability. Funded organizations also can promote capacity building by providing skills-based and leadership trainings (e.g., in grant writing). By diversifying funding sources to support program activities, community-based organizations can increase program maintenance and help sustain outcomes.

Although increasing community engagement and capacity to address disparities is essential, the glaring power imbalances between local communities and corporate or political entities cannot be dismissed, nor can it be effectively addressed by communities alone. By suggesting that solutions can be generated at the local level alone places unrealistic goals and an overwhelming burden on already disadvantaged communities. Funding from federal and state public health agencies for community-based projects can help to transform these power imbalances by creating partnerships with various institutional "goliaths" to promote participatory public health efforts. Agencies also can work together to address macro-level determinants that affect health disparities.

The Bronx Health REACH program encountered a range of internal and external influences that required it to be flexible and adapt its efforts appropriately. A clear, well-articulated plan is essential to successfully implementing an intervention and having a measurable impact on the target population. Additionally, community-based organizations must be flexible enough to adapt to the culture and needs of the community. Cultural tailoring should go beyond solely translating materials into different languages. It also should focus on incorporating cultural and spiritual beliefs, values, and traditions into the activities. Tailoring interventions to correspond to the cultural and spiritual beliefs and traditions of the participants is essential in adequately addressing the needs and realities of community members, and this approach will ensure greater responsiveness and potential impact.

Further qualitative and quantitative research is needed to examine the sociocultural and historical contexts that perpetuate disparities. Researchers also need to conduct mixed-method evaluations and disseminate findings on the effectiveness of other community-based participatory interventions. As more communities are attempting to address health disparities through multilevel interventions, intermediate outcomes that appropriately monitor policy and community change must be developed. In addition, policy and economic analyses of the impact of multiple health determinants on disparities would provide important information for public health professionals and community leaders to guide their interventions.

SUMMARY

This qualitative assessment validated previous research findings, suggesting that multiple health determinants are significantly impacting low-income, minority neighborhoods. Moreover, these findings also highlight a growing concern of how historical power imbalances between communities and social and political structures are perpetuating health disparities. Although local communities are fertile ground for developing and testing innovative strategies for eliminating disparities, to suggest that solutions can be generated at the local level alone places unrealistic goals and an overwhelming burden on already disadvantaged communities. Federal and state public health agencies can help address these macro-social determinants and transform such power imbalances between affected communities and institutional "goliaths." Further research is needed to examine the sociocultural and historical contexts that perpetuate disparities, as well as to assess intervention studies examining ecologically driven, community-based participatory efforts aimed at eliminating disparities in diabetes among racial and ethnic populations.

REFERENCES

Center for Health Workforce Studies. (2006). *The supply and distribution of physicians in New York, 2004*. University at Albany, State University of New York. Retrieved from http://chws.albany.edu/index.php?id=11,0,0,1,0,0

Centers for Disease Control and Prevention. (2006). *At a glance: Racial and ethnic approaches to community health (REACH) 2010: Addressing disparities in health 2006*. Atlanta: U.S. Department of Health and Human Services, Centers for Disease Control and Prevention. Retrieved from http://www.cdc.gov/reach/reach_2010/index .htm

Glanz, K., Lankenau, B., Foerster, S., Temple., S., Mullis, R., & Schmid, T. (1995). Environmental and policy approaches to cardiovascular disease prevention through nutrition: Opportunities for state and local action. *Health Education Quarterly, 22(4)*, 512–527.

Glanz, K., Sallis, J. F., Saelens, B. E., & Frank, L. D. (2005). Healthy nutrition environments: Concepts and measures. *American Journal of Health Promotion, 19(5)*, 330–333.

Glanz, K., & Yaroch, A. L. (2004). Strategies for increasing fruit and vegetable intake in grocery stores and communities: Policy, pricing and environmental change. *Preventive Medicine, 39*, S75–S80.

Jasek, J., Van Wye, G., Kerker, B., Thorpe, L., & Friedan, T. R. (2007). *Health care access among adults in New York City: The importance of having insurance and a regular care provider.* New York: New York City Department of Health and Mental Hygiene.

Karpati, A., Kerker, B., Mostashari, F., Singh, T., Hajat, A., Thorpe, L., Bassett, M., Henning, K., & Frieden, T. (2004). *Health disparities in New York City*. New York: New York Department of Health and Mental Hygiene. Retrieved from http://www .commonwealthfund.org/publications/publications_show.htm?doc_id=232638

Kim, M., Berger, D., & Matte, T. (2006). *Diabetes in New York City: Public health burden and disparities.* New York: New York City Department of Health and Mental Hygiene. Retrieved from http://www.nyc.gov/html/doh/html/diabetes/diabetes.shtml

Liburd, L. C., & Vinicor, F. (2003). Rethinking diabetes prevention and control in racial and ethnic communities. *Journal of Public Health Management and Practice, November(Suppl)*, S74–S79.

Moore, L. V., & Diez Roux, A. V. (2006). Associations of neighborhood characteristics with the location and type of food stores. *American Journal of Public Health, 96(2)*, 325–331.

National Center for Health Statistics. (2007). *Health, United States, 2007 with chartbook on trends in the health of Americans.* Hyattsville, MD: National Center for Health Statistics. Retrieved from http://www.cdc.gov/nchs/hus.htm

Olsen, E. C., Van Wye, G., Kerker, B., Thorpe, L., & Frieden, T. R. (2006a). Take Care Highbridge and Morrisania. *In Community health profiles* (2nd ed.). New York: New York City Department of Health and Mental Hygiene.

Olsen, E. C., Van Wye, G., Kerker, B., Thorpe, L., & Frieden, T. R. (2006b). Take Care Central Bronx. *In Community health profiles* (2nd ed.). New York: New York City Department of Health and Mental Hygiene.

Perdue, W. C., Stone, L. A., & Gostin, L. O. (2003). The built environment and its relationship to the public's health: The legal framework. *American Journal of Public Health, 94(9)*, 1390–1394.

U.S. Census Bureau. (2006). *2006 American community survey: Selected population profile in the United States.* Retrieved from http://factfinder.census.gov/servlet/DatasetMainPageServlet?_program=ACS&_submenuId=&_lang=en&_tss=

U.S. Census Bureau. (2008). *State and county quickfacts.* Retrieved from http://quickfacts.census.gov/qfd/states/36/36005.html

16

Diabetes Disparities Reduction Through Improvement in Healthy Eating: The Chicago Southeast Diabetes Community Action Coalition[1]

AIDA L. GIACHELLO, JOSE O. ARROM,
DINAH RAMIREZ, AND NEAL BOSANKO

Editor's Note: This case study describes one community's efforts to reduce determinants of diabetes disparities caused by lack of access to healthy foods in a declared "food desert." The Chicago Southeast Diabetes Community Action Coalition (CSeDCAC) uses the community participatory action research approach to address social determinants of diabetes among Hispanics/Latinos and African Americans in a southeastern Chicago community. This approach is an iterative process that actively involves the community in the research process and allows the

[1] The authors would like to acknowledge the hard work and commitment shown by members of the Chicago Southeast Diabetes Community Action Coalition (CSeDCAC), established as a result of funding from the Centers for Disease Control and Prevention (CDC) for Racial and Ethnic Approaches to Community Health (REACH) 2010, particularly the following key partners: the South Chicago Chamber of Commerce and its staff, Alicia Lopez, Community Health Worker (CHW); Healthy Southeast Chicago (formerly Healthy South Chicago) and its director, Dinah Ramirez; the staff of the Midwest Latino Health Research, Training and Policy Center, a unit of the Jane Addams College of Social Work at the University of Illinois at Chicago, particularly Ada Caranton, CHW and project manager of the REACH 2010 Community Diabetes Self-Care Center; Amparo Castillo, MD, REACH 2010 project director; Rosemary George, MA, REACH 2010 grant manager; and editorial consultants Judith Sayad, Eve Spiker, and Nancy Simon. The CSeDCAC was organized to address diabetes disparities in several underserved Chicago southeast communities with high concentration of Hispanics/Latinos and African Americans by assessing community problems and engaging in individual, community, and system change. The coalition is funded by CDC REACH 2010 Initiative Phases I and II Grant U50/CCU517388-01. Additional funds were obtained for the Eat Healthy South Chicago Project from the Chicago Community Trust, a local community foundation.

375

community to focus on actions that lead to change and improvements. Engaging community members and institutions in the research process from the beginning adds credibility to the research findings and facilitates action over time and across sectors of the community.

In an effort to understand the social factors that contribute to diabetes in this community, the CSeDCAC collaborated with community members and partners, collected and analyzed qualitative and qualitative data, disseminated the findings, and created an action plan. The primary objective of the action plan was to increase the demand for and supply of healthy foods in southeast Chicago, a community declared as a food desert. Being designated a food desert does not imply that people do not have access to any food in their community; it instead suggests that most of the available foods are high in calories and low in nutrition. In response, the Eat Healthy South Chicago project was created to improve the supply of healthy food in this southeastern Chicago community.

Like many other community coalitions, the CSeDCAC faced multiple challenges as it addressed the social determinants of diabetes. These challenges included limitations in being able to disseminate information, absence of a national health promotion campaign in Illinois, and lack of cooperation of some local grocers. Despite the challenges, the CSeD-CAC learned the importance of involving various sectors in the planning process, involving health professionals and academicians in changing social norms to healthier behaviors, and building capacity among nontraditional partners working in diverse communities.

As you read this selection, consider the following questions:

- What additional sectors (i.e., community members, local government, community-based organizations, and businesses) in southeast Chicago might work together with the CSeDCAC to increase access to and demand for healthy foods while creating local economic growth and employment opportunities?
- Why is it important for the CSeDCAC to build capacity among community-based organizations and business that are unfamiliar with federal and research-based food and nutrition guidelines?
- With which existing or potential coalition partners should the CSeDCAC begin to collaborate with to establish public policy for a healthy community environment?
- Dissemination and promotion of community-wide information and strategies might be challenging for coalitions addressing Eng-

lish- and non-English-speaking community members. What are effective modes of communicating information community-wide? How might the CSeDCAC use those modes of communication to share information and implement health promotion strategies community-wide?

■ The Eat Healthy South Chicago project will be sustained in the target community with new federal funds. Financial sustainability is only one resource that is used to bring about durable changes in a community. What are other resources the coalition will need to influence institutionalization and sustainability of the project?

BACKGROUND

In 1999 the Midwest Latino Health Research, Training and Policy Center (Latino Research Center) at the Jane Addams College of Social Work, University of Illinois at Chicago (UIC), initiated a partnership with African American and Hispanic/Latino (H/L) leaders in six communities in southeast Chicago to respond to a request for application from the Centers for Disease Control and Prevention (CDC) under the Racial and Ethnic Approaches to Community Health (REACH) 2010 initiative. The Latino Research Center is a 15-year-old center that conducts health disparities research in the areas of type 2 diabetes and other chronic diseases. In addition, the center engages in training minority students, community health workers (CHWs), and health professionals locally, nationally, and internationally. The research that emerges from the center informs the development of health policy.

Community Assessment

Following community participatory approaches described later in the case study, CSeDCAC community partners were trained on diverse community assessment methodologies, such as how to plan and facilitate focus group discussions, how to develop and conduct community surveys, how to write informed consent forms, and other data collection techniques. As a result, the coalition conducted 12 focus groups with African Americans and H/Ls living with or at risk for developing diabetes and a telephone health survey of about 400 participants based on a probability sample (stage 4 in the participatory action research [PAR] model). The 2000 REACH 2010 assessment provided sufficient evidence of the seriousness of type 2 diabetes and its risk factors, including unhealthy eating. For example, 16.2% of the telephone survey population had diabetes, with this percentage reaching as high as 22% among some segments of the target population (i.e., those with gestational diabetes). Close to 50% of the survey respondents reported being either overweight (22.3%) or obese (25.7%). About 73% reported eating outside their homes on a regular basis with respondents reporting eating in fast food restaurants 3.2 times per week on average.

Data on community inventory and mapping showed few public parks for physical activity and few grocery stores and food store chains in the area. Most of the available stores were geographically located one-half mile from each other and primarily in South Chicago's commercial strip (Commercial Avenue). The average distance for community residents to travel to reach a grocery/food store was found to be at least one-quarter mile. Even if residents desired to purchase healthy foods, the effort involved to do this was very time-consuming and costly. Because of the closing of the steel mills and other sources of employment, large chain supermarkets had abandoned the area, leaving only corner stores (e.g., small, local convenience stores and and liquor stores) (Ashman et al., 1993). These small stores do not tend to stock fresh fruits and vegetables, but instead more packaged goods and quick-fix snack items. Because of this lack of grocery/food stores within close geographical range, the South Chicago community has been classified as a "food desert" (Gallagher, 2006).

ORIGINS AND HISTORY OF THE PROJECT

REACH 2010 was a two-phase demonstration project that called for coalition building to engage in community mobilization and action to reduce health disparities. During the 12-month phase I funding period, a leading agency (UIC), working with representatives of the Illinois Diabetes Control Program (IDCP) and community residents, established and maintained an African American and H/L coalition, conducted a comprehensive community assessment following participatory action research methodologies, and developed a community action plan that was implemented during the phase II funding cycle. (See Giachello et al. [2003] for a specific description of the process followed in the formation of the CSeDCAC.)

The coalition targeted geographic areas, including six community areas in Chicago's southeast side. However, this case study focuses on one community area, South Chicago. In comparison to other neighborhoods in the city, South Chicago has lower levels of income, high poverty, high representation of female heads of households, and a high dependency on public assistance programs. The 2000 census counted 68% of the population as African American and 27% H/L (Salem, Hooberman, & Ramirez, 2005). Historically, the major sources of employment in the southeast communities were the steel mills and automotive industries, which provided great stability for working-class, blue-collar families. During the 1970s, these industries declined considerably and many closed in the early 1980s, causing severe unemployment and displacement in these areas. Mexicans/Mexican Americans began entering the South Chicago community in the early 1900s, and in the 1990s a second wave of Mexican immigrants began to arrive. Since 2000 additional African Americans and Caribbean and African immigrants have moved into the area.

The Southeast Chicago communities have a strong history of labor movements, and upon consultation with community leaders and based on limited community health data available, it was determined that these communities were seriously affected by problems of overweight and obesity and high hospitalization rates for type 2 diabetes. Moreover, the communities were surrounded by fast food restaurants and corner grocery stores that did not sell fresh fruits and vegetables or other healthy food items. Because there was no diabetes coalition, community leaders felt that the community could be mobilized around diabetes to reach a state of readiness, that is, to engage in targeted actions to reduce diabetes disparities.

COMMUNITY AND INSTITUTIONAL PARTICIPANTS

The UIC Latino Research Center's community entry into the Chicago Southeast communities was facilitated by local well-known and respected community leaders who participated in the initial city-wide dialogue that the UIC had with minority leaders in an attempt to identify target communities for interventions and collaborators for the REACH 2010 phase I grant application. Due to the seriousness of type 2 diabetes in Southeast Chicago, its leaders were able to get UIC attention and interest to focus on these communities. Specifically, they facilitated community relations and dialogues that led to community interest in diabetes and the formation of the CSeDCAC with a committed group of residents and community-based organizations (stage 1 in the PAR model in Giachello et al. [2003]).

The CSeDCAC had as principal partners the Healthcare Consortium of Illinois, a broad-based organization of community health advocates, hospitals, and health professionals with many years of experience in maternal and child health; the IDCP of the Illinois Department of Human Services; Centro Comunitario Juan Diego, a local community organization that primarily serves recent immigrants with trained CHWs; Healthy South Chicago (HSC) (renamed Healthy Southeast Chicago in 2007), a broadly-based local coalition that came together in 2001 in response to a Chicago Department of Public Health pilot project (Salem et al., 2005); and the South Chicago Chamber of Commerce (SCCC). These groups brought into the partnership a network of local hospitals, minority professional organizations (e.g., The Hispanic Nurses Association, the Chicago chapter of the Black Nurses Association, and the African American Dieticians Association), faith-based groups, community-based health and human services organizations, community members, and local businesses including the chamber of commerce, providing a broad and diverse base of support for planning and implementing a diabetes prevention and control strategy that included the healthy eating project. For organizations receiving financial support to assist with major coalition work, written memoranda of agreement were developed.

Capacity Building through Education and Training

In addition to addressing group dynamics involved in forming a coalition and educating members about type 2 diabetes, its associated risk factors, and diabetes self-management and control, it was also essential to build understanding about the socioeconomic, political, and environmental conditions associated with type 2 diabetes. These efforts are ongoing and reflected in stage 2 of the PAR model. Central to the development of the coalition and attention to group dynamics was insuring the coalition was successful in defining the mission, principles and values, leadership development, and opportunities to strengthen the coalition and achieve cohesiveness. The mission adopted by the group was "to assure and enhance access to quality health services and quality of life of persons 'at risk' and with diabetes in Chicago Southeast communities through the establishment and institutionalization of a Diabetes Coalition of community residents, health and human services providers, and persons living with diabetes, that will engage in community approaches to reduce diabetes and its consequences."

Through education, the connection between diabetes, healthy eating, and the demand for and supply of healthy foods in the neighborhood environment became evident to the collaborating organizations and community residents, leading to a commitment to joint action. This capacity building through training was facilitated by an average of 5–10 annual training sessions, planned and implemented by coalition members with UIC support, targeting diverse audiences. Participants included community residents and leaders, health professionals, and CHWs and health promoters. Training topics included diabetes, its risk factors, and the relationship of diabetes risk to sociocultural values and norms; strategies for community organizing and coalition building; community assessment methodologies (e.g., focus groups and community survey); ethical and social issues in research; action planning; dissemination strategies; program evaluation; and sustainability of coalition activities through grant writing. Training programs stressed community empowerment and learning by doing using methods of adult education.

STRATEGIES FOR COMMUNITY ENGAGEMENT

The community participatory action research (CPAR) approach was used for the CDC REACH 2010 project, including Eat Healthy South Chicago (EHSC). (See Giachello et al. [2003] for a detailed description of this CPAR model and its application to REACH 2010.) CPAR refers to a family of research methodologies that pursues research objectives (i.e., knowledge and understanding) with the meaningful involvement of community members (i.e., stakeholders) and an ultimate focus on social action leading to changes and improvements in social conditions (Stringer, 1999). The CPAR approach stresses increasing the knowledge and skills of community members (i.e., community capacity), so they can understand and be better equipped to address aspects of the sociopolitical and economic circumstances that may be associated with the health problem(s) in question. It also includes building community infrastructures, such as coalitions, to foster a united effort to collectively take action. The CPAR model (see Figure 16.1) developed by the UIC Latino Research Center has been applied to a diverse set of health issues,

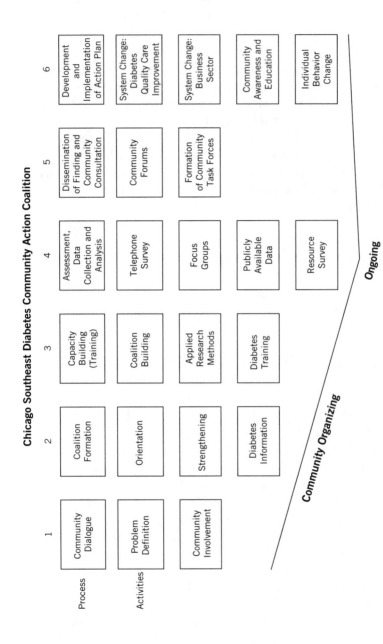

Figure 16.1 *Source:* A. L. Giachello, J. O. Arrom, M. Davis, et al. (2003). Reducing diabetes health disparities through community-based participatory action research: The Chicago Southeast Diabetes Community Action Coalition. *Public Health Reports, 118(4),* 309–323.

including environmental exposure, occupational health, cancer, tobacco, and diabetes prevention and control.

Data Dissemination and Development of Action Plan

Following PAR model stages 5 and 6, CSeDCAC engaged in diverse strategies to disseminate data collected during phases I and II of REACH 2010. Strategies included town hall meetings and community forums, with and without media coverage; distribution of selected fact sheets with results of findings from the community assessment; and presentations on the project that were given to other targeted community and professional audiences (e.g., APHA and public hearings). A number of peer-reviewed publications have also come out of this project. (Selected preliminary findings of REACH 2010 phase I are found in Giachello et al. [2003].) In some instances, bilingual community forums attracted over 50 persons. Members of the coalition presented selected findings and action plan strategies. The coalition members who were physicians used these forums to continue dialogue and education with the community about diabetes. Once the data were collected and disseminated, the information obtained in community forums was used to set priorities for the implementation of the community action plan.

The community action plan included the following areas for action: (a) training African Americans and H/L CHWs as diabetes educators, (b) developing a bilingual and culturally and educationally appropriate diabetes empowerment education program to educate the community on diabetes self-management and control based on reflective thinking and learning by doing[2], (c) establishment of three community diabetes self-care centers run by CHWs under the direction of the coalition, and (d) community mobilization and policy work to address a variety of community health and chronic disease control issues (e.g., diabetes and tobacco control) through community and systems change. These self-care centers served as resources for referrals and education on diverse topics (e.g., nutrition) and drop-in centers for social support and for the development of community programs like walking clubs. During these discussions, concerns about diabetes were linked to education

---

[2] The success of this local program led to the replication of our model in diverse communities nationwide in collaboration with local departments of public health and other community partners.

about healthy eating and increasing both the demand for and the supply of fresh fruits and vegetables in the community. Therefore, the EHSC project emerged as another target action included in the CSeDCAC community action plan.

PROGRAM COMPONENTS

The main objective of EHSC is to increase the demand for and the supply of healthy foods in southeast Chicago communities through several business and consumer-based interventions. Objectives for the program included (a) to increase H/L consumption of fruits and vegetables and promotion of other healthy eating guidelines; (b) to educate representatives of the local food industry about how they can impact the reduction of overweight and obesity, thereby delaying the onset of diabetes by increasing the supply of affordable, healthy foods within local stores; and (c) to improve promotion and visible placement of such items within stores through technical assistance and education to grocery store managers and owners.

Some additional objectives were to increase the number of partnerships for promoting healthy eating, establish linkages with food banks and other resources for food assistance to community members, promote the prevention of obesity in the community, and increase the number of programs and activities promoting healthy eating offered by organizations serving this community.

The CSeDCAC's EHSC project built on the earlier work of HSC, a CSeDCAC partner. HSC conducted a community health assessment following the community health improvement planning model adapted from the National Association for County and City Health Officials and the CDC called Mobilizing for Action through Planning and Partnerships (Salem et al., 2005). This model calls on community members' experiences and public health data to describe the community and the availability of local resources. HSC members conducted a block-by-block assessment through a community landscape asset mapping process that looked at a variety of quality of life indicators based on the observations of community residents. The coalition's assessments relevant to healthy eating included Grocery Shopping and Eating Out.

Some of the key Grocery Shopping Survey findings based on 28 grocery stores were: 11% had an aisle for low salt, sugar, or diabetic food; 7% displayed nutritional information; 21% sold alcoholic beverages; 86%

sold tobacco; 32% sold fresh fruit; and 36% sold fresh vegetables. Findings from the Eating Out survey of 32 restaurants indicated: 78% offered chicken, 63% offered fish, 72% offered beef, 34% offered salads, 50% were smoke-free, 9% had signs warning pregnant women about alcohol, and 50% were handicap-accessible (HSC Coalition, 2003).

CSeDCAC REACH 2010 engaged in additional assessments to obtain baseline data. Based on observations and qualitative methods, data were collected on the quantity, variety, access, affordability, and display characteristics of fruits, vegetables, and low-fat foods at 10 neighborhood grocery stores in July 2006. Ten store managers were also interviewed as part of this assessment.

Implementation of Eat Healthy South Chicago

Following are key implementation steps for the EHSC Project:

1. The EHSC Project involved representatives of the South Chicago Food Industry. HSC and the SCCC received seed funding from REACH 2010 and the Chicago Community Trust. SCCC involved its members from the local food industry in the project by holding bi-monthly meetings to educate them about their unique role in insuring healthy communities and the specific problems related to community residents accessing affordable and quality fruits and vegetables. The SCCC's executive director's strong commitment and passion about this project was extremely valuable in motivating its members.
2. The SCCC distributed free boxes of fruits and vegetables. To increase the supply of fruits and vegetables, the SCCC provided to selected members in the food industry free and/or subsidized boxes of fruits and vegetables preferred by the H/L community.
3. The EHSC Project provided technical assistance and support to grocery managers. Specifically, the UIC and SCCC provided assistance to grocery managers on how to display fruits and vegetables in an attractive and visible place to promote sales.
4. The project sponsored food testing and sampling and food of the month events to introduce community members to a broad range of healthy and tasty food options. With financial support from REACH 2010, the SCCC executive director hired a CHW to engage in consumer education through food testing and sampling in local grocery stores. This allowed the consumers to learn

how they can integrate fruits and vegetables into the everyday preparation of ethnic food and snacks like *pico de gallo*. A key element in this intervention was a fruits and vegetables of the month promotion. Some of the fruits and vegetables offered by SCCC and HSC to its members and/or promoted to the community included *nopales* (prickly cactus), jicama, cucumbers, green tea, tomatoes, and kiwi. About 60–80 hours each month was devoted to taste tests and food sampling, consumer education, and making referrals to healthy food sources by the community health promoters and volunteers at participating food stores in the South Chicago community and at major community events (e.g., health fairs, coalition meetings, and school report card pickup days) in 2007. Nutrition education materials and recipe cards were provided during individual and group education sessions conducted with consumers.

5. The project implemented a restaurant intervention. The UIC Latino Research Center conducted two surveys that highlighted the important role restaurants play in the dietary intake of people living in Southeast Chicago. During 2007, the coalition partners launched a healthy menu option initiative at Roma's Restaurant. A key feature of this initiative was the provision of a healthy meal at a reasonable price. Parallel to this project, the SCCC developed a restaurant healthy menu initiative with its restaurant membership. The healthy menu option of Roma's (chicken breast, steamed vegetables, brown rice, wheat roll, and green tea), available at a subsidized cost by the chamber of commerce of $3.99, was featured the week of June 25–28, 2007. A total of 81 individuals tried this healthy menu option, of which 48 persons completed a modified consumer survey. Of these 48, most reported trying the healthy menu option because of the health benefit, whereas a smaller percentage decided to order the menu item for both cost and health benefits. Subsequently, the restaurant made changes in its regular menu, and additional restaurants followed suit.

Findings from the Eat Healthy South Chicago Consumer Food Survey

Survey questions asked of participants in the food sampling intervention included: Did the participant intend to use or cook the food item within the next month?, How many servings of vegetables did the participant eat on a typical day?, What was their preference for buying vegetables (i.e., fresh/raw, cooked, frozen, or canned)?, How often did they shop at the store per week or month?, and How far do they go to grocery shop? Demographic data were collected (i.e., gender, age group, race, and ethnicity). Other data included the date, location, and food sampled. The data were collected from a series of repeat taste samplings in four small food stores in the South Chicago/East Side area and twice each at two public schools (e.g., on report card days). The data below represent a sampling of the total number of events and persons reached.

Who Was Reached?

During the test period, we analyzed 385 consumer food surveys. For those persons whose data were available:

- 91.3% were from the local community zip code (60617) and 1.8% ($n = 7$) were from Chicago area suburbs;
- 74.9% were females and 24.7% were males;
- the self-reported race/ethnicity was predominantly H/L (63.4%, $n = 244$), followed by African American (28.6%, $n = 110$), other Black (e.g., Caribbean or West African origin) (1.8%, $n = 7$), and non-Hispanic Whites (4.4%, $n = 17$); and
- younger age groups predominated in the survey.

Selected key findings from the survey included:

- only 13.8% prefer canned vegetables to other alternatives;
- most persons reported eating two or three servings per day of vegetables (29% in each category);
- males in this sample were more likely than females to eat fewer vegetables; and
- H/Ls were more likely than African Americans to eat more vegetable servings.

Intention to Use or Consume Promoted Food Products

The response categories were: "I am using it regularly," "I intend to try it," "I am not sure," and "I don't think I will try it." For each food item surveyed, more than 50% of respondents fell in the "I intend to try it" category with green tea (71.2%), and cucumbers (69.9%) generated the greatest intention to "try it."

Other findings include:

- people who eat more vegetables reported using or having more intentions to try the target food products, and
- people who were ambivalent or "non-tryers" were more likely to be consuming three or fewer vegetable servings per day.

PROGRAM EVALUATION

The participatory process led to an increased awareness of the complexities of diabetes in the community, the importance of healthy eating, and strategies for engaging key community sectors (e.g., the business sector) in the work of the local coalition in improving community health. The support given to small grocery stores played an essential role in shaping community nutritional consumption. The program's consumer education component proved to be effective, because it was characterized by culturally, linguistically, and health appropriate approaches. Based on the preliminary findings, this program appears to be a promising practice that is grounded in the centrality of a community coalition, building capacity of coalition members through education and training, utilizing community participatory action research methods, information dissemination and action planning, and the implementation and evaluation of the CAP, using the expertise of the coalition's Evaluation Committee. The short-term impact of the program provides evidence of an increase in demand for fruits and vegetables, based on the purchase of items in participating stores, increases in community knowledge about fruits and vegetables, and greater consumption of fruits and vegetables promoted by the program. Based on grocers' sales records, we learned that they had sold three times more of foods used in the food sampling intervention during and after the intervention. Use and acceptance of specific food products varied by ethnicity; the number of other Blacks and Whites was too small for analysis. For local people, there was no statistical correlation between the distance people had to travel to shop and the level of fruits and vegetables consumption.

Other impressive outcomes of the EHSC project included one grocer becoming a local wholesaler of fruits and vegetables and opening another mid-size grocery store on the same block. We now have a Sav-a-Lot, six local mid-size stores, and six bodegas that sell fruits and vegetables. In addition, there are now three local urban vegetable gardens feeding over 100 families.

CHALLENGES TO PROGRAM IMPLEMENTATION

In terms of information resources, the South Chicago area has very little community media. At this time, community media is limited to a monthly newspaper, the Observer. This limits our ability to disseminate information and strategies that encourage healthy eating to a larger audience, such as promoting the food of the month and culturally appropriate recipes for these foods.

The absence of a formal 5-a-Day Fruit and Vegetable/Healthy Produce Program in Illinois is a barrier to accessing educational materials at a low cost. As a result, there is not a broad Illinois or Chicago area 5-a-Day produce media campaign. The absence of this campaign has increased our confidence in data documenting the impact of REACH 2010 interventions, but with this campaign, we could do even more in terms of creating awareness of the benefits of healthy eating.

We observed that community-based and business organizations do not always follow federal and research-based food and nutrition guidelines recommendations. First, these guidelines are not easily available to the community in simple formats that can be applied to fresh produce in grocery stores and restaurants in terms of labeling. In addition, dietary guidelines are subject to change, most recently in 2005. Community organizations need ongoing training and support to assure that they are promoting appropriate foods, portions, and recipes.

Chain food stores require central office approval before being surveyed and to host food demonstration interventions. The one medium-sized chain store approached during the summer of 2006 failed to obtain this approval for undisclosed reasons.

Although it was expected that many stores would be able to share sales statistics on specific food items, most small stores did not have the systems in place to collect this data. Some other grocery stores with the needed technology and systems to do this did not want to share their sales data.

LESSONS LEARNED

We learned that multiple partners are required to improve healthy eating in the community. Changes in supply and demand are linked, and therefore the business sector (e.g., grocers) as well as the consumer sector (i.e., community residents) must be involved in the planning and education about connections between health and eating. There is also a key leadership role for health professionals and universities in changing social norms toward healthier diets.

Food market researchers must learn how to work with community stakeholders to identify social, economic, and cultural factors that support grocers in these neighborhoods. In addition, the shelves of local stores must reflect community health needs, including a new view of what a "big box" means in urban America. (Gallagher, 2008).

Further Observations on Lessons Learned

Another outcome of this coalition-based project has been to improve the quality of food and snack offerings in public meetings and events. Providing hospitality in the form of meals and snacks has been the norm at public events and meetings in Chicago for many years. In the past, donuts, cookies, and salty snacks were offered. Today at South Chicago community events, fruits and lower fat products are offered and expected.

Multiple sets of partners were important to this project, since the ultimate goal is to make systems changes. In addition to the partnership with the grocers, restaurant operators, and wholesalers of produce, another set of partners were community-based service organizations. Regularly occurring community events, such as the Chicago Police Department beat meetings, school-parent events, and senior activities, are important for introducing basic healthy foods and reinforcing the messages of healthy eating and foods to the largest segment of the community possible.

The food sampling outreach component also created an opportunity to dialogue with the community about its health and food practices. Persons who completed the consumer survey became aware of how few fruits and vegetables they were eating. Given that the healthy eating project was coordinated by the CSeDCAC, people with diabetes were also reached by the community health promoter. As a result of their participation in the consumer survey, they received referrals to appropriate clinical services, as well as diabetes self-management education programs supported by CSeDCAC.

From a systems or socioecological perspective, this project has begun to impact the food system and the community's communication system through referrals. While major immediate changes are not to be expected with the small scale of the interventions, continuity over several years will result in positive change in community food norms and habits. One major barrier is the broader economic environment, which presents cost barriers to many lower-income residents. However, as noted above, we are observing the re-introduction of medium-sized food stores in the area and increased produce availability through local wholesaling to the smaller stores. Another facilitator of change is the willingness of the SCCC and other coalition organizations to sustain the championing of these efforts and prioritizing the concepts of healthy eating and healthy food in their business practices through food sampling and other strategies.

PROGRAM SUSTAINABILITY

In 2007 the UIC competed successfully for a CDC REACH U.S. grant to be designated a Center of Excellence for the Elimination of Health Disparities (CEED). There are 18 such centers funded across the U.S. and charged to disseminate innovative strategies developed in REACH communities like the EHSC project and train and mentor new communities. In 2007 the CDC also funded 22 Action Communities to continue to implement successful local community interventions. Chicago received funding for both a CEED and an Action Community. Through the CDC Action Community grant, this project will continue to be implemented in the target community. Additionally, through the CDC UIC CEED, the EHSC project will be one of the legacy projects disseminated locally and nationwide.

SUMMARY

Transforming an urban, low-income community from a food desert to a place where access to healthy food options are available and affordable requires the committed involvement of a wide range of community partners. Using methods of community participatory action research and innovative community interventions, we are documenting much-needed changes in the knowledge, attitudes, and behaviors of community members in tandem with changes in the food environment of southeast Chicago that tend toward positive health outcomes. Our program is demonstrating the health benefits of coupling economic development through increased supply and demand for fresh fruits and vegetables with a community concern to eliminate diabetes disparities. While there are challenges to meeting our goals, we have the foundation, broad-based community participation and investment in systems changes, for overcoming these challenges. With sustained leadership, financial support, and improvements in economic opportunities for members of this community, we expect to see greater health equity in southeast Chicago.

REFERENCES

Ashman, L., de La Vega, J., Dohan, M., Fisher, A., Hippler, R., & Romain, B. (1993). *Seeds of change: Strategies for food security for the inner city.* Los Angeles: Southern California Interfaith Hunger Coalition.

Gallagher, M. (2006). *MG food desert definition.* Mari Gallagher Research and Consulting Group, LaSalle Bank Chicago Food Desert Project. Retrieved July 18, 2006, from http://www.marigallagher.com

Gallagher, M. (September 15, 2008). *Grocer, can you make a profit?* Comment posted by "SCOrganizer" [Dinah Ramirez]. Retrieved September 18, 2008, from http://www.huffingtonpost.com/mari-gallagher/grocer-can-you-make-a-pro_b_126306.html

Giachello, A. L., Arrom, J. O., Davis, M., et al. (2003). Reducing diabetes health disparities through community-based participatory action research: The Chicago Southeast Diabetes Community Action Coalition. *Public Health Reports, 118(4),* 309–323.

Healthy South Chicago Coalition. (2003). *Executive summary: Strategic plan for community health improvement.* Retrieved September 19, 2008, from http://www.cchsd.org/chicagohealthpartners.org/pdfs/HSCExecSumm.pdf

Salem, E., Hooberman, J., & Ramirez, D. (2005). MAPP in Chicago: A model for public health systems development and community building. *Journal of Public Health Management Practice, 11(5),* 393–400.

Stringer, E. (1999). *Action research* (2nd ed.). Thousand Oaks, CA: Sage Publications.

Epilogue[1]

LEANDRIS C. LIBURD

To create a truly healthy republic requires us to address health disparities on many fronts, recognizing its root causes in social inequities that are amenable to change through intersectional policy changes. Economic policy is health policy. Education policy is health policy. Housing policy is health policy. Transportation policy is about health policy. And make no bones about it, agricultural policy is truly health policy.

>   —*Dr. Robert Valdez, Executive Director of the Robert Wood*
>   *Johnson Foundation for Health Policy (Valdez, 2008)*

As this text goes to press in the spring of 2009, our nation is facing an economic downturn, the likes of which have not been seen since the Great Depression of the 1930s. According to the Current Employment Statistics, the national unemployment rate was 8.1% in February 2009, seasonally adjusted, up from 7.6% the prior month and from 4.8% a year earlier (Bureau of Labor Statistics, 2009).

The loss of jobs has implications for a host of factors affecting the well-being of people with and at risk for type 2 diabetes, including health insurance coverage, medications compliance, housing, the tax base that

---

[1] The findings and conclusions in this chapter are those of the author and do not necessarily represent the views of the Centers for Disease Control and Prevention.

supports schools and other services in communities, and access to healthy foods. Communities of color that have historically lagged behind economically, politically, and in other social indicators that influence health can expect to experience higher rates of poorer health outcomes if supportive policies are not enacted and enforced to combat these effects of joblessness. Economic policy, argues Kaplan (2001), *is* health policy.

Diabetes is a complex biomedical condition caused by a complex interaction of genetics and environmental factors. In *Diabetes and Health Disparities: Community-Based Approaches for Racial and Ethnic Populations,* we call for greater attention to the social determinants of diabetes in efforts to reverse the tide of type 2 diabetes in communities of color in the United States. Our goal was to balance conceptual and applied approaches to expanding community-based public health practice for diabetes prevention and control in racial and ethnic communities. We intentionally focused on the outer rings of the socioecological model where supporting science, policy, and environmental change interventions are still emerging. This text is a primer for addressing the social determinants of type 2 diabetes and, while it is far from complete, we are hopeful that it will spur new knowledge, innovative community-based strategies, and added confidence in our ability to reduce the burden of diabetes in disproportionately affected populations.

We began with an overview of the different types of diabetes and a description of the epidemiology of diabetes in racial and ethnic groups in chapter 2. Understanding the burden of the disease and its associated risk factors and complications is a crucial first step for developing a population-based plan of action. Type 2 diabetes and its principle risk factor, obesity, have emerged as twin epidemics in communities of color. We described the relationship between obesity and type 2 diabetes in chapter 3, including the influence of what has been described as an "obesogenic" environment (Brown & Krick, 2001; Critser, 2000) in obesity rates observed within communities of color, particularly among African American women. Reducing the incidence of type 2 diabetes, therefore, is linked to reducing rates of obesity, a public health priority of the Centers for Disease Control (http://www.cdc.gov/obesity).

Chapter 4 examined meanings of body size expressed by a group of college-educated, professional African American women to explore the paradox of why advanced education and higher incomes (>\$50,000 annually) do not appear to protect African American women from obesity as they appear to protect their White counterparts. Culture, which is never static, is commonly reinforced through structures, even though those structures are not always as palpable and visible as are physical structures. Understanding the structural influences of mainstream White culture on the lifestyles and perceptions of other racial and ethnic communities is particularly important in any examination of health disparities. We hope additional research examining the intersection of race, class, and gender in diabetes prevention and control is inspired in response to chapter 4.

Throughout the text, we were careful to provide definitions of key concepts upon which our primary arguments and approaches are based. For example, as I travel and give talks on community health, I am frequently asked "what is a community?" There is increasing effort among scholars to articulate theories of community in public health research and practice. In chapter 5, we began with a consideration of the range of definitions of community and our understanding of it as reflected through community-based research and practice. At a minimum, public health researchers and practitioners are encouraged to more clearly delineate socioeconomic, political, and historical characteristics of the community with which they are working beyond race and ethnicity and to give voice and share power in determining the scope and breadth of community-based diabetes programs. Navarro in chapter 6 adds residential segregation and the cascading impact of the resulting inequalities in particularly urban, low-income communities of color to the discourse on community. Among the critical ideas discussed are the social construction of health disparities and the need for greater attention to broader arenas for policy change to eliminate health disparities.

Rivera and Tucker in chapter 7 challenge the reader to invert the evaluation lens from one that solely documents changes in people's behaviors and metabolic profiles who live in the community to one that also assesses changes in community institutions and resources that support diabetes prevention and control where people live. We believe measuring community change is a meaningful outcome for determining the effectiveness of community-based diabetes programs.

Lastly, since the rise in the burden of type 2 diabetes is global, we are hopeful that nation-states around the world will find some utility in the experience of communities represented in the case studies in chapters 8–16. There is much more work to be done across all sectors, including federal, state, and local governments; community-based organizations; institutions of higher learning; and the business sectors.

There is a growing discourse around the globe about the necessity of addressing social inequities as we seek to eliminate health disparities and achieve health equity for all segments of our society. The task ahead is daunting and will require policy makers to make a long-term commitment (i.e., beyond political election cycles or traditional funding periods of 5–7 years) to achieving health equity, along with a sound base of science, intervention research, and evaluation. Additional resources are needed to advance work in the social epidemiology of diabetes. We must take advantage of opportunities to foster linkages between academic institutions, state and local health departments, and communities of color to develop a cadre of public health workers with the skills needed to work with communities and health agencies to effectively address the social determinants of health. In the interim, we must continue to build awareness across sectors of our society of the relationship between social inequalities, broadly understood, and health.

As communities mobilize to address disparities in health, we can develop and sustain strategic actions that lead to change. The journey will not be a straight or uninterrupted one, as we will continue to have economic booms and busts, changes in community structures and composition, and the unforeseen opportunities and challenges that characterize contemporary life. Our vision is that 60 years from now, evidence-based strategies that effectively address the social determinants of health in eliminating disparities in the burden of diabetes experienced by communities of color will compare with, if not exceed, that found in the biomedical literature. We invite the reader to join us in working to achieve this vision.

REFERENCES

Bureau of Labor Statistics. (2009). Mass Layoffs in April 2009. Retrieved from http://www.bls.gov/news.release/mmls.nr0.htm

Brown, P. J., & Krick, S. V. (2001). The etiology of obesity: Diet, television and the illusion of personal choice. In F. Johnson & G. D. Foster (Eds.), *Obesity, growth and development* (pp. 111–127). London: Smith-Gordon.

Centers for Disease Control and Prevention. (2009). Obesity and Overweight for Professionals: Causes. Retrieved from http://www.cdc.gov/obesity

Critser, G. (March 2000). Let them eat fat: The heavy truths about American obesity. *Harper's Magazine*, 41–47.

Kaplan, G. A. (2001). Economic policy is health policy: Findings from the study of income, socioeconomic status, and health. In J. A. Auerbach & B. K. Krimgold (Eds.), *Income, socioeconomic status, and health: Exploring the relationships* (pp. 13137–13149). Washington, DC: National Policy Association.

Valdez, R. (December 16–18, 2008). *Keynote address delivered during the National Institutes of Health Summit on the Science of Eliminating Health Disparities.* National Harbor, MD.

Index